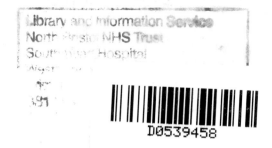

OXFORD MEDICAL PUBLICATIONS

Drugs in Anaesthesia and Intensive Care

THIRD EDITION

Oxford University Press makes no representation, express or implied, that the drug dosages in this book are correct. Readers must therefore always check the product information and clinical procedures with the most up to date published product information and data sheets provided by the manufacturers and the most recent codes of conduct and safety regulations. The authors and the publishers do not accept responsibility or legal liability for any errors in the text or for the misuse or misapplication of material in this work.

Drugs in Anaesthesia and Intensive Care

THIRD EDITION

MARTIN SASADA

Consultant Anaesthetist
Royal United Hospital
Bath

and

SUSAN SMITH

Consultant Anaesthetist
Cheltenham General Hospital
Cheltenham

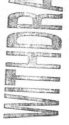

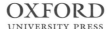

OXFORD

UNIVERSITY PRESS

OXFORD
UNIVERSITY PRESS

Great Clarendon Street, Oxford OX2 6DP

Oxford University Press is a department of the University of Oxford.
It furthers the University's objective of excellence in research, scholarship, and
education by publishing worldwide in

Oxford New York

Auckland Bangkok Buenos Aires Cape Town Chennai
Dar es Salaam Delhi HongKong Istanbul Karachi Kolkata
Kuala Lumpur Madrid Melbourne Mexico City Mumbai
Nairobi São Paulo Shanghai Taipei Tokyo Toronto

Oxford is a registered trade mark of Oxford University Press
in the UK and in certain other countries

Published in the United States
by Oxford University Press Inc., New York

First edition (published by Castle House Publications) 1990
Second edition 1997 (reprinted 1998 (twice), 1999, 2000)
Third edition 2003

A catalogue record for this book is available from the British Library

Library of Congress Cataloging in Publication Data
(Data available)
ISBN 0 19 852616 4

Typeset by Newgen Imaging Systems (P) Ltd., Chennai, India

Printed in China

Preface to the third edition

This book continues in its original structured format. Advances in pharmacology and medicine have required some rewriting and we hope it continues to be useful for anaesthetists in training, operating department personnel, and for examination purposes. Any comments or criticisms would be gratefully received via email (susan.smith@egnhst.org.uk).

M.P.S.
S.P.S.
March 2003

Preface to the second edition

In this edition we have retained the format of the original; the major changes being the removal of a number of less important or defunct agents. The text for the remainder has been updated to encompass significant developments since 1990.

The first edition proved popular and hopefully useful for preparation for postgraduate examinations in anaesthesia; we trust that this will remain true for the new examinations format.

Cheltenham   M.P.S.
February 1997   S.P.S.

Preface to the first edition

The aim of this book is twofold: firstly to summarise concisely the main pharmacodynamic and pharmacokinetic properties of the drugs with which the practising anaesthetist might be expected to be familiar. Secondly, it seeks to introduce the candidate for the FRCAnaes (and in particular for the second part of this examination) to an ordered scheme for the presentation of information, which we have found to be of value in both the written and oral sections of the examinations. Examiners are more likely to turn a blind eye to minor errors or omissions of knowledge if they are in the context of a clear and well-ordered presentation. A further advantage of this scheme of presentation is that it allows rapid access to specific information. It is our hope that this compendium will prove to be a useful rapid source of reference for clinical anaesthetists in their day-to-day endeavours, both in the theatre and intensive care unit.

This book is intended to complement, rather than to replace, the standard texts on pharmacology for anaesthetists, since it includes no discussion of the principles of pharmacology, an understanding of which is essential for the clinical use of drugs. We feel that these aspects are very satisfactorily covered elsewhere.

Although our research has been as comprehensive as possible, there will obviously remain some information that will have eluded us, or perhaps remains to be discovered. Many practitioners will disagree with our choice of 172 drugs. Any comments or suggestions will be most gratefully and humbly received, in order that further editions of this book may hopefully prove to be more useful.

Finally, we should like to thank the members of the Oxford Regional Drug Information Unit, the many drug company information departments and all our colleagues for their help and support in this venture. In particular, we should like to thank Professor Roy Spector and Drs John Sear and Tim Peto for their invaluable advice on the manuscript.

Oxford   M.P.S.
1990   S.P.S.

Foreword

The ever-increasing size of pharmacological textbooks bears witness to the increased number of drugs on the market and to the greater knowledge of their properties. It is no longer possible for the average doctor to memorise all the information relevant to clinical practice and there is, therefore, a need for a concise handbook which contains the essential information in an easily accessible form.

This book satisfies that need. The authors have been closely concerned with the teaching of pharmacology to junior doctors and have evolved a standardised format for the description of each drug which not only facilitates reference but also aids learning.

They have included most of the drugs commonly used in anaesthesia and intensive care so that the information should prove particularly valuable to junior doctors working in these fields. However, I suspect that this volume will soon become the first source of reference for their senior colleagues as well!

M.K. Sykes
Emeritus Nuffield Professor of Anaesthetics
Oxford, UK

How to use this book

The layout of this book requires some explanation in order for the reader to gain the maximum benefit. The 181 drugs we have included are arranged in alphabetical order to obviate both reference to an index and artificial categorisation of some drugs. Each drug is presented in an identical format and confined to one or two pages under the following headings:

Uses The main clinical uses are listed.

Chemical A brief chemical classification is given.

Presentation The formulation of the commercially available preparations are described.

Main Action The fundamental pharmacological properties are briefly indicated.

Mode of Action The mode of action at a cellular or molecular level (where known) is described.

Routes of Administration/Doses The manufacturer's recommended dose ranges are listed in this section; alternative clinical uses are also mentioned.

Effects The pharmacodynamic properties are systematically reviewed. Where a drug has no specific or known action on a particular physiological system, the relevant section has been omitted.
The systems described are:
CVS   Cardiovascular system.
RS   Respiratory system.
CNS   Central nervous system.
AS   Alimentary system.
GU   Genito-urinary system.
Metabolic/Other   Metabolic, endocrine and miscellaneous.

Toxicity/Side Effects The major side effects are listed, with particular reference to the practice of anaesthesia and intensive care.

Kinetics The available pharmacokinetic data are provided. Quantitative data are not available for all drugs, particularly the long-established ones. Where information on the absorption, distribution, metabolism or excretion is unavailable for a particular drug, the relevant section has been omitted.

Absorption Details of the absorption and bioavailability are given.

Distribution This section provides information on the volume of distribution and degree of protein binding of the drug, together, where appropriate, with details of central nervous penetration, transplacental passage etc.

Metabolism   The site and route of metabolic transformation and nature and activity of metabolites are described.

Excretion   The excretory pathways, clearance and elimination half-life are listed. Although clearances are usually expressed in ml/min/kg, this has not always been possible, due to inadequacies in the original source material.

Special Points   This section describes points of relevance to the practice of anaesthesia and intensive care; in particular, significant drug interactions are reviewed.

This standard format offers great advantages; it enables specific questions to be answered very rapidly. For example, the question 'How is fentanyl metabolised?' may be answered simply by locating the drug alphabetically and then consulting the Metabolism section of the text. This principle holds true for all possible permutations of queries.

Glossary of terms used in this book

ACE	Angiotensin converting enzyme
ADH	Antidiuretic hormone
ARDS	Adult respiratory distress syndrome
ATP	Adenosine triphosphate
AS	Alimentary system
AV	Atrio-ventricular
cAMP	Cyclic adenosine monophosphate
CNS	Central nervous system
COX	Cyclo-oxygenase
CSF	Cerebrospinal fluid
CVS	Cardiovascular system
cGMP	Cyclic guanine monophosphate
DNA	Deoxyribonucleic acid
DVT	Deep vein thrombosis
ECG	Electrocardiogram
EEG	Electroencephalogram
ESR	Erythrocyte sedimentation rate
FEV_1	Forced expiratory volume in 1 second
FiO_2	Inspired oxygen concentration
FVC	Forced vital capacity
GABA	Gamma-aminobutyric acid
GU	Genito-urinary
HIV	Human immunodeficiency virus
5-HT	5-hydroxytryptamine
INR	International normalised ratio
LMA	Laryngeal mask airway
MAC	Minimum alveolar concentration
MAOI	Monoamine oxidase inhibitor
MIC	Minimum inhibitory concentration
mRNA	Messenger ribonucleic acid
MRSA	Methicillin-resistant *Staphylococcus aureus*
NMDA	N-methyl-D-aspartate
NSAID	Non-steroidal anti-inflammatory drug
P_aCO_2	Arterial carbon dioxide tension
PEFR	Peak expiratory flow rate
PVR	Pulmonary vascular resistance
REM	Rapid eye movement
RS	Respiratory system
SA	Sinoatrial
tRNA	Transfer ribonucleic acid
V_D	Volume of distribution

Drugs in Anaesthesia and Intensive Care

Acetazolamide

Uses Acetazolamide is used in the treatment of:
1. glaucoma
2. petit mal epilepsy
3. Menière's disease
4. familial periodic paralysis and
5. the prophylaxis and treatment of mountain sickness.

Chemical A sulphonamide.

Presentation As 250 mg tablets of acetazolamide and in vials containing 500 mg of the sodium salt of acetazolamide for reconstitution with water prior to injection.

Main Actions Diuresis and a decrease in intraocular pressure.

Mode of Action Acetazolamide is a reversible, non-competitive inhibitor of carbonic anhydrase situated within cell cytosol and on the brush border of the proximal convoluted tubule. This enzyme catalyses the conversion of bicarbonate and hydrogen ions into carbonic acid and then carbonic acid to carbon dioxide and water. Under normal circumstances, sodium ions are reabsorbed in exchange for hydrogen ions in the proximal and distal renal tubules; acetazolamide decreases the availability of hydrogen ions and therefore sodium and bicarbonate ions remain in the renal tubule, leading to a diuresis.

Routes of Administration/Doses The adult oral and intravenous dose is 250–1000 mg 4-hourly.

Effects
RS Acetazolamide produces a compensatory increase in ventilation in response to the metabolic acidosis and increased tissue carbon dioxide that the drug causes.
CNS Acetazolamide has demonstrable anticonvulsant properties, possibly related to an elevated carbon dioxide tension within the central nervous system. The drug decreases the pressure of both the cerebrospinal fluid and the intraocular compartment by decreasing the rate of formation of cerebrospinal fluid and aqueous humour (by 50–60%).
AS The drug inhibits gastric and pancreatic secretion.
GU Acetazolamide produces a mild diuresis, with retention of sodium ions and a subsequent increase in plasma sodium ion concentration. The drug also decreases renal excretion of uric acid.
Metabolic/Other The excretion of an alkaline urine results in the development of a hyperchloraemic metabolic acidosis in response to the administration of acetazolamide. The drug also interferes with iodide uptake by the thyroid gland.

Toxicity/Side Effects   Occur rarely, and include gastro-intestinal and haemopoietic disturbances, rashes, renal stones and hypokalaemia.

Kinetics

Absorption   Acetazolamide is rapidly and well absorbed when administered orally; the bioavailability by this route is virtually 100%.

Distribution   The drug is 70–90% protein-bound in the plasma.

Metabolism   Acetazolamide is not metabolised in man.

Excretion   The drug is excreted unchanged in the urine; the clearance is 2.7 l/hour and the elimination-half-life is 1.7–5.8 hours.

Special Points   The use of acetazolamide is contraindic-ated in the presence of hepatic or renal failure, as the drug will worsen any metabolic acidosis and may also cause urolithiasis. Pretreatment with the drug will obtund the increase in intraocu-lar pressure produced by the administration of suxamethonium; however, the use of acetazolamide is of dubious value during eye surgery as it simultaneously increases intrachoroidal vascu-lar volume. Acetazolamide has been used effectively for the correction of metabolic alkalosis in the critically ill.

Acetazolamide is removed by haemodialysis.

Acyclovir

Uses Acyclovir is used in the treatment of:
1. *Herpes simplex* infections of the skin and eye
2. *Herpes simplex* encephalitis
3. recurrent *Varicella zoster* virus infections and
4. for the prophylaxis of *Herpes simplex* infections in immunocompromised patients.

Chemical An analogue of the nucleoside 2'-deoxyguanosine.

Presentation As 200/400/800 mg tablets, a suspension containing 40 mg/ml, a white lyophilised powder in vials containing 250 mg of acyclovir sodium which is reconstituted prior to injection in water and as a 3% and 5% w/w cream for topical application.

Main Actions Acyclovir is an antiviral agent active against *Herpes simplex* (I and II) and *Varicella zoster* virus.

Mode of Action Acyclovir is activated within the viral cell via phosphorylation by a virus-coded thymidine kinase and thus has a low toxicity for normal cells. Acyclovir triphosphate inhibits viral DNA polymerase by becoming incorporated into the DNA primer template, effectively preventing further elongation of the viral DNA chain.

Routes of Administration/Doses The adult oral dose is 200–400 mg 2–5 times daily, initially for a period of 5 days. The corresponding intravenous dose is 5–10 mg/kg 8-hourly infused over a period of one hour. A higher dose is used for zoster than for simplex infections. Topical application should be performed 5 times daily, again for an initial period of 5 days.

Effects
Metabolic/Other Increases in plasma levels of urea and creatinine may occur if the drug is administered intravenously too rapidly.

Toxicity/Side Effects Acyclovir is generally well tolerated. Central nervous system disturbances (including tremors, confusion and seizures) and gastrointestinal upsets may occur. Precipitation of the drug in the renal tubules leading to renal impairment may occur if the drug is administered too rapidly or if an adequate state of hydration is not maintained. The drug is irritant to veins and tissues.

Kinetics

Absorption Oral absorption of the drug is erratic; the bioavailability by this route is 15–30%.

Distribution The drug is 9–33% protein-bound in the plasma; the V_D is 0.32–1.48 l/kg.

Metabolism The major metabolite is 9-carboxymeth-oxymethyl guanine, which is inactive.

Excretion The drug is excreted by active tubular secretion in the urine, 45–80% unchanged. The elimination half-life is 2–3 hours.

Special Points A reduced dose should be used in the presence of renal impairment; haemodialysis removes 60% of the drug.

Adenosine

Uses Adenosine is used in the diagnosis and treatment of paroxysmal supraventricular tachycardia.

Chemical A naturally occurring purine nucleoside.

Presentation As a clear, colourless solution containing 3 mg/ml adenosine in saline.

Main Action Evanescent depression of SA and AV nodal activity. The drug also antagonizes cAMP-mediated catechol stimulation of ventricular muscle. Both actions result in negative chronotropic and dromotropic effects.

Mode of Action Adenosine acts as a direct agonist at specific cell membrane receptors, classified into A1 and A2 subsets. A1 receptors are coupled to potassium channels by a guanine nucleotide-binding protein in supraventricular tissue.

Routes of Administration/Doses Adenosine is administered as a rapid intravenous bolus, followed by a saline flush. The initial adult dose is 3 mg, followed if necessary by a 6 mg and then a 12 mg bolus at 1–2 minute intervals until an effect is observed. The paediatric dose is 0.0375–0.25 mg/kg. The drug acts within 10 seconds and has a duration of action of 10–20 seconds.

Effects

CVS Depression of SA and AV nodal activity leads to termination of paroxysmal supraventricular tachycardia. Atrial dysrhythmias are revealed by AV nodal block leading to transient slowing of ventricular response. Adenosine has no clinically important effects on blood pressure when administered as a bolus. Continuous high-dose infusion may result in a decrease in systemic vascular resistance and decreased blood pressure. When administered as an infusion adenosine causes a dose-dependent reflex tachycardia and an increase in cardiac output. The drug also causes a dose-dependent increase in myocardial blood flow secondary to coronary vasodilation mediated via endothelial A2 receptors. Adenosine decreases PVR in patients with pulmonary hypertension.

RS Bolus administration of adenosine leads to an increase in both the depth and rate of respiration, probably mediated by A2 receptor stimulation in the carotid body. Infusion of the drug results in a fall in PCO_2. Bronchospasm may occur.

CNS Infusion of adenosine results in increased cerebral blood flow. Low-dose adenosine induces neuropathic pain, hyperalgesia and ischaemic pain.

GU Hypotensive doses of adenosine stimulate A2 receptors, resulting in renal and hepatic arterial vasoconstriction, although low doses have no effect on the glomerular filtration rate or sodium excretion.

Metabolic/Other   Adenosine inhibits lipolysis and stimulates glycolysis.

Toxicity/Side Effects   The most common side effects are transient facial flushing, dyspnoea and chest discomfort. Bronchospasm has also been reported. The induced bradycardia predisposes to ventricular excitability and may result in ventricular fibrillation. Profound bradycardia requiring pacing may occur.

Kinetics   Data are incomplete.

Absorption   Adenosine is inactive when administered orally.

Metabolism   Exogenous adenosine is absorbed from the plasma into red blood cells and vascular endothelium, where it is phosphorylated to AMP or deaminated to inosine and hypoxanthine. The plasma half-life is less than 10 seconds.

Special Points   No dose adjustment is necessary in the presence of renal or hepatic impairment. Adenosine has been used to induce hypotension peri-operatively.

Intraoperative use of adenosine decreases the MAC of isoflurane and decreases postoperative analgesic requirements.

Alcuronium

Uses   Alcuronium is used to facilitate intubation and controlled ventilation.

Chemical   A semi-synthetic alkaloid which is a derivative of toxiferine.

Presentation   As a clear, colourless solution for injection (in brown ampoules) containing 5 mg/ml of alcuronium chloride.

Main Action   Competitive neuromuscular blockade.

Mode of Action   Alcuronium acts by competitive antagonism of acetylcholine at nicotinic (N2) receptors at the post-synaptic membrane of the neuromuscular junction; it also has some pre-junctional action.

Route of Administration/Doses   Alcuronium is administered intravenously; the normal intubating dose is 0.2–0.25 mg/kg with subsequent doses of one-quarter this amount. Satisfactory intubating conditions are produced within 2 minutes; a single dose lasts 20–40 minutes. The recovery index of the drug is 11–17 minutes.

Effects
CVS   Alcuronium may cause a slight decrease in blood pressure due to blockade of nicotinic receptors in autonomic ganglia and the adrenal medulla; with the use of higher doses, histamine release may contribute to this effect.
RS   Neuromuscular blockade results in apnoea. High doses may cause histamine release leading to bronchospasm. The drug also tends to increase bronchial secretions.
CNS   Alcuronium has no effect on the intraocular pressure.
AS   The mild propensity of the drug to cause ganglion blockade may lead to a decrease in gut motility and oesophageal sphincter tone. Salivary secretion may increase after the administration of alcuronium.

Toxicity/Side Effects   Severe anaphylactoid reactions have been reported following the use of alcuronium. Malignant hyperpyrexia has been reported in association with the use of the drug.

Kinetics

Absorption   The drug is poorly and erratically absorbed and is inactivated after oral administration.

Distribution   Alcuronium is 40% protein-bound, predominantly to albumin in the plasma; the V_D is 0.37 l/kg. The drug does cross the placenta in significant amounts; the fetal: maternal concentration gradient is 0.6.

Metabolism   No detectable metabolites of the drug have been found in man.

Excretion   70–90% of an administered dose of alcuronium is excreted in the urine unchanged; the remainder is excreted via the bile and faeces. The clearance is 1.3 ml/kg/min and the elimination half-life is 2–4.3 hours. The drug should be used with caution in the presence of renal impairment.

Special Points   The duration of action of alcuronium, in common with other non-depolarising relaxants, is prolonged by hypokalaemia, hypocalcaemia, hypermagnesaemia, hypo-proteinaemia, dehydration, acidosis and hypercapnia. The following drugs, when co-administered with non-depolarising relaxants, increase the effect of the latter: volatile and induction agents, fentanyl, suxamethonium, diuretics, calcium antagonists, alpha- and beta-adrenergic antagonists, protamine, metronidazole and the aminoglycoside antibiotics.

Infusion of alcuronium may cause fixed, dilated pupils.

Alcuronium is pharmaceutically incompatible with thiopentone.

Alfentanil

Uses Alfentanil is used to provide:
1. the analgesic component of general anaesthesia and
2. sedation regimes for intensive care.

Chemical A synthetic anilinopiperidine derivative.

Presentation As a clear, colourless solution for injection containing 0.5/5 mg/ml of alfentanil hydrochloride.

Main Actions Analgesia and respiratory depression.

Mode of Action Alfentanil is a highly selective mu agonist; the mu opioid receptor appears to be specifically involved in the mediation of analgesia. Opioids appear to exert their effects by increasing intracellular calcium concentration which, in turn, increases potassium conductance and hyperpolarisation of excitable cell membranes. The decrease in membrane excitability that results may decrease both pre- and post-synaptic responses.

Route of Administration/Dose Alfentanil is administered intravenously in boluses of 10–50 µg/kg and may be infused at a rate of 0.5–1 µg/kg/minute, The peak effect of the drug occurs within 90 seconds of intravenous administration and the duration of effect is 5–10 minutes.

Effects
CVS The most significant cardiovascular effect that alfentanil demonstrates is bradycardia of vagal origin; the cardiac output, mean arterial pressure, pulmonary and systemic vascular resistance and pulmonary capillary wedge pressure are usually unaffected by the administration of the drug, although hypotension may occur. Doses of 5 mg/kg increase left ventricular contractility and cardiac output in animal models. Alfentanil obtunds the cardiovascular responses to laryngoscopy and intubation.
RS Alfentanil is a potent respiratory depressant, causing a decrease in both the respiratory rate and tidal volume; it also diminishes the ventilatory response to hypoxia and hypercapnia. The drug is a potent antitussive agent. Chest wall rigidity (the 'wooden chest' phenomenon) may occur after the administration of alfentanil – this may be an effect of the drug on mu-receptors located on GABA-ergic interneurones. Alfentanil causes minimal release of histamine; bronchospasm is thus rarely precipitated by the drug.
CNS Alfentanil is 10–20 times more potent as an analgesic than morphine and has little hypnotic or sedative activity. Miosis is produced as a result of stimulation of the Edinger-Westphal nucleus.
AS Alfentanil decreases gastrointestinal motility and decreases gastric acid secretion; it also increases the common bile duct pressure by causing spasm of the sphincter of Oddi.

GU The drug increases the tone of the ureters, bladder detrusor muscle and sphincter.

Metabolic/Other High doses of alfentanil will obtund the metabolic 'stress response' to surgery; the drug appears to be even more effective than fentanyl in this respect.

Toxicity/Side Effects Respiratory depression, bradycardia and nausea and vomiting may complicate the use of alfentanil.

Kinetics

Distribution The drug is 85–92% protein-bound in the plasma; the V_D is 40–70l.

Metabolism Alfentanil is predominantly metabolised in the liver by N-dealkylation to noralfentanil; the remainder of the drug is metabolised by a variety of pathways, including aromatic hydroxylation, demethylation and amide hydrolysis followed by acetylation. The major phase II pathway is by conjugation to glucuronide. There is some evidence for genetic polymorphism in the metabolism of the drug.

Excretion 90% of the dose appears in the urine ($<1\%$ unchanged). The clearance is 300–500 ml/min and the elimination half-life is 100 minutes. The relatively brief duration of action of a single dose of alfentanil in comparison to that of fentanyl is due to the smaller volume of distribution and shorter elimination half-life of the former.

Special Points Alfentanil decreases the apparent MAC of co-administered volatile agents. The concomitant use of erythromycin, fluconazole and diltiazem significantly inhibits the clearance of alfentanil.

It is unknown whether alfentanil is removed by haemodialysis.

Alimemazine

Uses   Alimemazine is used:
1. for premedication and sedation in children
2. for the relief of pruritus and
3. as an antiemetic.

Chemical   A phenothiazine.

Presentation   As 10 mg tablets and an elixir containing 1.5/6mg/ml of alimemazine tartrate.

Main Action   Antihistaminergic (H1 receptors), sedative and antiemetic.

Mode of Action   Alimemazine acts primarily as a reversible competitive antagonist at H1 histaminergic receptors; it also has some anticholinergic and antidopaminergic activity.

Route of Administration/Dose   The recommended oral does for premedication is 2 mg/kg administered 1–2 hours pre-operatively.

Effects
CVS   When normal therapeutic doses are used, alimemazine has no significant cardiovascular effects. The drug may cause reversible ECG changes, including prolongation of the Q-T interval and S-T depression.
RS   Alimemazine causes a decrease in respiratory tract secretions and has antitussive properties. Delayed respiratory depression may occur.
CNS   The drug is a potent sedative and anxiolytic; it is also antiemetic by an inhibitory action at the chemoreceptor trigger zone.
AS   Alimemazine potentiates opioid-induced biliary smooth muscle contraction.
Metabolic/Other   In common with other phenothiazines, the chronic use of alimemazine may result in hyperprolactinaemia.

Toxicity/Side Effects   The drug exhibits predictable anticholinergic side effects and may produce extra-pyramidal reactions (including the neuroleptic maligant syndrome) when used in high doses. Jaundice, photosensitivity, gastrointestinal and haemopoietic disturbances may complicate the use of trimeprazine.

Kinetics   Data are incomplete.

Absorption   The drug is well absorbed when administered orally; the bioavailability by this route is 70–100%, dependent upon the formulation.

Distribution   Alimemazine is 90% protein-bound in the plasma.

Metabolism   The drug is extensively metabolised; 50% of the dose undergoes hydroxylation to a sulphone.

Excretion   The elimination half-life is 4–5 hours.

Special Points   The depressant effects of the drug on the central nervous system are additive with those produced by anaesthetic agents.
   Alimemazine is not removed by dialysis.

Allopurinol

Uses Allopurinol is used:
1. for the prophylaxis of gout
2. to prevent renal stone formation in patients with xanthin-uria and
3. in the prophylaxis of the tumour lysis syndrome.

Chemical A hypoxanthine analogue.

Presentation As 100/300 mg tablets of allopurinol.

Main Action Xanthine oxidase inhibitor and free-radical scavenger.

Mode of Action Allopurinol and its active metabolite oxipurinol inhibit xanthine oxidase, the enzyme responsible for the conversion of hypoxanthine and xanthine to uric acid. The drug has no anti-inflammatory, analgesic or uricosuric actions.

Route of Administration/Dose The adult oral dose is 100–900 mg daily, adjusted according to the serum uric acid level. The serum urate levels begin to decrease 24–48 hours after initiation of treatment; the maximum effect is observed after 1–3 weeks.

Effects
GU Allopurinol decreases the urinary excretion of uric acid and calcium.

Toxicity/Side Effects Allopurinol is generally well toler-ated. Rashes, gastrointestinal and haemopoietic disturbances, jaundice and interstitial nephritis may complicate the use of the drug. Allopurinol may precipitate an acute attack of gout during the early stages of treatment.

Kinetics

Absorption Allopurinol is well absorbed when admin-istered orally; the bioavailability by this route is 80–90%.

Distribution The drug is not protein-bound in the plasma; the V_D is 0.6 l/kg.

Metabolism Allopurinol is rapidly converted to an active metabolite, oxipurinol.

Excretion Occurs of both allopurinol and oxipurinol pre-dominantly in the urine; some 20% is excreted in faeces. The clearance of allopurinol is 680 ml/min/kg and the elimination half-life is 1–3 hours.

Special Points An adequate urine output should be ensured during treatment with the drug; the dose of allopurinol should be reduced in the presence of severe renal impairment.

Allopurinol may protect against stress-induced gastric mucosal injury by scavenging oxygen-derived free radicals.

The drug and its metabolites are removed by haemodialysis.

Alteplase

Uses Alteplase is used in the treatment of acute myocardial infarction occurring as a result of coronary artery thrombosis.

Chemical A recombinant DNA-derived version of a naturally occurring glycoprotein.

Presentation As a dry powder in vials containing 10 mg (5.8 million IU) and 50 mg (29 million IU) of alteplase, which is reconstituted in water prior to injection.

Main Action Thrombolysis.

Mode of Action Alteplase binds to clots and selectively converts fibrin-bound plasminogen to plasmin, which then acts to lyse the fibrin clot. Systemic fibrinogenolysis occurs to a lesser extent than occurs after the administration of streptokinase.

Route of Administration/Dose The drug should be administered intravenously within 6 hours of the onset of the thrombotic episode. The adult dose is 100 mg (1.5 mg/kg) administered over a period of three hours. 10% of the total dose should be administered as a bolus over 1–2 minutes, 50% of the total dose should be administered as an infusion over the next hour and the remainder over the subsequent two hours. Coronary artery reperfusion occurs within 15–30 minutes and is complete within one hour. The fibrinolytic action of alteplase lasts several hours.

Effects
CVS The ejection fraction increases and the left ventricular end-diastolic pressure decreases after administration of the drug to patients with acute coronary artery thrombosis; the incidence of dysrhythmias is also decreased. The drug significantly improves survival in patients with acute myocardial infarction if administered within 6 hours.
Metabolic/Other Clot lysis occurs more rapidly after the administration of alteplase than after streptokinase and reperfusion is achieved in 65–75% of patients; the drug thus appears to be more effective than streptokinase in this respect. The commercial preparation of alteplase contains arginine which may impair glucose tolerance.

Toxicity/Side Effects The drug is usually well tolerated. Bleeding may occur at the injection site and intracerebral haemorrhage occurs in 0.5%. No serious allergic reactions have been reported. The drug occasionally causes nausea and vomiting.

Kinetics Data are incomplete.

Distribution   The V_D is 0.09–1.2 l/kg.

Metabolism   Occurs primarily in the liver.

Excretion   The clearance is 10 ml/min/kg and the elimination half-life is 14–38 minutes. A reduced dose should be used in the presence of renal impairment.

Special Points   The drug should not be used after traumatic cardiopulmonary resuscitation or within 10 days of major surgery.

Amikacin

Uses   Amikacin is used in the treatment of serious infections caused by sensitive Gram-negative bacteria.

Chemical   A semi-synthetic aminoglycoside.

Presentation   As a clear solution for injection containing 50/250 mg/ml of amikacin sulphate.

Main Actions   Amikacin is a broad spectrum antibiotic that is effective against the Gram-negative organisms *Pseudomonas*, indole-positive and negative *Proteus, Klebsiella, Salmonella* and *Shigella* sp. and *Escherichia coli*. The Gram-positive *Staphylococcus aureus* (including some MRSA) is also sensitive to the drug. Acquired bacterial resistance occurs less commonly with amikacin that with other aminoglycosides.

Mode of Action   Amikacin binds irreversibly to specific bacterial ribosomal proteins and inhibits protein synthesis by interfering with initiation of the polypeptide chain and by inducing misreading of mRNA.

Routes of Administration/Doses   The adult intramuscular and intravenous dose is 500 mg 8–12 hourly.

Toxicity/Side Effects   Ototoxicity (with vestibular and auditory components) and nephrotoxicity (a form of acute tubular necrosis occurring 5–7 days after exposure) are the most serious side effects and both are correlated with high trough concentrations of the drug. Rashes, nausea and vomiting and drug fever may also occur with the use of amikacin.

Kinetics

Absorption   The drug is not absorbed orally.

Distribution   Amikacin is 21% protein-bound in the plasma; the V_D is 0.21–0.33 l/kg.

Metabolism   The drug is not metabolised in man.

Excretion   Amikacin is excreted unchanged in the urine. The clearance is 0.7–1.9 ml/min/kg and the elimination half-life is 1.9–2.7 hours. A reduced dose and/or an increased dosage internal should be used in patients with renal impairment.

Special Points   Monitoring of plasma concentrations should commence after 3–5 doses of amikacin and 24 hours after any change in dose. Trough samples are taken immediately before a dose and peak samples should be taken one hour after intramuscular and 10 minutes after intravenous administration. The optimum peak concentrations are 15–25 mg/1 and the corresponding trough concentrations are <4–6 mg/ml. The drug is removed by both haemodialysis and haemofiltration.

Aminolycosides prolong the action of non-depolarising muscle relaxants by inhibiting pre-synaptic acetylcholine release and by stabilisation of the post-synaptic membrane at the neuromuscular junction. This effect may be reversed by the intravenous administration of calcium.

Amiloride

Uses   Amiloride is used in the treatment of:
1.   oedema of cardiac, renal or hepatic origin
2.   hypertension and
3.   in combination with loop or thiazide diuretics to conserve potassium.

Chemical   A pyrazinoylguanidine.

Presentation   As 5 mg tablets of amiloride hydrochloride and in various fixed-dose combinations with thiazide or loop diuretics.

Main Action   Diuretic.

Mode of Action   Amiloride selectively blocks sodium reabsorption in the distal convoluted tubule. As a result of the inhibition of sodium ion transport, the electrical potential across the tubular epithelium decreases and potassium ion excretion is inhibited. The net result is a slight increase in renal sodium ion excretion and a decrease in excessive potassium ion excretion.

Route of Administration/Dose   The adult oral dose is 10–20 mg daily. The diuretic effect, commences within 2 hours and lasts 24 hours.

Effects
CVS   With chronic use, amiloride causes a slight decrease in the systolic and diastolic blood pressure, probably due to a reduction in the sodium ion content of arteriolar smooth muscle producing a decrease in the systemic vascular resistance.
GU   The principal effect is diuresis, with an increased rate of sodium and bicarbonate ion excretion, and a decreased rate of potassium, calcium, ammonium and hydrogen ion excretion. The drug has no effect on free water clearance.
Metabolic/Other   The inhibition of hydrogen ion excretion leads to slight alkalinisation of the urine; serum uric acid concentrations are also increased following the administration of amiloride. A metabolic acidosis may occur.

Toxicity/Side Effects   The most significant side effect of the drug is hyperkalaemia; other reported side effects, although legion, occur infrequently. These include nausea and vomiting, abdominal pain, diarrhoea, rashes, cramps, central nervous system and haemopoietic disturbances, impotence and interstitial nephritis.

Kinetics

Absorption   Amiloride is incompletely absorbed when administered orally; the bioavailability by this route is 50%.

Distribution The drug is <5% protein-bound in the plasma; the V_D is 5 l/kg.

Metabolism No metabolism of the drug occurs in man.

Excretion 50% of the dose is excreted unchanged in the urine; the remainder in the faeces. The clearance is 264–372 ml/min and the elimination half-life is 18–24 hours (this is prolonged to 140 hours in the presence of renal failure).

Special Points Amiloride inhibits the excretion of co-administered digoxin; concurrent NSAID therapy tends to obtund the diuretic and antihypertensive effects of the drug.

Aminophylline

Uses Aminophylline is used in the treatment of:
1. asthma
2. chronic obstructive airways disease and
3. heart failure.

Chemical The ethylenediamine salt of theophylline (a methylated xanthine derivative).

Presentation As tablets containing 100/225/350 mg of aminophylline, as 180/360 mg suppositories and as a clear solution for injection containing 25 mg/ml of aminophylline.

Main Actions Bronchodilatation, associated with an increased ventilatory response to hypoxia and hypercapnia.

Mode of Action Aminophylline acts by inhibiting a magnesium-dependent phosphodiesterase, the enzyme responsible for the degradation of cAMP. The drug has a synergistic effect with those catecholamines which directly activate adenyl cyclase and lead to an increase in the intracellular concentration of cAMP. In addition, aminophylline interferes with the influx of calcium ions into smooth muscle cells and stabilises mast cells by antagonising the action of adenosine.

Routes of Administration/Doses The adult daily oral dose is 900 mg administered in 2–3 divided doses, and the rectal dose 360 mg daily, titrated according to response. The loading dose by the intravenous route is 5 mg/kg over 10–15 minutes; this may be followed by a maintenance infusion of 0.5 mg/kg/hr. An intravenous loading dose should be administered with extreme caution to patients already receiving oral or rectal aminophylline. The therapeutic range is narrow (10–20 μg/ml) and estimations of the plasma concentration of aminophylline are of value during chronic therapy.

Effects
CVS The drug has mild positive inotropic and chronotropic effects, producing an increase in cardiac output and a decrease in systemic vascular resistance, leading to a decrease in arterial blood pressure. The left ventricular end-diastolic pressure and pulmonary capillary wedge pressure tend to decrease with the use of the drug. Aminophylline is arrhythmogenic at the upper extremes of its therapeutic range; it is synergistic with halothane in this respect.
RS Aminophylline causes bronchodilatation, leading to an increase in vital capacity. It also increases the sensitivity of the respiratory centre to CO_2 and increases diaphragmatic contractility. Intravenous administration of the drug inhibits hypoxic pulmonary vasoconstriction and necessitates the administration of oxygen during therapy.

CNS Aminophylline is a central nervous system stimulant and lowers the seizure threshold. The cerebral blood flow tends to decrease.

AS Intravenous aminophylline increases gastric acid and pepsin output and decreases small and large bowel motility. The drug counteracts opioid-induced spasm of the sphincter of Oddi.

GU Aminophylline increases the renal blood flow and glomerular filtration rate and decreases renal tubular sodium absorption, leading to a diuretic effect.

Metabolic/Other Hypokalaemia may occur secondary to the diuretic effect and also to increased cellular uptake of potassium. Abnormalities of liver function tests and inappropriate ADH secretion are also recognised effects of the drug.

Toxicity/Side Effects Gastrointestinal and central nervous system disturbances (including convulsions after rapid intravenous administration), and cardiac dysrhythmias (including ventricular fibrillation) may occur, especially with plasma concentrations in excess of 20 μg/ml.

Kinetics

Absorption Aminophylline is rapidly absorbed when administered orally and has a bioavailability by this route of 88–96%. Rectal absorption is slow and erratic.

Distribution The drug is 50–60% protein-bound in the plasma; the V_D is 0.4–0.5 l/kg.

Metabolism Occurs in the liver by demethylation and oxidation; a 3-methyl xanthine derivative is active.

Excretion Demethylated metabolites are excreted in the urine; 10–13% of the dose is excreted unchanged. The clearance is 0.83–1.16 ml/min/kg; this is decreased in the presence of heart failure, liver disease and in the elderly. Saturation of the metabolic pathways occurs near the therapeutic range; whilst obeying zero-order kinetics, the elimination half-life varies with the dose. Under conditions of first-order kinetics, the elimination half-life is 8 hours.

Special Points Co-administration of cimetidine, propranolol or erythromycin will elevate plasma concentrations of aminophylline; conversely, co-administration of barbiturates, alcohol or phenytoin will decrease plasma concentrations of aminophylline. The site of these interactions appears to be cytochrome P450. In high concentrations, the drug will antagonise non-depolarising neuromuscular blockade caused by pancuronium or tubocurarine.

Aminophylline infusion shortens the recovery time from enflurane–nitrous oxide anaesthesia.

Amiodarone

Uses   Amiodarone is used in the treatment of:
1.   tachydysrhythmias inappropriate for, or resistant to, other drugs and
2.   those associated with the Wolff-Parkinson-White syndrome.

Chemical   An iodinated benzofuran derivative.

Presentation   As 100/200 mg tablets of amiodarone hydrochloride and in ampoules containing 30/50 mg/ml of amiodarone hydrochloride for injection.

Main Actions   A class III antiarrhythmic agent.

Mode of Action   Amiodarone acts by partial antagonism of alpha- and beta-agonists by reducing the number of receptors or by inhibiting the coupling of receptors to the regulatory subunit of the adenylate cyclase system. In addition, the drug has a direct action in isolated myocardial preparations to decrease the delayed slow outward potassium current and, in higher doses, additionally depresses the fast and slow inward currents, which are due to sodium and calcium respectively.

Routes of Administration/Doses   The initial intravenous dose is 5 mg/kg, administered by infusion diluted in 250 ml of 5% dextrose over 20–120 minutes via a central vein (the drug carrier is highly irritant). Most patients respond to an intravenous loading dose within 1 hour. Subsequently, 15 mg/kg/day may be administered intravenously if oral administration is not desirable or feasible. The adult oral dose is initially 200 mg 8-hourly, reducing to 100–200 mg daily after 1 week. The therapeutic level is 0.1 µg/ml.

Effects
CVS   Sinus rhythm is slowed by 15% secondary to a reduction in the slow diastolic depolarisation in nodal cells after the administration of amiodarone. Atrio-ventricular nodal automaticity is depressed and atrio-ventricular nodal conduction is slowed by 25% in the face of atrial tachycardia due to a decreased speed of depolarisation of cells and an increase in the duration of the action potential. Amiodarone has no effect on conduction in the His bundle or ventricular myocardium. After oral administration, little effect is seen on the blood pressure or left ventricular contractility; the systemic vascular resistance decreases and coronary sinus blood flow increases. After intravenous administration, left ventricular contractility may decrease; the effects are otherwise similar to those observed after oral administration.
Metabolic/Other   Abnormalities of liver function tests occur in up to 50% of patients; abnormalities of thyroid function

tests may also occur due to inhibition of triiodothyronine and enhancement of reverse-triiodothyronine production.

Toxicity/Side Effects Almost all patients receiving amiodarone develop corneal microdeposits and one-third develop signs of central nervous system toxicity. Pneumonitis, cirrhosis, peripheral neuropathy, photosensitivity and gastrointestinal upsets are well recognised complications. Hypotension, cardiovascular collapse and atrio-ventricular block have been reported after intravenous injection. Other dysrhythmias may arise, especially in the presence of hypokalaemia.

Kinetics

Absorption The drug is incompletely absorbed after oral administration and has a bioavailability of 22–86%.

Distribution Amiodarone is 96–98% protein-bound in the plasma; the V_D is 1.3–65.8 l/kg according to the dose.

Metabolism The metabolic pathways of amiodarone have not been fully elucidated – it appears to be extensively metabolised in the liver, the major metabolite being desethyl-amiodarone which has antiarrhythmic properties and is cumulative.

Excretion 1–5% of the dose appears in the urine, the drug appears to be extensively excreted in the bile and faeces. The clearance is 0.14–0.6 l/min and the elimination half-life has been estimated at 4 hours–52 days, depending on the dose and route of administration.

Special Points Modification of the dose is not required in the presence of renal impairment; amiodarone is not removed by haemodialysis. The actions of digoxin, calcium antagonists, oral anticoagulants and beta-adrenergic antagonists may be potentiated by amiodarone, due to displacement from plasma proteins. Bradycardia, complete and atrio-ventricular heart block resistant to atropine, adrenaline and noradrenaline have been reported in patients receiving amiodarone undergoing general anaesthesia; it has been suggested that such patients may require temporary pacing in the peri-operative period.

The drug is contraindicated in porphyria.

Amitriptyline

Uses   Amitriptyline is used for the treatment of:
1. depression
2. nocturnal enuresis and can be used
3. as an adjunct in the treatment of chronic pain syndromes including chronic tension headache, post-herpetic neuralgia, painful neuropathies and chronic spinal syndromes.

Chemical   A dibenzocycloheptadiene derivative.

Presentation   As tablets containing 10/25/50 mg and a clear, colourless solution for injection containing 10 mg/ml of amitriptyline hydrochloride. A syrup containing 2 mg/ml of amitriptyline embonate is also available.

Main Actions   Antidepressant, sedative and analgesic.

Mode of Action   Tricyclic antidepressants potentiate the action of biogenic amines within the central nervous system by preventing their re-uptake at nerve terminals. They also antagonise muscarinic cholinergic, alpha-1 adrenergic and H1 and H2 histaminergic receptors.

Routes of Administration/Doses   The adult oral dose is initially 75–150 mg/day, decreasing to 50–100 mg/day for maintenance. The corresponding parenteral dose is 10–20 mg 6-hourly. The drug takes from 3–30 days to become fully effective.

Effects
CVS   In high doses, amitriptyline may cause postural hypotension, sinus tachycardia, dysrhythmias and an increase in the conduction time through the atrio-ventricular node. The PR and QT intervals may be prolonged.
RS   The drug may cause respiratory depression when administered in toxic doses.
CNS   The predominant effect of the drug is an antidepressant action, which may take several weeks to develop; sedation, weakness and fatigue are also commonly produced.

Toxicity/Side Effects   A wide spectrum of cardiovascular, central nervous system, gastrointestinal and haematological disturbances may complicate the use of amitriptyline. Anticholinergic side effects (blurred vision, dryness of the mouth, constipation and urinary retention) tend to predominate.

Kinetics

Absorption   The drug is rapidly absorbed when administered orally; the bioavailability is 45% by this route.

Distribution   Amitriptyline is 95% protein-bound in the plasma; the V_D is 18–22 l/kg.

Metabolism   Occurs by N-demethylation and hydroxylation with subsequent conjugation to glucuronide and sulphate.

Excretion   The conjugates are excreted in the urine. The clearance is 9.7–15.3 ml/min/kg and the elimination half-life is 12.9–36.1 hours.

Special Points   Scopolamine and the phenothiazines displace tricyclic antidepressants from their binding sites on plasma proteins and thus increase the activity of the latter; barbiturates increase the rate of hepatic metabolism of tricyclic antidepressants and decrease their activity. Amitriptyline accentuates the cardiovascular effects of epinephrine; care should be exercised when local anaesthetic agents containing epinephrine are used in patients receiving the drug. Amitriptyline also increases the likelihood of dysrhythmias and hypotension occurring during general anaesthesia.

Amitriptyline is not removed by haemodialysis.

Amphotericin

Uses Amphotericin is used in the treatment of life-threatening systemic fungal infections, especially disseminated candidosis, coccidiomycosis, histoplasmosis, aspergillosis and crytococcosis.

Chemical Amphotericin is a mixture of two polyene macrolides (amphotericin A and B) produced by *Streptomyces nodosus*.

Presentation As 100 mg tablets and a yellow powder in vials containing 50 000 units of amphotericin (with sodium desoxycholate which solubilises amphotericin); the mixture forms a colloidal suspension in water.

As a yellow opaque suspension of 5 mg/ml of amphotericin B complexed with two phospholipids is a 1:1 drug to lipid molar ratio, pH 5–7 – a ribbon-like structure. As liposomal amphotericin, a lyphophilised 50 mg product presentation where the 100 nm liposomes are created so that the amphotericin is intercalated within the unilamellar bilayer structure. As an elongated disc structure 100 nm in diameter of 1:1 molar ratio of amphotericin B and cholesteryl sulphate is 50 and 100 mg vials, presented in lypholised powder for reconstitution to form a colloidal dispersion.

Main Actions Amphotericin is a fungistatic antibiotic which is active against a wide range of yeasts and yeast-like fungi, including *Candida albicans*.

Mode of Action The drug binds to cell membrane sterols, leading to altered membrane permeability to univalent ions, water and small non-electrolyte molecules. Leakage of intracellular components occurs, cell growth is inhibited and cell death may result. Amphotericin binds preferentially to sterols (especially ergosterol) in fungal cell membranes, although it does bind to sterols (especially cholesterol) in animal cell membranes, where it exerts similar effects.

Route of Administration/Dose Amphotericin is administered by slow intravenous infusion (via a dedicated vein) diluted in 5% dextrose over 6 hours; the daily dose is 0.25–1.5 mg/kg and treatment will usually be required for a period of several weeks. Intrathecal, topical and nebulised administration of the drug have also been described. Amphotericin may also be administered orally for selective decontamination of the gut.

Effects
GU Deterioration of renal function leading to hypokalaemia, renal tubular acidosis or nephrocalcinosis occurs in more than 80% of patients who receive the drug; this is usually reversible but is not necessarily so.

Metabolic/Other   The drug may decrease serum magnesium levels. Amphotericin may alter immune function (especially that of T cells and monocytes) and thereby potentiate host defences.

Toxicity/Side Effects   The list of side effects reported with the use of amphotericin is lengthy. Gastrointestinal upsets (anorexia, nausea and vomiting, loss of weight), haematological impairment (anaemia, thrombocytopenia, leucopenia) and disturbances of the central nervous system (headache, muscle pains, vision disturbances, hearing loss, convulsions, peripheral neuropathy) may occur. The drug may also cause fever and phlebitis; acute dysrhythmias have also been reported.

Kinetics   The assay only distinguishes amphotericin B.

Absorption   The drug is poorly absorbed when administered orally.

Distribution   Amphotericin is 90–95% bound in the plasma to lipoproteins; the V_D is 3.6–4.4 l/kg.

Metabolism   The metabolic pathway of amphotericin has not been established; the liver appears to be the principal site of metabolism.

Excretion   The drug is predominantly excreted in the urine, 2–5% unchanged. The dose should be reduced in the presence of renal impairment as continued use of the drug may lead to further renal impairment. The clearance is 0.35–0.51 ml/min/kg and the elimination half-life is 15 days. The high clearance and large V_D indicate tissue uptake and the long half-life indicates slow redistribution from tissues. Non-linear behaviour occurs with increasing dosage.

Special Points   Liposomal encapsulation or incorporation into a lipid complex can substantially affect amphotericin's action compared to the free drug. There is a theoretical risk of amphotericin enhancing the effect of non-depolarising relaxants and digoxin secondary to the hypokalaemia that the former produces. Liposomal amphotericin (amphotericin incorporated into unilamellar liposomes) is safe, effective and better tolerated, but may cause disordered liver function tests. The drug is, poorly dialysable.

Ampicillin

Uses   Ampicillin is used in the treatment of:
1. ear, nose, and throat and respiratory tract infections
2. urinary tract infections, including gonorrhoea
3. septicaemia
4. endocarditis and
5. meningitis.

Chemical   A semi-synthetic aminopenicillin.

Presentation   As 250/500 mg capsules and a suspension containing 25/50/100 mg/ml of ampicillin trihydrate and in vials containing 250/500 mg of ampicillin sodium.

Main Actions   Ampicillin is bactericidal against a wide range of organisms including some strains of the Gram-negative *Haemophilus influenzae* and *Escherichia coli* (benzylpenicillin showing lower activity against these species), *Proteus mirabilis, Bordetella pertussis* and *Neisseria, Salmonella* and *Shigella* sp. The drug is nearly always effective against the Gram-positive *Streptococcus, Staphylococcus* and *Clostridium* sp. It is ineffective against *Pseudomonas* and *Klebsiella* sp. and penicillinase-producing organisms.

Mode of Action   Ampicillin acts in the manner typical of penicillins; it binds to penicillin-binding proteins in the bacterial cell wall and inhibits pentapeptide cross-linking during its formation, resulting in cell wall disruption.

Routes of Administration/Doses   The adult oral dose is 250 mg–1 g 6-hourly and the corresponding parenteral dose is 500 mg–2 g 6-hourly.

Toxicity/Side Effects   Allergic phenomena, gastrointestinal upsets, interstitial nephritis and haemopoietic disturbances may complicate the use of the drug. Intracranial hypertension has been reported in association with the use of ampicillin. An erythematous rash generally specific to ampicillin has been described.

Kinetics

Absorption   The drug is rapidly but incompletely absorbed when administered orally; the bioavailability by this route is 20–60%.

Distribution   Ampicillin is 18% protein-bound in the plasma, predominantly to albumin; the V_D is 0.28 l/kg.

Metabolism   12–21% is metabolised in the liver by hydrolysis to penicilloic acid.

Excretion   After intravenous injection, 90% appears as unchanged ampicillin in the urine. The drug is also excreted in the bile; enterohepatic recycling occurs and an appreciable quantity appears in the faeces. The clearance is 3.9 ml/min/kg and the elimination half-life is 1–1.3 hours.

Special Points A reduced dose should be used if the creatinine clearance is less than 50 ml/min; haemodialysis removes about 40% of an administered dose.

There is an increased incidence of dermatological reactions in patients with cytomegalovirus infections, infectious mononucleosis and leukaemias who receive ampicillin.

Amoxicillin is similar to ampicillin but has the advantage of an improved bioavailability (70–98%) – it is used in an oral dose of 3 g for the prophylaxis of subacute bacterial endocarditis.

Aprotinin

Uses   Aprotinin is used for:
1. life-threatening haemorrhage due to hyperplasminaemia and has been used for
2. the treatment of acute pancreatitis
3. the reduction of blood loss during cardiopulmonary bypass, transurethral resection of the prostate gland and liver transplantation and
4. the prevention of post-operative deep vein thrombosis.

Chemical   A single chain polypeptide which occurs naturally in bovine lung and other tissues.

Presentation   As a clear solution containing 1.4 mg/ml (10 000 kallikrein inactivator units) in 0.9% sodium chloride.

Main Action   Inhibition of fibrinolysis.

Mode of Action   Aprotinin acts as an inhibitor of human trypsin, plasmin and plasma and tissue kallikreins by forming reversible enzyme-inhibitor complexes. Haemostasis is thus re-established by the inactivation of free plasmin.

Route of Administration/Doses   Aprotinin is administered intravenously as an adult loading dose of 500 000–1 000 000 KIU, followed by an infusion of 200 000 KIU/hour until bleeding stops.

Effects
GU   The glomerular filtration rate is decreased by the drug.
Metabolic/Other   The drug inhibits platelet aggregation and prevents microaggregate formation in stored blood. High doses may limit complement activation.

Toxicity/Side Effects   Side effects are rare with the use of aprotinin; thrombophlebitis and hypersensitivity reactions (including anaphylaxis) have occasionally been reported.

Kinetics

Absorption   Being a protein, aprotinin is destroyed when taken orally.

Distribution   The drug is highly protein-bound in the plasma to acidic glycoproteins.

Metabolism   The drug is virtually completely metabolised in lysosomes within the kidney to small peptides and amino acids.

Excretion   Occurs in the urine; the elimination half-life is 0.7–2 hours.

Special Points   There have been isolated reports of prolongation of the duration of action of suxamethonium and tubocurarine by aprotinin.

Aspirin

Uses Aspirin is used:
1. for the treatment of pain of mild to moderate severity and severe bone pain
2. as an anti-inflammatory agent in e.g. rheumatoid and osteoarthritis
3. as an antipyretic
4. for the prevention of recurrence after myocardial infarction
5. for the prevention of graft occlusion after coronary artery surgery
6. in the treatment of pre-eclampsia
7. for the prevention of transient ischaemic attacks and
8. DVT prophylaxis post joint replacement or fractured neck of femur.

Chemical An aromatic ester of acetic acid.

Presentation As 75/100/300/600 mg tablets of aspirin and in a variety of fixed-dose combinations.

Main Actions Antipyretic, analgesic and anti-inflammatory.

Mode of Action Aspirin acetylates and thereby inhibits the enzyme cyclo-oxygenase which converts arachidonic acid to cyclic endoperoxides, thus preventing the formation of prostaglandins and thromboxanes. Prostaglandins are involved in the sensitisation of peripheral pain receptors to noxious stimuli. It may also inhibit the lipo-oxygenase pathway by an action on hydroperoxy fatty acid peroxidase. The drug inhibits cyclo-oxygenase irreversibly in platelets, but not in endothelium.

Route of Administration/Dose The adult oral dose is 300–900 mg 6–8 hourly; aspirin is not recommended for use in children under 12 years of age.

Effects
CVS Aspirin has minimal haemodynamic effects at normal doses; however, platelet aggregation is inhibited and the bleeding time is increased by a decrease in thromboxane A_2 production (with large doses, the concentration of prothrombin is decreased).
RS Therapeutic doses of aspirin increase oxygen consumption and carbon dioxide production by uncoupling oxidative phosphorylation. Overdosage may lead to hyperventilation (by a direct action of the drug on the respiratory centre), pulmonary oedema and respiratory failure.
CNS The analgesic effect of the drug appears to be exerted by both central and peripheral mechanisms; the antipyretic effect may be a manifestation of inhibition of prostaglandin synthesis at the hypothalamic level.

AS Aspirin increases gastric acid production.

GU The drug may cause proteinuria and an increase in the number of renal tubular casts appearing in the urine. Aspirin is uricosuric in high doses but paradoxically decreases urate excretion at low doses.

Metabolic/Other Blood sugar tends to decrease with low doses, and increase with high doses of aspirin. Transient elevation of serum urea concentrations and elevation of liver enzymes may occur. Lipogenesis is decreased; very large doses of aspirin stimulate steroid secretion.

Toxicity/Side Effects Gastrointestinal upsets occur in 2–6%; haemorrhage and gastric ulceration occur in about 1 in 10 000 of habitual users of aspirin. Large doses of the drug taken over a prolonged period may cause hepatic impairment and renal papillary necrosis leading to chronic renal failure. Allergic response (including bronchospasm), central nervous system disturbances and aplastic anaemia may also occur. The use of aspirin is associated with the development of Reye's syndrome in children.

Kinetics

Absorption Aspirin is rapidly and completely absorbed from the upper gastrointestinal tract and has a bioavailablity of 70% due to an extensive first-pass metabolism.

Distribution Aspirin is rapidly hydrolysed to salicylic acid – the pharmacokinetics are of this compound. Salicylic acid is 80–90% protein-bound in the plasma, primarily to albumin. The V_D is 9.6–12.71. The drug has only a limited ability to cross the blood–brain barrier.

Metabolism/Excretion At therapeutic doses 50% of salicylic acid is metabolised to salicylurate in the liver via a saturable enzyme pathway. A further 20% is metabolised to salicylphenolic glucuronide, which is also a saturable pathway. First-order kinetics occur with the metabolic pathways of salicylacyl glucuronide (10%) and gentisic acid (5%) production and with the urinary excretion of salicylic acid (15%). Due to the two saturable metabolic pathways, the elimination of salicylic acid obeys non-linear kinetics, i.e. the half-life varies with the dose administered.

Special Points Salicylates may increase the effect of co-administered oral anticoagulants and sulphonylureas due to displacement from plasma proteins. Overdosage with aspirin has a 1–2% mortality and may result in respiratory alkalosis or metabolic acidosis according to the age of the patient and the time of ingestion. Alkalisation of the urine increases the excretion of free salicylic acid – the fraction of free drug may increase from 5 to 85%. This principle is used in forced alkaline diuresis and aspirin is removed by haemodialysis.

Aspirin

A normal bleeding time should be demonstrated before embarking upon spinal or epidural anaesthesia in patients receiving aspirin.

Pre-operative ingestion of aspirin is associated with increased blood loss during open heart surgery and prostatectomy.

Atenolol

Uses   Atenolol is used in the treatment of:
1. hypertension
2. angina
3. tachydysrhythmias
4. both in the acute phase of myocardial infarction and in the prevention of reinfarction

Chemical   A phenoxypropanolamine.

Presentation   As 25/50/100 mg tablets (and in fixed-dose combinations with nifedipine, amiloride and chlorthalidone), a 0.5% syrup and as a clear, colourless solution for injection containing 0.5 mg/ml of atenolol.

Main Actions   Atenolol is negatively inotropic and chronotropic, leading to a fall in myocardial oxygen consumption; it also has antihypertensive and antiarrhythmic properties.

Mode of Action   Atenolol acts by reversible competitive blockade of cardiac beta-1 receptors, and also has some action at beta-2 receptors.

Routes of Administration/Doses   The adult oral dose is 50–100 mg daily. Intravenously, 2.5–10 mg may be administered at a rate of 1 mg/min until the desired effect is achieved.

Effects

CVS Sinus node automaticity and atrio-ventricular nodal conduction are decreased. Atrial and atrio-ventricular node effective refractory periods are all increased by the administration of atenolol. No effect is seen on conduction in the His-Purkinje system or the effective refractory period of the ventricles. The ensuing negative inotropic and chronotropic effects lead to a decrease in myocardial oxygen consumption. Atenolol has no intrinsic sympathomimetic activity. The drug has a prolonged antihypertensive effect and can lead to regression of left ventricular hypertrophy in hypertensive patients.

RS Little effect is seen on lung function due to the cardio-selectivity of atenolol.

CNS Poor central nervous system penetration means that little effect is seen; however, sleep disturbances and vivid dreams have been reported.

GU A clinically insignificant elevation in serum urea or creatinine may be produced by the drug.

Metabolic/Other   The plasma triglyceride levels may increase and HDL cholesterol levels may decrease following the use of atenolol.

Toxicity/Side Effects   The side effects are predictable manifestations of the drug's pharmacological effects: exacerbation of peripheral vascular disease, bronchospasm, masking of the signs of hypoglycaemia, depression, impotence and altered bowel habit. The precipitation of heart failure by atenolol is rare.

Kinetics

Absorption   The oral bioavailability is 50%.

Distribution   Atenolol is 3% protein-bound in the plasma; the V_D is 0.7 l/kg.

Metabolism   Less than 10% is metabolised in the liver.

Excretion   The drug is excreted largely unchanged in the urine. The clearance is 77 ml/min/kg (which is decreased in the presence of renal failure) and the elimination half-life is 6–9 hours.

Special Points   The dosage should be reduced in renal failure if the glomerular filtration is less than 35 ml/min; the drug is readily dialysable.

Beta-blockade should be continued throughout the peri-operative period; a single pre-operative dose of atenolol may be as valuable as chronic treatment in the anaesthetic management of patients with borderline hypertension, and in decreasing the hypertensive response to intubation and subsequent dysrhythmias.

Atracurium

Uses   Atracurium is used to facilitate intubation and controlled ventilation.

Chemical   A benzyl isoquinolinium ester.

Presentation   As a clear, colourless solution for injection containing 10 mg/ml of atracurium besilate needing to be stored at 4–10 °C.

Main Action   Competitive neuromuscular blockade.

Mode of Action   Atracurium acts by competitive antagonism of acetylcholine at nicotinic (N2) receptors at the post-synaptic membrane of the neuromuscular junction.

Route of Administration/Dose   The drug is administered intravenously; the normal intubating dose is 0.3–0.6 mg/kg with subsequent doses of one-third this amount. Satisfactory intubating conditions are produced within 90 seconds; there is a linear relationship between the dose and the duration of action. The recovery rate following administration by infusion is similar to that observed after bolus administration; the recovery index is 10–16 minutes, independent of dose. 95% recovery of twitch height occurs in 35 minutes. The drug is non-cumulative with repeated administration.

Effects
CVS   Atracurium has minimal cardiovascular effects; there is a change of $< 5\%$ in the heart rate, mean arterial pressure, systemic vascular resistance, central venous pressure and pulmonary capillary wedge pressure following administration of the drug.
RS   Bronchospasm may occasionally occur secondary to histamine release.
CNS   The drug has no effect on intracranial or intraocular pressure.
AS   Lower oesophageal sphincter pressure is unaffected by administration of atracurium.

Toxicity/Side Effects   Histamine release may occur if doses of $> 600\,\mu g/kg$ are used, leading to cutaneous flushing, hypotension and bronchospasm. Bradycardia has been reported following administration of atracurium.

Kinetics   The pharmacokinetic model of atracurium is unusual, as Hofmann degradation occurs in both the central and peripheral compartments.

Distribution   Atracurium is 82% protein-bound in the plasma; the V_D is 162–182 ml/kg. The drug does not cross the placental or blood–brain barrier.

Metabolism   Occurs by two pathways; the major pathway is via Hofmann degradation (cleavage of the link between the quaternary nitrogen ion and the central chain) to laudanosine and a quaternary monoacrylate. Laudanosine is cleared primarily by the liver. The minor degradative pathway is via hydrolysis by non-specific esterases in the blood to a quaternary alcohol and a quaternary acid. The metabolites have insignificant neuromuscular-blocking activity.

Excretion   The clearance is 5.1–6.1 ml/kg/min and the elimination half-life is 17–21 minutes; these parameters are altered little by renal or hepatic impairment and no alteration in dose is necessary in such patients.

Special Points   The duration of action of atracurium, in common with other non-depolarising relaxants, is prolonged by hypokalaemia, hypocalcaemia. hypermagnesaemia, hypoproteinaemia, dehydration, acidosis and hypercapnia. The following drugs, when co-administered with non-depolarising relaxants, increase the effect of the latter: volatile and induction agents, fentanyl, suxamethonium, diuretics, calcium antagonists, alpha- and beta-adrenergic antagonists, protamine, metronidazole and the aminoglycoside antibiotics.

The use of atracurium appears to be safe in patients susceptible to malignant hyperpyrexia.

Laudanosine (in concentrations >17 μg/ml) has been shown to cause seizures in animal models and becomes measurable in patients who have received atracurium by infusion for 6 days – the clinical significance of this is unclear.

A number of stereoisomers of atracurium exist which have less propensity to cause histamine release.

Cisatracurium besilate is now available commercially.

Atracurium is pharmaceutically incompatible with thiopentone.

Atropine

Uses Atropine is used:
1. traditionally, to dry secretions prior to ether or chloroform anaesthesia (nowadays when a dry airway is desirable, especially in children under one year of age)
2. to counter bradycardia due to increased vagal tone
3. to counter the muscarinic effects of anticholinergic agents
4. during cardiopulmonary resuscitation
5. as a cycloplegic
6. as a constituent of cold cures and in the treatment of
7. organophosphorus poisoning and
8. tetanus.

Chemical An alkaloid from *Atropa belladona*; atropine is a tertiary amine which is the ester of tropic acid and tropine. Commercial atropine is the racemic mixture of D- and I-hyoscyamine (I-form is active).

Presentation As a clear, colourless solution for injection containing 500/600 µg/ml of atropine sulphate; it is also available as 600 µg tablets.

Main Actions Anticholinergic.

Mode of Action Atropine exerts its effects by competitive antagonism of acetylcholine at muscarinic receptors (having little effect at nicotinic receptors except at high doses).

Routes of Administration/Doses Atropine may be administered intramuscularly or intravenously in a dose of 0.015–0.02 mg/kg. The adult oral dose is 0.2–0.6 mg. 3 mg is needed for complete vagal blockade in adults.

Effects
CVS In low doses, atropine may produce an initial bradycardia (Bezold-Jarisch reflex) followed by a tachycardia (the usual effect). The cardiac output is increased, but there is little effect on blood pressure. Atropine decreases atrio-ventricular conduction time and may produce dysrhythmias. Dilatation of facial capillaries may occur with the use of high doses.

RS Atropine produces bronchodilation with an increase in physiological dead space. Bronchial secretions are reduced by the drug. The respiratory rate is increased and a decreased incidence of laryngospasm has been reported following administration of the drug.

CNS Central excitation or depression may occur (central anticholinergic syndrome). The syndrome is characterised by somnolence, confusion, amnesia, agitation, hallucinations, dysarthria, ataxia or delirium. Atropine also has antiemetic and anti-Parkinsonian actions.

AS   The drug reduces salivation, the volume of gastric secretions and tone and peristalsis throughout the gut. Atropine has a mild antispasmodic action on the biliary tree. Lower oesophageal tone is reduced by the drug.

GU   Tone and peristalsis in the urinary tract are decreased.

Metabolic/Other   Cycloplegia, mydriasis and an increase in intraocular pressure may be produced by the drug. Sweating is inhibited and the basal metabolic rate is increased. The drug suppresses ADH secretion. Atropine has local anaesthetic properties.

Toxicity/Side Effects   Atropine is painful when injected intramuscularly and the sensation of a dry mouth is unpleasant. The central anticholinergic syndrome may occur in the elderly and inhibition of sweating may lead to hyperpyrexia in children. Urinary retention may be precipitated by the drug. Glaucoma may result from ocular (but not intravenous or intramuscular) administration.

Kinetics

Absorption   Atropine is rapidly absorbed from the gut; the bioavailability by the oral route is 10–25%.

Distribution   Atropine is 50% protein-bound in the plasma, the V_D is 2.0–4.0 l/kg. The drug crosses the placenta and blood–brain barrier.

Metabolism   Atropine is hydrolysed in the liver and tissues to tropine and tropic acid.

Excretion   94% of the dose is excreted in the urine in 24 hours, some unchanged. The clearance is 70 l/hour and the elimination half-life is 2.5 hours.

Special Points   Atropine reduces the incidence and morbidity of oculocardiac crises.

Bendroflumethiazide

Uses Bendroflumethiazide is used in the treatment of:
1. hypertension
2. oedema due to heart failure or the nephrotic syndrome
3. diabetes insipidus
4. renal tubular acidosis
5. hypercalcuria and for
6. the inhibition of lactation.

Chemical A thiazide.

Presentation As 2.5/5 mg tablets of bendroflumethiazide and in a variety of fixed-dose combinations with beta-adrenergic antagonists.

Main Actions Diuretic and antihypertensive.

Mode of Action Thiazide diuretics inhibit Na^+Cl^- co-transport in the distal convoluted tubule. They inhibit sodium ion reabsorption, which results in an increased urinary excretion of sodium, potassium and water.

Route of Administration/Dose The adult oral dose is 2.5–10 mg daily. Bendroflumethiazide has a duration of action of 12–18 hours.

Effect
CVS Bendroflumethiazide exerts its antihypertensive effect by decreasing the plasma volume and as a vasodilator. It also causes a slight decrease in the cardiac output.
CNS In toxic doses, the drug causes depression of the central nervous system.
GU Bendroflumethiazide decreases the renal blood flow and may also cause a reduction in the glomerular filtration rate. The drug decreases the urinary excretion of calcium and increases that of sodium, potassium and magnesium.
Metabolic/Other Thiazide diuretics may increase the blood sugar concentration by enhancing glycogenolysis and decreasing the rate of glycogenesis and insulin secretion. They may also increase the serum urate, triglyceride and cholesterol concentrations and give rise to a hypochloraemic acidosis.

Toxicity/Side Effects Central nervous system and haemopoietic disturbances, rashes, impotence and acute pancreatitis may complicate the use of the drug. Bendroflumethiazide may interfere with diabetic control and produce hypercholesterolaemia and gout and it may aggravate renal or hepatic insufficiency.

Kinetics

Absorption Bendroflumethiazide is completely absorbed when administered orally.

Distribution The drug is 94% protein-bound in the plasma; the V_D is 1.18 l/kg.

Metabolism Occurs to a variety of metabolites which may be active.

Excretion Occurs predominantly in the urine, 30% unchanged. The clearance is 3.68 ml/min/kg and the elimination half-life is 2.7–4.1 hours.

Special Points The drug may cause hypokalaemia and hypercalcaemia, which may precipitate digoxin toxicity, potentiate the effect of non-depolarising muscle relaxants and increase the likelihood of dysrhythmias occurring during general anaesthesia.

The hypotension occurring secondary to the administration of opioids, barbiturates and halothane is reportedly exaggerated in patients receiving thiazide diuretics.

Bretylium tosylate

Uses   Bretylium is used in the treatment of ventricular dysrhythmias refractory to other drugs.

Chemical   A quaternary ammonium compound.

Presentation   As a clear, colourless solution for injection containing 50 mg/ml of bretylium fosylate.

Main Action   A class III antiarrhythmic.

Mode of Action   The precise mode of action of the drug has not been fully elucidated. It initially stimulates the release of noradrenaline from adrenergic nerve endings but subsequently becomes concentrated in adrenergic nerve terminals and exerts a local anaesthetic effect, thereby inhibiting further noradrenaline release. It also inhibits uptake-1 in adrenergic nerve terminals and thus potentiates the actions of circulating catecholamines. It may terminate ventricular fibrillation by a direct action on the myocardium.

Routes of Administration/Doses   The intramuscular dose is 5 mg/kg, repeated after 6–8 hours if necessary. The drug may also be administered by slow intravenous injection (over 8–10 minutes) in a loading dose of 5–10 mg/kg, followed by a maintenance infusion of 1–2 mg/min. The drug acts in 20–40 minutes and has a duration of action of 6–12 hours.

Effects
CVS   Bretylium initially causes the release of noradrenaline, which results in a transient increase in blood pressure, heart rate and ventricular excitability. Subsequently, adrenergic blockade results in vasodilation, with little attendant change in cardiac output, although orthostatic hypotension may occur. The antiarrhythmic effects of the drug are similarly biphasic; the duration of the action potential and effective refractory period initially decreases and subsequently increases.
CNS   The drug has weak local anaesthetic effects.
AS   Bretylium causes slight inhibition of gastrointestinal tract motility.

Toxicity/Side Effects   The use of bretylium may be complicated by postural hypotension, parotid pain, sweating, diarrhoea and nausea and vomiting. Repeated intramuscular administration may result in tissue necrosis.

Kinetics

Absorption   The drug is poorly and erratically absorbed when administered orally; the bioavailability by this route is 18–23%.

Distribution   Bretylium is <10% protein-bound in the plasma; the V_D is 8.2 l/kg.

Metabolism   No metabolites of the drug have been detected in man.

Excretion   The drug is predominantly excreted in the urine, 70–80% unchanged. The clearance is 47 l/hour and the elimination half-life is 4–17 hours. The elimination half-life is markedly prolonged in the presence of renal failure, requiring alteration of dosage.

Special Points   Bretylium is ineffective in patients concurrently receiving MAOIs or tricyclic antidepressants; the drug should be avoided in patients with fixed cardiac output disorders.

Bretylium is removed by haemodialysis.

Bupivacaine

Uses Bupivacaine is used as a local anaesthetic.

Chemical An amide which is a structural homologue of mepivacaine.

Presentation As a clear, colourless solution containing 0.25/0.5% bupivacaine hydrochloride – the 0.25/0.5% solutions are available combined with 1:200 000 adrenaline. A 0.5% ('heavy') solution containing 80 mg/ml of glucose (with a specific gravity of 1.026) is also available.

Main Action Local anaesthetic.

Mode of Action Local anaesthetics diffuse in their uncharged base form through neural sheaths and the axonal membrane to the internal surface of cell membrane sodium ion channels; here they combine with hydrogen ions to form a cationic species which enters the internal opening of the sodium ion channel and combines with a receptor. This produces blockade of the sodium ion channel, thereby decreasing sodium ion conductance and preventing depolarisation of the cell membrane.

Routes of Administration/Doses Bupivacaine may be administered topically, by infiltration, intrathecally or epidurally; the toxic dose of bupivacaine is 2 mg/kg (with or without adrenaline). The drug acts within 10–20 minutes and has a duration of action of 5–16 hours.

Effects
CVS Bupivacaine is markedly cardiotoxic; it binds specifically to myocardial proteins. In toxic concentrations, the drug decreases the peripheral vascular resistance and myocardial contractility, producing hypotension and possibly cardiovascular collapse.
CNS The principal effect of bupivacaine is reversible neural blockade; this leads to a characteristically biphasic effect in the central nervous system. Initially, excitation (lightheadedness, dizziness, visual and auditory disturbances and fitting) occurs, due to the blockade of inhibitory pathways in the cortex. With increasing doses, depression of both facilitatory and inhibitory pathways occur, leading to central nervous system depression (drowsiness, disorientation and coma). Local anaesthetic agents block neuromuscular transmission when administered intra-arterially; it is thought that a complex of neurotransmitter, receptor and local anaesthetic is formed which has negligible conductance.

Toxicity/Side Effects Allergic reactions to the amide-type local anaesthetic agents are extremely rare. The side effects are predominantly correlated with excessive plasma concentrations of the drug, as described above. The use of the drug for intra-venous regional blockade is no longer recommended, as refract-ory cardiac depression leading to death has been reported when it is used for this purpose.

Kinetics

Absorption The absorption of local anaesthetic agents is related to:
1. the site of injection (intercostal > epidural > brachial plexus > subcutaneous)
2. the dose – a linear relationship exists between the total dose and the peak blood concentrations achieved and
3. the presence of vasoconstrictors, which delay absorption.
The addition of adrenaline to bupivacaine solutions does not influence the rate of systemic absorption as:
1. the drug is highly lipid soluble and therefore uptake into fat is rapid and
2. the drug has a direct vasodilatory effect.

Distribution Bupivacaine is 95% protein-bound in the plasma; the V_D is 41–103 l.

Metabolism Occurs in the liver by N-dealkylation, primarily to pipcolyloxylidine. N-desbutyl bupivacaine and 4 hydroxy bupivacaine are also formed.

Excretion 5% of the dose is excreted in the urine as pip-colyloxylidine; 16% is excreted unchanged. The clearance is 0.47 l/min and the elimination half-life (after intravenous administration) is 0.31–0.61 hours.

Special Points The onset and duration of conduction blockade is related to the pKa, lipid solubility and extent of protein binding of the drug. A low pKa and a high lipid solu-bility are associated with a rapid onset time; a high degree of protein binding is associated with a long duration of action. The pKa of bupivacaine is 8.1 and the heptane: buffer partition coefficient is 27.5. In infants under 6 months of age, the low level of albumin and alpha-l-acid glycoprotein results in an increase in the free fraction of bupivacaine. Local anaesthetic agents significantly increase the duration of action of both depolarising and non-depolarising relaxants.

Levobupivacaine is a S(-) enantiomer of racemic bupiva-caine, which differs in having less CNS and CVS toxicity and less prolonged motor blockade but longer sensory blockade after epidural administrator.

Buprenorphine

Uses   Buprenorphine is used:
1. in the treatment of moderate to severe pain and has been used
2. in sequential analgesia.

Chemical   A synthetic derivative of the alkaloid thebaine.

Presentation   As a clear, colourless solution containing 300 µg/ml buprenorphine hydrochloride and 200/400 µg tablets.

Main Action   Analgesia.

Mode of Action   The mode of action of buprenorphine remains to be fully elucidated. The drug acts as a partial agonist at mu-opioid receptors, but dissociates slowly from the latter, leading to prolonged analgesia. Buprenorphine appears also to have a high affinity for (but a low intrinsic activity at) kappa-opioid receptors.

Routes of Administration/Doses   The adult intramuscular and intravenous dose is 0.3–0.6 mg 6–8 hourly; the corresponding sublingual dose is 0.2–0.4 mg 6–8 hourly. The drug is also effective when administered by the epidural route; a dose of 0.3 mg has been recommended. Buprenorphine has a significantly longer latency period and duration of action than morphine.

Effects
CVS   Buprenorphine has minimal cardiovascular effects; the heart rate may decrease (by up to 25%) and the systolic blood pressure may fall by 10% following administration of the drug.
RS   The drug produces respiratory depression and an antitussive effect, similar to that produced by morphine. Buprenorphine may cause histamine and tryptase release from lung parenchymal mast cells and may increase pulmonary vascular resistance.
CNS   The drug is 25 times as potent an analgesic as morphine. In common with other opioids, buprenorphine produces miosis. The drug decreases cerebral glucose metabolism by up to 30%.
AS   Buprenorphine delays the rate of gastric emptying and has an emetic effect.
GU   The drug has been shown to reduce the rate of urine output in animals.
Metabolic/Other   Buprenorphine decreases the release of luteinising hormone and increases the release of prolactin.

Toxicity/Side Effects   Side effects are similar in nature and incidence to those produced by morphine. Drowsiness, dizziness, headache, confusion, dysphoria and nausea and vomiting may be produced by the drug. Buprenorphine appears to be less liable to produce dependence than pure mu-agonists.

Kinetics

Absorption The drug is absorbed when administered orally, but undergoes a significant first-pass metabolism and the sublingual route is therefore preferred. The bioavailability is 40–90% when administered intramuscularly and 44–94% when administered sublingually.

Distribution Only unchanged buprenorphine appears to reach the central nervous system. The drug is 96% protein-bound *in vitro*; the V_D is 3.2 l/kg.

Metabolism Occurs in the liver by dealkylation with subsequent conjugation to glucuronide – the polar conjugates then appear to be excreted in the bile and hydrolysed by bacteria in the gastrointestinal tract.

Excretion Occurs predominantly via the faeces as unchanged buprenorphine; the remainder is excreted in the urine as conjugated buprenorphine and dealkylated derivatives. The clearance is 1 l/min (this is decreased by 30% under general anaesthesia) and the elimination half-life is 5 hours.

Special Points Being a partial agonist, buprenorphine antagonises the effects of morphine and other opioid agonists and may precipitate abstinence syndromes in opiate-dependent subjects. The respiratory depressant effects of the drug are not completely reversed by even large doses of naloxone; doxapram, however, will do so. Severe respiratory depression has occurred when benzodiazepines have been co-administered with buprenorphine.

Buprenorphine is not removed by haemodialysis.

The addition of buprenorphine to local anaesthesia for brachial plexus blockade triples the length of post-operative analgesia compared to local anaesthesia alone.

Captopril

Uses   Captopril is used for the treatment of:
1. essential and renovascular hypertension
2. congestive heart failure and
3. diabetic nephropathy.

Chemical   A mercapto alkanoyl derivative.

Presentation   As 12.5/25/50 mg tablets of captopril and in a fixed dose combination with hydrochlorothiazide.

Main Action   Antihypertensive.

Mode of Action   Captopril is an angiotensin-converting enzyme inhibitor that binds to angiotensin-converting enzyme (with an affinity 30 000 times greater than that of angiotensin I) so preventing the formation of angiotensin II from angiotensin I. Part of its action may also be exerted through modulation of sympathetic tone or of the kallikren-kinin-prostaglandin system.

Route of Administration/Dose   The adult oral dose is 12.5–50 mg 8–12 hourly; the drug should be introduced with caution as profound hypotension may occur on initial exposure ('first-dose effect') to captopril.

Effects
CVS   The systemic vascular resistance decreases by 18–40% leading to a decrease in the systolic and diastolic blood pressure; cardiac output may increase by up to 20%, especially in patients in heart failure. The heart rate may increase or decrease; baroreceptor reflexes remain unaffected by captopril.
RS   The drug may produce a persistent dry cough; bronchospasm occurs on occasion.
CNS   Captopril appears to have a beneficial effect in restoring cerebral flow.
GU   The drug produces a decrease in renal vascular resistance; natriuresis may ensue.
Metabolic/Other   Plasma renin activity increases in patients maintained on captopril; the drug causes a decrease in aldosterone concentration which may lead to hyperkalaemia, especially in patients with a degree of renal impairment. The serum creatinine and urea concentrations may also increase in these patients.

Toxicity/Side Effects   Captopril is generally well tolerated. Loss of taste, cough and rashes occur commonly; agranulocytosis (which is probably dose-dependent), aphthous ulceration and cholestatic jaundice may also occur with the use of the drug.

Kinetics

Absorption   The drug is rapidly absorbed when administered orally; the bioavailability by this route is 75%.

Distribution   Captopril is 30% protein-bound in the plasma; the V_D is 0.61–0.79 l/kg.

Metabolism   The drug is metabolised to a disulphide dimer and cysteine disulphide.

Excretion   95% of an administered dose is excreted in the urine, 50% as the unchanged drug and the remainder as polar metabolites. The clearance is 9.7–15.7 ml/min/kg and the elimination half-life is 1.9 hours. The dose should be reduced in the presence of renal impairment.

Special Points   The hypotensive effect of captopril is additive with that of anaesthetic agents; it does not, however, protect against the cardiovascular responses to laryngoscopy. Rebound hypertension may occur if the drug is discontinued abruptly.

Captopril is readily removed by haemodialysis.

In the presence of hypovolaemia, the co-administration of captopril and NSAIDs produces a high incidence of renal failure.

Carbamazepine

Uses Carbamazepine is used in the treatment of:
1. epilepsy, especially temporal lobe and tonic-clonic seizures.
2. trigeminal neuralgia and
3. prophylaxis of bipolar disorder.

Chemical An iminostilbene derivative structurally related to the tricyclic antidepressants.

Presentation As 100/200/400 mg tablets, 125/250 mg suppositories and as a white syrup containing 20 mg/ml of carbamazepine.

Main Actions Anticonvulsant and analgesic.

Mode of Action The mode of action of carbamazepine is unknown: it may act via alterations in adenosine disposition within the central nervous system. It does not appear to act in the same manner as tricyclic antidepressants.

Routes of Administration/Dose The adult oral dose is 100–1600 mg daily in divided doses.

Effects
CVS Carbamazepine has antiarrhythmic properties and depresses atrio-ventricular conduction.
CNS The drug is more effective than phenytoin in raising the threshold for minimal electroshock seizures. Carbamazepine also has analeptic properties.
GU Carbamazepine has an antidiuretic effect that may lead to water intoxication.

Toxicity/Side Effects Diplopia, nausea and vomiting, drowsiness and ataxia are relatively common side effects of the drug. Rashes occur in 3% of patients. Carbamazepine may also cause renal and liver damage. Mild neutropenia occurs commonly; fatal aplastic anaemia is extremely rare.

Kinetics

Absorption The drug is well absorbed when administered orally; the bioavailability by this route is nearly 100%.

Distribution Carbamazepine is 75% protein-bound in the plasma; the V_D is 1 l/kg.

Metabolism Occurs via oxidation in the liver to an epoxide which is active. With chronic use, the drug induces its own metabolism.

Excretion The drug is predominantly excreted in the urine as unconjugated metabolites; the clearance is 20 ml/kg/hr and the elimination half-life is 16–36 hours.

Special Points   Sodium valproate and calcium antagonists may increase the plasma concentrations of free carbamazepine if administered concurrently. The efficacy of both pancuronium and vecuronium is reportedly decreased in patients receiving carbamazepine. Regular liver function tests and estimation of white cell counts need to be performed during chronic carbamazepine therapy.

The drug is not removed by haemodialysis.

Carbon dioxide

Uses   Carbon dioxide is used:
1. to reverse apnoea due to passive hyperventilation
2. to facilitate the inhalational induction of anaesthesia and blind nasal intubation
3. to speed the onset of action of local anaesthetics
4. to increase cerebral blood flow during carotid artery surgery
5. for the insufflation of body cavities during endoscopy
6. for cryotherapy and
7. in the treatment of hiccups.

Chemical   An organic gas.

Presentation   As a liquid in cylinders at a pressure of 50 bar at 15 °C; the cylinders are grey and are available in three sizes (C–E, containing 450–1800 l respectively). Carbon dioxide is a colourless gas with a pungent smell in high concentrations; it is non-flammable and does not support combustion. The specific gravity of the gas is 1.98, the critical temperature −31 °C and the critical pressure 73.8 atmospheres.

Main Actions   Respiratory and sympathetic stimulation.

Routes of Administration   The gas is generally administered by inhalation, but may be insufflated into e.g. the peritoneal cavity. Any concentration that is desired may be employed; concentrations of up to 5% are generally administered by inhalation.

Effects
CVS   *In vitro*, the gas has negative inotropic and chronotropic effects; *in vivo* these effects are offset by sympathetic stimulation. The overall effect of the administration of 5% carbon dioxide is to increase the heart rate, systolic and diastolic blood pressure and cardiac output. Dysrhythmias may occur *in vivo*, although *in vitro* the gas increases the threshold for catecholamine-induced dysrhythmias. The peripheral vascular resistance is decreased *in vivo*; carbon dioxide is a potent coronary arterial vasodilator.
RS   Carbon dioxide (in a concentration of 5%) stimulates respiration by an action on the respiratory centre and peripheral chemoreceptors, leading to an increase in tidal volume and respiratory rate; bronchodilatation is also produced. At high concentrations, respiratory depression occurs. The presence of an increased partial pressure of carbon dioxide in the blood shifts the oxygen dissociation curve to the right; the Bohr effect.
CNS   A P_aCO_2 of 8–11 kPa will increase the cerebral blood flow by 100% and lead to an increase in intracranial pressure and progressive narcosis. A P_aCO_2 of 3.5 kPa will reduce cerebral blood flow by 30%.

Metabolic/Other The administration of exogenous carbon dioxide causes a respiratory acidosis which may, in turn, lead to hyperkalaemia. The plasma concentrations of adrenaline, noradrenaline, angiotensin and 15-hydroxy-corticosteroid are increased by the administration of carbon dioxide.

Toxicity/Side Effects When administered in concentrations >10%, the gas may cause dyspnoea, headache, dizziness, restlessness, paraesthesiae, diaphoresis and dysrhythmias.

Kinetics

Absorption The gas is freely permeable through normal alveolar tissue.

Distribution Carbon dioxide is transported in the blood in solution, in the form of bicarbonate ions and in combination with plasma proteins and haemoglobin.

Metabolism/Excretion The gas is transformed in the blood to the forms described above.

Excretion Predominantly by exhalation and some as renally excreted bicarbonate.

Special Points A respiratory acidosis may alter drug action by altering both the degree of ionisation and protein binding of drugs; an increased dose of thiopentone and a decreased dose of tubocurarine are required in the face of an uncompensated respiratory acidosis.

Ceftazidime

Uses Ceftazidime is used in the treatment of infections of:
1. the lower respiratory tract
2. the urinary tract
3. skin and soft tissues and in
4. intra-abdominal, gynaecological and obstetric sepsis
5. meningitis and
6. septicaemia.

Chemical A third-generation aminothiazolyloximino cephalosporin.

Presentation As a white powder in vials containing 0.25/0.5/1/2 g of ceftazidime pentahydrate (with sodium carbonate) for dilution in water prior to use, and as eye drops.

Main Actions Ceftazidime is a broad spectrum bactericidal antibiotic which is resistant to hydrolysis by beta-lactamases. It is effective against the Gram-negative *Pseudomonas, Klebsiella, Proteus, Salmonella, Shigella and Neisseria* sp., *Haemophilus influenzae* and *Escherichia coli*. The Gram-positive *Staphylococcus* (not MRSA) and *Streptococcus* sp. (not *Strep. faecalis*) and the anaerobes *Clostridium perfringens* and *Bacteroides* sp. are also sensitive to the drug.

Mode of Action Ceftazidime acts by binding to penicillin-binding proteins on the bacterial cytoplasmic membrane, thereby blocking-peptidoglycan synthesis and thus cell wall synthesis.

Routes of Administration/Doses The drug may be administered intravenously or intramuscularly; the adult daily dose is 1–6 g in 2–3 divided doses.

Toxicity/Side Effects Ceftazidime is generally well tolerated. Rashes, fever, diarrhoea, transient eosinophilia and abnormalities of liver function tests may occur with the use of the drug. If administered in high doses to patients concurrently receiving other nephrotoxic drugs, further deterioration in renal function may result.
  Clostridium difficile infection may complicate the administration of this drug.

Kinetics

Absorption The drug is not absorbed when administered orally; it is well absorbed via the intramuscular route.

Distribution Ceftazidime is 5–23% protein-bound in the plasma; the V_D is 0.22–0.29 l/kg.

Metabolism The drug is not metabolised in man.

Excretion   Ceftazidime is excreted unchanged, predominantly in the urine, with <1% appearing in the bile. The clearance is 1.05–2.07 ml/min/kg and the elimination half-life is 1.5–2.8 hours. The dose should be reduced and/or the dose interval increased in patients with a creatinine clearance <50 ml/min.

Special Points   5% of patients receiving ceftazidime develop a positive Coombs' test; this may interfere with blood cross-matching.

The drug is readily removed by haemodialysis.

Cefuroxime

Uses Cefuroxime is used in the treatment of infections of:
1. the respiratory tract
2. the urinary tract
3. bone, joint and soft tissues and of
4. meningitis
5. gonorrhoea and for
6. surgical prophylaxis.

Chemical A second-generation semi-synthetic cephalosporin.

Presentation As a white powder in vials containing 250/750/1500 mg of cefuroxime and as 125/250 mg tablets of cefuroxime axetil. Cefuroxime axetil is an ester pro-drug of cefuroxime; after absorption, it is immediately de-esterified in the gut-wall and blood to form free cefuroxime.

Main Actions Cefuroxime is a broad spectrum bactericidal antibiotic resistant to the action of most beta-lactamases. It is effective against *Staphylococcus*, *Salmonella*, *Shigella*, *Clostridium*, *Klebsiella*, *Haemophilus*, *Pseudomonas*, *Neisseria* and *Streptococcus* sp. (except *enterococci*), *Escherichia coli* and *Bordetella pertussis*.

Mode of Action Cefuroxime acts by binding to penicillin-binding proteins on the bacterial cytoplasmic membrane, thereby blocking peptidoglycan synthesis and thus cell wall formation.

Routes of Administration/Doses The adult oral dose is 125–500 mg 12-hourly, the corresponding intramuscular or intravenous dose is 750–1500 mg 6–8 hourly.

Effects
Metabolic/Other Transient alterations of liver enzymes and hyperbilirubinaemia may occur with the use of the drug.

Toxicity/Side Effects Hypersensitivity reactions, haematological disturbances (including a positive Coombs' test which may interfere with the cross-matching of blood) may occur. Gastrointestinal disturbances, including pseudomembranous colitis have been reported following the use of cefuroxime.

Kinetics

Absorption The bioavailability of orally administered cefuroxime is 36–52%.

Distribution The drug is 35% protein-bound in the plasma; the V_D is 0.22 l/kg. The drug penetrates into the cerebrospinal fluid well if the meninges are inflamed.

Metabolism   Cefuroxime is not metabolised to any significant extent *in vivo*.

Excretion   The drug is excreted unchanged in the urine by tubular secretion and glomerular filtration. The clearance is 1.91 ml/min/kg and the elimination half-life is 1.3 hours.

Special Points   The dose of cefuroxime should be reduced in patients with a creatinine clearance <20 ml/min if it is to be administered intravenously or intramuscularly; the drug is removed by haemodialysis.

Chloramphenicol

Uses   Chloramphenicol is used in the treatment of:
1. meningitis in children under school age
2. serious *Haemophilus influenzae* infections, e.g. epiglottitis and osteomyelitis
3. brain abscess
4. typhoid and
5. eye infections.

Chemical   A nitrobenzene derivative.

Presentation   As 250 mg tablets of chloramphenicol palmitate; in ampoules containing 1 g of chloramphenicol succinate (a powder which is reconstituted in water prior to use) for intravenous injection and as eye drops and a 1% ointment.

Main Actions   Chloramphenicol is a broad spectrum antibiotic that is bactericidal to *Haemophilus influenzae, Neisseria meningitidis* and *Streptococcus pneumoniae* and bacteriostatic to other susceptible organisms, including *Salmonella typhi, Treponema pallidum, Legionella* sp., *Mycoplasma*, rickettsiae, *Chlamydia* and a variety of anaerobes.

Mode of Action   The drug is a protein synthesis inhibitor which binds reversibly to the 50S subunit of the bacterial ribosome, thereby inhibiting the formation of peptide chains.

Routes of Administration/Doses   The adult oral dose is 500 mg 6-hourly; the corresponding intravenous dose is 50 mg/kg daily in divided doses. The therapeutic range of plasma concentrations is 5–10 µg/ml (trough) and 15–20 µg/ml (peak).

Toxicity/Side Effects   The most important tend to occur at plasma concentrations exceeding 25 µg/ml and include reversible bone marrow depression, idiosyncratic irreversible aplastic anaemia and the 'grey syndrome' in neonates (a complex of vomiting, abdominal distension, respiratory distress, hypotension and an ashen appearance which is due to either failure of conjugation or inadequate renal excretion of the unconjugated drug). Other side effects of the drug include gastrointestinal disturbances, optic neuritis and allergic reactions.

Kinetics

Absorption   The bioavailability of chloramphenicol is 80% when administered orally and 70% when administered intravenously.

Distribution   Chloramphenicol diffuses well into body fluids and CSF levels are 50% of that in serum; the drug is concentrated nine-fold in brain tissue. Chloramphenicol is 60% protein-bound in the plasma; the V_D is 0.6–1 l/kg.

Metabolism The drug is metabolised to an active form when administered either intravenously (metabolism occurring predominantly in the liver) or orally (metabolism occurring predominantly in the small bowel); it is inactivated in the liver by conjugation to glucuronide.

Excretion 90% is excreted in the urine, 5–10% in the active form. The elimination half-life is 4 hours.

Special Points The dose of chloramphenicol should be reduced in patients with hepatic impairment.

The drug is removed by haemodialysis.

Chlorphenamine

Uses Chlorphenamine is used in the treatment of:
1. allergic rhinitis
2. urticaria
3. pruritus and
4. anaphylactic and anaphylactoid reactions.

Chemical An alkylamine.

Presentation As 4 mg tablets, a syrup containing 0.4 mg/ml and a clear, colourless solution for injection containing 10 mg/ml of chlorphenamine maleate.

Main Actions Antihistaminergic (H1 receptors) and anticholinergic.

Mode of Action Chlorphenamine acts by reversible competitive antagonism of histamine H1 receptors.

Routes of Administration/Doses The adult oral dose is 4 mg 6–8 hourly. The drug may also be administered intravenously (over a period of 1 minute), intramuscularly or subcutaneously as a stat dose of 10 mg.

Effects
CVS The drug inhibits, histamine-induced vasodilation and increased capillary permeability.
RS Chlorphenamine decreases bronchial secretions; it does not completely reverse anaphylactic bronchospasm in man, since leukotrienes are involved in the mediation of allergic bronchoconstriction.
CNS The drug has a sedative effect and local anaesthetic properties.
Metabolic/Other Chlorphenamine has anticholinergic properties.

Toxicity/Side Effects The predominant side effect of the drug is drowsiness, but it may also produce gastrointestinal disturbances (including nausea and vomiting) and anticholinergic side effects.

Kinetics

Absorption The drug is slowly absorbed when administered orally; the bioavailability by this route is 25–50% due to an extensive first-pass metabolism in the gut wall and liver.

Distribution The drug is 70% protein-bound in the plasma; the V_D is 7.51–7.65 l/kg.

Metabolism Occurs via demethylation and oxidative deamination in the liver.

Excretion The mono- and didesmethyl-derivatives are excreted predominantly in the urine; 1–27% (dependent upon the urinary pH) of an administered dose is excreted unchanged in the urine. The clearance is 4.4–7.92 ml/min/kg and the elimination half-life is 2–43 hours.

Special Points The sedative effect of the drug is additive with that produced by anaesthetic agents.

The drug is not removed by dialysis.

Chlorpromazine

Uses Chlorpromazine is used in the treatment of:
1. schizophrenia and related psychoses
2. nausea and vomiting associated with terminal illness and
3. intractable hiccup.

Chemical A phenothiazine (with an aliphatic side chain).

Presentation As 10/25/50/100 mg tablets, a syrup containing 5 mg/ml, 100 mg suppositories and as a straw-coloured solution for injection containing 25 mg/ml of chlorpromazine hydrochloride.

Main Actions Antipsychotic, antiemetic and sedative.

Mode of Action The antiemetic and neuroleptic effects of the drug appear to be mediated by central dopaminergic (D_2-) blockade leading to an increased threshold for vomiting at the chemoreceptor trigger zone. The other pharmacological effects are mediated by antagonism of serotoninergic, histaminergic, muscarinic cholinergic and alpha-adrenergic receptors.

Routes of Administration/Doses The adult oral dose is 10–50 mg 6–8 hourly; the corresponding dose by the intramuscular route is 25–50 mg 6–8 hourly.

Effects
CVS Chlorpromazine is negatively inotropic; in combination with the decrease in systemic vascular resistance mediated by alpha-adrenergic blockade that it produces, postural hypotension with a reflex tachycardia are the main effects observed. The drug increases coronary blood flow and has a mild quinidine-like action on the heart. Chlorpromazine may produce ECG changes, including prolongation of the P-R and Q-T intervals, T-wave flattening and S-T segment depression.
RS The drug is a respiratory depressant; it also diminishes bronchial secretions.
CNS The main central effect of the drug is neurolepsis, but sedation and anxiolysis are also produced Chlorpromazine enhances the effect of co-administered analgesics and lowers the seizure threshold; it also has local anaesthetic properties. The drug causes skeletal muscle relaxation via a central effect. Miosis occurs due to alpha-adrenergic blockade. It increases sleep time, but decreases the time spent in the REM phase. The characteristic EEG changes associated with the use of chlorpromazine are slowing with an increase in theta- and delta-wave activity and a decrease in alpha- and beta-wave activity, associated with some increase in burst activity.
AS Chlorpromazine increases appetite and may cause weight gain; it tends to decrease salivation, gastric secretion and gastrointestinal motility.

GU The drug increases renal blood flow and has a weak diuretic action. Ejaculation and micturition may be inhibited secondary to the drug's anticholinergic effect.

Metabolic/Other Chlorpromazine impairs temperature regulation by both central and peripheral mechanisms; anaesthetised subjects receiving the drug show a tendency to become poikilothermic. The phenothiazines increase prolactin secretion and tend to decrease adrenocorticotrophic and antidiuretic hormone release. Insulin release and thus glucose tolerance may also be impaired by the drug.

Toxicity/Side Effects Chlorpromazine is generally a well-tolerated and safe drug, despite its panoply of effects. The drug may produce a variety of extrapyramidal syndromes, including the rare neuroleptic malignant syndrome (a complex of symptoms that include catatonia, cardiovascular lability, hyperthermia and myoglobinaemia) which has a mortality in excess of 10%. A variety of anticholinergic effects, jaundice, blood dyscrasias and allergic phenomena may also complicate the use of the drug.

Kinetics

Absorption Chlorpromazine is well absorbed when administered orally, but has a bioavailability by this route of 30% due to an extensive first-pass metabolism in the liver and gut-wall.

Distribution The drug is 95–98% protein-bound in the plasma; the V_D is 12–30 l/kg.

Metabolism Chlorpromazine is extensively metabolised in the liver by oxidation, dealkylation, demethylation and hydroxylation with subsequent conjugation to glucuronide; at least 168 metabolites have been described, many of which are active.

Excretion Occurs in equal quantities in the urine and faeces; less than 1% is excreted unchanged. The clearance is 5.7–11.5 ml/min/kg and the elimination half-life is 30 hours.

Special Points The depressant effects of chlorpromazine are additive with those produced by general anaesthetic agents.
  The drug is not removed by haemodialysis.

Chlorpropamide

Uses   Chlorpropamide is used:
1. in the treatment of non-insulin-dependent (type II) diabetes mellitus and may be of use
2. in the management of diabetes insipidus.

Chemical   An arylsulphonylurea.

Presentation   As 100/250 mg tablets of chlorpropamide.

Main Action   Hypoglycaemia.

Mode of Action   Chlorpropamide acts by liberating insulin from pancreatic beta-cells; it appears to act by binding to the plasma membrane of the beta-cell and producing prolonged depolarisation, reducing the permeability of the membrane to potassium. This in turn leads to opening of calcium channels; the resulting influx of calcium causes triggering of insulin release. Sulphonylureas may also act by altering peripheral insulin-receptor number and sensitivity.

Route of Administration/Dose   The adult oral dose is 100–500 mg daily. The hypoglycaemic effect is maximal 3–6 hours after administration and persists for at least 24 hours.

Effects
GU   Chlorpropamide appears to sensitise the renal tubules to the action of endogenous ADH; it consequently impairs free water clearance.
Metabolic/Other   The principal effect of chlorpropamide is to decrease the blood sugar concentration; healthy subjects show a smaller decrease than do diabetic subjects. Sulphonylureas are ineffective in pancreatectomised patients and insulin-dependent diabetics. The drug also causes a decrease in the plasma cholesterol, triglyceride and free fatty acid concentrations. Hyponatraemia may occur in a small number of patients.

Toxicity/Side Effects   Occur in about 6% of patients who receive the drug. Hypoglycaemia, gastrointestinal disturbances, cholestatic jaundice and alterations in liver function tests may occur. Chlorpropamide has a disulfiram-like interaction when taken with alcohol. Rashes, reversible leucopenia, haemolytic anaemia and thrombocytopenia have also been reported.

Kinetics

Absorption   The drug is rapidly absorbed when administered orally; the bioavailability by this route is 90%.

Distribution   Chlorpropamide is 87% protein-bound in the plasma, predominantly to albumin; the V_D is 0.08–0.10 l/kg.

Metabolism   The drug is extensively metabolised in the liver by hydroxylation, hydrolysis and side chain cleavage to a variety of active and inactive metabolites.

Excretion   Occurs predominantly in the urine, 6–60% unchanged. The clearance is 0.025–0.035 ml/min/kg and the elimination half-life is 27–39 hours, which is increased in the presence of renal impairment.

Special Points   Chlorpropamide therapy should ideally be stopped 48 hours prior to elective surgery; failing this, close supervision of the patient in the peri-operative phase is necessary. The drug should not be used in patients with hepatic or renal impairment.

The following drugs may potentiate the effect of sulphonylureas either by displacement from plasma proteins or by inhibition of their hepatic metabolism and result in hypoglycaemia: NSAIDs, salicylates, sulphonamides, oral anticoagulants, MAOIs and beta-adrenergic antagonists. Conversely, the following drugs tend to counteract the effect of sulphonylureas and lead to loss of diabetic control: thiazide and other diuretics, steroids, phenothiazines, phenytoin, sympathomimetic agents and calcium antagonists.

Chlorpropamide is not removed by haemodialysis.

Cimetidine

Uses Cimetidine is used in the treatment of:
1. peptic ulcer disease
2. reflux oesophagitis
3. the Zollinger-Ellison syndrome
4. pancreatic insufficiency to reduce the degradation of enzyme supplements
5. malabsorption and fluid loss in the short-bowel syndrome and in the prophylaxis of
6. stress ulceration in the critically ill (especially in patients with liver disease) and
7. acid aspiration pneumonitis, especially during pregnancy and labour.

Chemical An imidazole derivative.

Presentation As 200/400/800 mg tablets, a syrup containing 40 mg/ml and as a solution for injection containing 100 mg/ml of cimetidine. Fixed-dose combinations with sodium alginate are also available.

Main Action Inhibition of gastric acid secretion.

Mode of Action Cimetidine acts by reversible competitive antagonism of H_2 receptors. Histamine appears to be necessary to potentiate the action of gastrin and acetycholine on the gastric parietal cell, as well as acting directly as a secretogogue.

Routes of Administration/Doses The normal adult dose is 400 mg 12-hourly or 800 mg as a single nocturnal dose. The adult intravenous dose is up to 2.4 gm/day as required to maintain the gastric pH above 4. Intravenous administration should be slow.

Effects
CVS Bradycardias and dysrhythmias may occur after rapid intravenous administration of the drug.
AS Cimetidine inhibits all phases of physiological gastric acid secretion leading to a decrease in the volume and acidity of gastric acid secretion and pepsin output. No consistent effect of the drug on the lower oesophageal sphincter tone or rate of gastric emptying has been demonstrated.
GU The drug may cause altered renal tubular transport of creatinine leading to a clinically insignificant elevation of serum creatinine.
Metabolic/Other Cimetidine has a weak antiandrogenic effect which may occasionally lead to gynaecomastia, impotence and a fall in the sperm count in males.

Toxicity/Side Effects Central effects such as headaches, dizziness, confusion and hallucinations may occur, especially in the elderly and those with impaired renal function. Muscle pains, rashes and leucopenia have also been described following the use of the drug.

Kinetics

Absorption Cimetidine is rapidly absorbed when administered orally, the bioavailability by this route is 60–75%.

Distribution Cimetidine is 20% protein-bound in the plasma; the V_D 1–1.2 l/kg.

Metabolism 30–40% is metabolised in the liver by cytochrome P-450, primarily to a sulphoxide.

Excretion 40–55% of an oral dose is excreted unchanged in the urine. The clearance is 9–12 ml/min/kg and the elimination half-life is 1.5–2.3 hours.

Special Points The dosage of cimetidine should be reduced in renal failure; the drug is removed by haemodialysis. Cimetidine inhibits the metabolism of drugs biotransformed by the mixed function oxidase system, e.g. lignocaine, diazepam, phenytoin, propranolol and oral anticoagulants. Caution should be used if the drug is administered concurrently with other drugs that are metabolised by the cytochrome P-450 system, in particular aminophylline, warfarin and phenytoin, as the toxicity of the latter may be enhanced.

Routine H_2 receptor blockade prophylaxis for patients receiving intensive care is not warranted.

Ciprofloxacin

Uses Ciprofloxacin is used in the treatment of infections of:
1. the urinary, respiratory and gastrointestinal tracts
2. bone, joint, skin and soft tissue
3. eye, ear, nose and throat and
4. pelvic and intra-abdominal infections
5. gonorrhoea and
6. septicaemia.

Chemical A fluorinated quinolone related to nalidixic acid.

Presentation As tablets containing 250/500/750 mg ciprofloxacin hydrochloride, an oral suspension containing 50 mg/ml, a clear, pale yellow solution for injection containing 2 mg/ml of ciprofloxacin lactate and an ophthalmic solution.

Main Actions Ciprofloxacin is bactericidal against a wide range of Gram-positive and Gram-negative organisms and anaerobes, including *Escherichia coli, Salmonella, Shigella, Klebsiella, Proteus, Haemophilus, Pseudomonas, Neisseria, Staphylococcus, Clostridium, Bacteroides and Brucella* sp. Ciprofloxacin markedly reduces Enterobacteriaceae with little effect on the anaerobic population of the gut. There is little evidence of bacterial overgrowth or of superinfection with the use of the drug. There is emerging resistance to ciprofloxacin from *Pseudomonas* and *Acinetobacter* sp.

Mode of Action Ciprofloxacin acts by inhibition of bacterial DNA gyrase, the enzyme responsible for introducing negative supercoils into bacterial DNA.

Routes of Administration/Doses The adult oral dose is 250–750 mg daily in divided doses; the corresponding intravenous dose is 200–400 mg daily.

Toxicity/Side Effects Gastrointestinal disturbances occur in 5–10% and disturbances of the central nervous system, including anxiety, insomnia, seizures and hallucinations, in 1–4% of patients receiving the drug. Allergic reactions, photosensitivity, transient elevations of liver enzymes and ruptured tendo Achillis have also been reported.

Kinetics

Absorption The oral bioavailability of the drug is 52–84%.

Distribution Ciprofloxacin is 16–40% protein-bound in the plasma; the V_D is 2–3 l/kg.

Metabolism Four active metabolites have been identified.

Excretion The drug is excreted in the urine and faeces, 70%

in an unchanged form. Active tubular secretion of the drug occurs. The clearance is 416–650 ml/min and the elimination half-life is 3–6.9 hours.

Special Points   The dose of ciprofloxacin should be reduced if the creatinine clearance is less than 20 ml/min; 25–30% of an administered dose is removed during haemodialysis.

The drug significantly increases the half-life of co-administered theophylline, necessitating monitoring of plasma concentrations of the latter.

Clomethiazole

Uses Clomethiozole is used:
1. in the management of alcohol withdrawal states
2. as an anticonvulsant (emergency use only)
3. as a hypnotic for the elderly
4. in the treatment of eclampsia and pre-eclampsia and
5. for sedation in patients undergoing surgery under regional blockade or intensive care.

Chemical A thiamine derivative.

Presentation As a clear aqueous solution containing 8 mg/ml of clomethiazole edisylate and in 192 mg capsule and 50 mg/ml syrup form.

Main Actions Anticonvulsant, sedative and anxiolytic.

Mode of Action The anticonvulsant and sedative actions are due to enhancement of central GABA-ergic transmission and possibly inhibition of central dopaminergic transmission.

Routes of Administration/Doses For the control of convulsions in adults, 40–100 ml of the 0.8% solution are infused intravenously over 5–10 minutes; subsequently, the infusion rate is tailored to the response. For sedation, 25 ml/min are administered intravenously for 1–2 minutes, followed by a maintenance infusion of 1–4 ml/mm. As a hypnotic, 1–2 capsules or 5–10 ml of the syrup are administered orally.

Effects
CVS Tachycardia and hypotension are the only clinically significant effects of the drug.
RS No effects are seen with the use of clomethiazole until, at high doses, airway obstruction may occur.
CNS Clomethiazole has anticonvulsant, sedative and hypnotic properties. It is also powerfully amnesic.

Toxicity/Side Effects Nasal and conjunctival irritation, headache and increased bronchial secretions may occur. Prolonged intravenous infusion of clomethiazole may lead to volume overload and electrolyte abnormalities due to the water load involved. Renal failure has been reported after prolonged use associated with hypotension. Physical dependence and withdrawal states have been reported following chronic use of the drug.

Kinetics

Absorption Clomethiazole is well absorbed when administered orally; the bioavailability by this route is 25–34% due to a high hepatic clearance.

Distribution   The drug is 65–70% protein-bound in the plasma, predominantly to albumin; the V_D is 3–5 l/kg.

Metabolism   Occurs predominantly by oxidation in the liver; there is an extensive first-pass effect. 10–20% is metabolised in the lung; there may also be some renal extraction of the drug.

Excretion   0.1% is excreted unchanged in the urine. The clearance is 2.1 l/min and the elimination half-life is 1–6 hours.

Special Points   Clomethiazole is absorbed by plastic giving-sets.

   It is removed by haemodialysis but this may not significantly affect the degree of sedation.

Clonidine

Uses Clonidine is used in the treatment of:
1. all grades of essential and secondary hypertension
2. hypertensive crises and in the management of
3. migraine
4. menopausal flushing and may be of use in
5. chronic pain
6. during opiate and alcohol withdrawal and
7. for intravenous regional analgesia for chronic regional pain syndromes

Chemical An aniline derivative.

Presentation As 0.1/0.25/0.3 mg tablets and as a clear, colourless solution for injection containing 0.15 mg/ml of clonidine hydrochloride.

Main Action Antihypertensive, analgesic, sedative and anxiolytic.

Mode of Action Clonidine acts acutely by stimulating alpha-2 (pre-synaptic) adrenoceptors, thereby decreasing nor-adrenaline release from sympathetic nerve terminals and consequently decreasing sympathetic tone; it also increases vagal tone. The drug acts chronically by reducing the responsiveness of peripheral vessels to vasoactive substances and to sympathetic stimulation. The analgesic effects are also mediated by activation of alpha-2 adrenoceptors in the dorsal horn of the spinal cord.

Routes of Administration/Doses The adult oral dose is 50–600 μg 8-hourly; the corresponding intravenous dose is 0.15–0.3 mg. When administered by the epidural route, a dose of 0.15 mg has been used. The drug acts within 10 minutes and lasts for 3–7 hours when administered intravenously.

Effects
CVS When administered intravenously, clonidine causes a transient increase in the blood pressure (due to stimulation of vascular alpha-1 receptors) followed by a sustained decrease. The heart rate and venous return may decrease slightly; the drug has no effect on cardiac contractility and cardiac output is well maintained. The coronary vascular resistance is decreased by clonidine; the systemic vascular resistance is decreased with long-term treatment.
CNS Clonidine decreases cerebral blood flow and intraocular pressure. It exerts a depressant effect on both spontaneous sympathetic outflow and afferent A delta- and C-fibre-mediated somatosympathetic reflexes
AS Clonidine decreases gastric and small bowel motility and is an antisialogogue.

GU Clonidine reduces renovascular resistance; however, little alteration in the glomerular filtration rate occurs.

Metabolic/Other The drug causes a decrease in plasma catecholamine concentrations and plasma renin activity. Blood sugar concentration may increase secondary to alpha-adrenergic stimulation.

Toxicity/Side Effects Drowsiness and a dry mouth may occur in up to 50% of patients who receive the drug. Central nervous system disturbances, fluid retention, impotence and constipation have also been reported. Rapid withdrawal of the drug may lead to life-threatening rebound hypertension and tachycardia.

Kinetics

Absorption The drug is rapidly and well absorbed when administered orally; the oral bioavailability is 100%.

Distribution Clonidine is very lipid-soluble and penetrates the central nervous system. The drug is 20% protein-bound in the plasma; the V_D is 1.7–2.5 l/kg.

Metabolism Less than half of an administered dose is metabolised in the liver to inactive metabolites.

Excretion 65% of the dose of clonidine is excreted unchanged in the urine; some 20% is excreted in the faeces. The clearance is 1.9–4.3 ml/min/kg and the elimination half-life is 6–23 hours. The latter is markedly increased in the presence of renal impairment; the dose of clonidine should be reduced if the glomerular filtration rate is <10 ml/min.

Special Points Clonidine decreases the MAC of co-administered volatile agents. It decreases the incidence of post-anaesthetic shivering and post-operative nausea and vomiting.

Clonidine decreases the dose of propofol needed for LMA insertion.

It obtunds tourniquet-induced hypertension.

Clonidine decreases post-operative agitation in children undergoing sevoflurane anaesthesia.

It prolongs the duration of local anaesthesia when co-administered for neural and retrobulbar blockade.

The drug is not removed by haemodialysis.

Cocaine

Uses   Cocaine is used as a topical vasoconstrictor.

Chemical   An ester of benzoic acid (a naturally occurring alkaloid derived from the leaves of *Erythroxylon coca*).

Presentation As   1–4% solutions and as a non-proprietary paste of varying concentration.

Main Actions   Local anaesthesia, vasoconstriction and euphoria.

Mode of Action   Local anaesthetics diffuse in their uncharged base form through neural sheaths and the axonal membrane to the internal surface of cell membrane sodium ion channels; here they combine with hydrogen ions to form a cationic species which enters the internal opening of the sodium ion channel and combines with a receptor. This produces blockade of the sodium ion channel, thereby decreasing sodium ion conductance and preventing depolarisation of the cell membrane. Cocaine also produces blockade of the uptake-1 pathway of noradrenaline and dopamine, leading to vasoconstriction and central nervous system excitation.

Route of Administration/Dose   Cocaine is administered topically; the toxic dose is 3 mg/kg. The drug has a duration of action of 20–30 minutes.

Effects
CVS   The usual effect of cocaine is to produce hypertension and tachycardia due to a combination of central sympathetic stimulation and the blockade of noradrenaline re-uptake at peripheral adrenergic nerve terminals, leading to intense peripheral vasoconstriction. Large doses produce myocardial depression and may precipitate ventricular fibrillation.
RS   Therapeutic concentrations of the drug cause stimulation of the respiratory centre and an increase in ventilation.
CNS   The principal effect of cocaine is reversible neural blockade; this leads to a characteristically biphasic effect in the central nervous system. Initially, excitation (euphoria, lightheadedness, dizziness, visual and auditory disturbances and fitting) occurs, due to the blockade of inhibitory pathways in the cortex; with increasing doses, depression of both facilitatory and inhibitory pathways occur, leading to central nervous system depression (drowsiness, disorientation and coma). Cocaine may also cause hyperreflexia, mydriasis and an increase in intraocular pressure.
AS   The drug produces hyperdynamic bowel sounds and marked nausea and vomiting (a central effect).
Metabolic/Other   Cocaine causes a marked increase in body temperature, due to increased motor activity combined with

cutaneous vasoconstriction and a direct effect of the drug on the hypothalamus.

Toxicity/Side Effects   Allergic phenomena occur occasionally with the use of cocaine. The side effects are predominantly correlated with excessive plasma concentrations of the drug. These include confusion, hallucinations, seizures, cerebral haemorrhage and infarction and medullary depression leading to respiratory arrest. Chest pain, pulmonary oedema, gut infarction, rhabdomyolysis and disseminated intravascular coagulation may also occur. Cocaine is a drug of dependence; maternal use may result in neonatal dependence.

Kinetics

Absorption   The drug is well absorbed from mucosae, including that of the gut. The bioavailability when administered intranasally is 0.5%.

Distribution   Cocaine is 98% protein-bound in the plasma; the V_D is 0.9–3.3 l/kg.

Metabolism   In common with the other ester-type local anaesthetic agents, cocaine is predominantly degraded by plasma esterases, predominantly to benzoylecgonine.

Excretion   The metabolites are excreted in the urine; 10% unchanged. The clearance is 26–44 ml/min/kg and the elimination half-life is 25–60 minutes.

Codeine phosphate

Uses   Codeine is used for the treatment of:
1.   pain of mild to moderate severity
2.   diarrhoea and excessive ileostomy output and
3.   as an antitussive agent and
4.   traditionally, to provide analgesia for head-injured patients.

Chemical   A naturally occurring phenanthrene alkaloid which is a methylated morphine derivative.

Presentation   As 15/30/60 mg tablets, a syrup containing 5 mg/ml and as a clear, colourless solution for injection containing 60 mg/ml of codeine phosphate. A number of fixed dose preparations containing paracetamol, ibuprofen or aspirin in combination with codeine phosphate are also available.

Main Actions   Analgesic, antitussive and a decrease in gastrointestinal motility.

Mode of Action   Codeine has a very low affinity for opioid receptors; 10% of the drug is metabolised to morphine and the analgesic and constipating effects are due to the morphine metabolite. The antitussive effects of codeine appear to be mediated by specific, high affinity codeine receptors.

Routes of Administration/Doses   The adult oral and intramuscular dose is 30–60 mg 4–6 hourly. Rectal administration in a dose of 1 mg/kg can be used in paediatrics. It should not be given intravenously due to hypotension probably due to histamine release.

Effects
RS   The principal effect of the drug is an antitussive effect; it also produces some respiratory depression, with a decreased ventilatory response to hypoxia and hypercapnia.
CNS   Codeine is 10 times less potent an analgesic compared to morphine and produces few of the central effects associated with opioids.
AS   The drug markedly inhibits gastrointestinal motility, leading to constipation.

Toxicity/Side Effects   Nausea and vomiting, dizziness and excitatory phenomena may complicate the use of the drug; cardiovascular collapse may occur when codeine is taken in overdose or administered intravenously. Codeine has a low propensity to cause dependence.

Kinetics

Absorption   Codeine phosphate is well absorbed when administered orally and rectally; the bioavailability by these routes is 60–70% as little first-pass metabolism of the drug occurs. Absorption is faster after intramuscular absorption (0.5 hours). Peak concentration occurs at 1 hour.

Distribution   Codeine is 7% protein-bound in the plasma; the V_D is 5.4 l/kg.

Metabolism   Codeine is extensively metabolised in the liver by three methods: principally (10–20%) by glucuronidation to codeine-6-glucuronide; by N-demethylation (10–20%) to nor-codeine and by O-demethylation to morphine (5–15%).

Other minor metabolites, normorphine, norcodeine-6-glucuronide, have been found.

Genetic variability occurs with the cytochrome P-450 enzyme CYP2D6 which causes conversion to morphine, so 'fast' metabolisers produce more morphine.

Excretion   Occurs predominantly in the urine as free and conjugated codeine, norcodeine and morphine; <17% of the dose is excreted unchanged. The clearance is 98 l/hour after oral administration and the elimination half-life is 2.8 hours. The dose should be reduced in the presence of renal failure.

Special Points   There are no published data to support the use of codeine in the management of head-injured patients. The drug has traditionally been used in these circumstances due to its low potency and consequent relative lack of respiratory and neurological depressant effects.

Cotrimoxazole

(Trimethoprim 1 sulphamethoxazole)

Uses   Cotrimoxazole should be used in the treatment of:
1. *Pneumocystis carinii* infections
2. toxoplasmosis and
3. nocardiasis.

Chemical   Trimethoprim is a diaminopyrimidine and sulpha-methoxazole a sulphonamide.

Presentation   All preparations contain trimethoprim and sulphamethoxazole in the ratio of 1:5. The tablets contain 20/80/160 mg of sulphamethoxazole in a fixed dose combination with 100/400/800 mg of sulphamethoxazole respectively. A suspension for oral administration is also available. A pale yellow preparation of cotrimoxazole is available for intravenous use and contains 16 mg of trimethoprim and 80 mg of sulphamethoxazole per ml. The intramuscular preparation contains 160 mg of trimethoprim and 800 mg of suiphamethoxazole in 3 ml.

Main Actions   Cotrimoxazole is bactericidal against a broad spectrum of Gram-positive and Gram-negative aerobic bacteria, including the Gram-positive *Staphylococcus* and *Streptococcus* sp.; the Gram-negative *Proteus, Salmonella, Shigella* and *Klebsiella* sp., and *Escherichia coli*. It is also effective against some protozoa, *Chlamydia* sp., and some anaerobic species. Bacterial resistance to the drug is widespread.

Mode of Action   Cotrimoxazole inhibits the synthesis of tetrahydrofolic acid, which is needed for the synthesis of nucleic acids and amino acids. The two components of the drug act at separate stages in the biosynthetic pathway of tetrahydrofolic acid; sulphamethoxazole inhibits the synthesis of dihydrofolic acid and trimethoprim is a competitive inhibitor of dihydrofolate reductase. Mammalian dihydrofolate reductase is minimally affected by cotrimoxazole; in any case, mammalian cells utilise preformed folate derived from-the diet.

Routes of Administration/Doses   The adult oral dose is 2–3 of the 80/400 mg tablets 12-hourly. The corresponding dose by the intravenous or intramuscular route is 160/800 to 240/1200 mg 12-hourly. The intravenous preparation should be diluted in a crystalloid prior to use and infused over a period of 90 minutes.

Effects
Metabolic/Other   Serum creatinine concentrations may increase with the use of the drug due to competition for tubular secretory mechanisms and to an effect on the assay of creatinine. The plasma concentration of thyroid hormone may also decrease.

Toxicity/Side Effects The use of cotrimoxazole may be complicated by allergic phenomena, gastrointestinal and haematological disturbances, especially neutropenia. Patients known to be deficient in vitamin B_{12} or folate are at increased risk for the latter complication.

Kinetics

Absorption Both components of the drug are well absorbed; the bioavailability of both sulphamethoxazole and trimethoprim is 100%.

Distribution The plasma ratio of trimethoprim:sulphamethoxazole is 1:20, which appears to be optimal for synergistic activity. Trimethoprim is 45% protein-bound in the plasma; its V_D is 1.6–2.0 l/kg. Sulphamethoxazole is 66% protein-bound in the plasma; its V_D is 0.19–0.23 l/kg.

Metabolism 5–15% of the dose of trimethoprim is metabolised to inactive products; sulphamethoxazole is extensively metabolised, the major metabolite being an acetyl derivative.

Excretion Both components are excreted predominantly in the urine; 80% of the dose of trimethoprim is excreted unchanged, whereas sulphamethoxazole is excreted predominantly as inactive metabolites. The clearance of trimethoprim is 1.6–2.8 ml/min/kg and the elimination half-life is 11 hours. The clearance of sulphamethoxazole is 0.28–0.36 ml/min/kg and the elimination half-life is 9 hours. The dose of cotrimoxazole should be reduced if the creatinine clearance is < 30 ml/min; hepatic impairment has no effect on the kinetics of the drug.

Special Points Cotrimoxazole potentiates the anticoagulant effect of co-administered warfarin and the hypo-glycaemic effect of co-administered sulphonylureas. The drug has a theoretically synergistic action with nitrous oxide on folic acid metabolism. Both components of the drug are haemodialysable.

Cyclizine

Uses Cyclizine is used in the treatment of nausea and vomiting due to:
1. opioid or general anaesthetic agents
2. motion sickness
3. radiation sickness and
4. Ménière's disease.

Chemical A piperazine derivative.

Presentation As tablets containing 50 mg of cyclizine hydrochloride and as a clear, colourless solution for injection containing 50 mg/ml of cyclizine lactate. Fixed dose combinations with morphine, caffeine and dipipanone are available.

Main Action Antiemetic.

Mode of Action Cyclizine is a competitive antagonist of histamine at H1 receptors; it is unknown how the drug exerts its antiemetic effect. It is postulated that this effect is mediated via blockade of central histamine (H1) and muscarinic receptors.

Effects
CVS The drug has a mild anticholinergic action and may produce a slight tachycardia.
RS Cyclizine, although it has antihistaminergic properties, does not completely reverse anaphylactic bronchospasm as leukotrienes are involved in the mediation of allergic bronchoconstriction.
CNS The principal effect of the drug is an antiemetic effect, with a slight degree of sedation.
AS Cyclizine increases the tone of the lower oesophageal sphincter.

Toxicity/Side Effects The predominant side effects are anticholinergic: drowsiness, dryness of the mouth and blurred vision.

Kinetics Data are incomplete.

Absorption The drug is well absorbed when administered orally; the bioavailability by this route is 80%.

Metabolism In animal models, metabolism of cyclizine occurs by N-demethylation to norcyclizine.

Excretion The elimination half-life in animals is 10 hours.

Special Points Cyclizine appears to be as effective as perphenazine in counteracting the nausea and vomiting associated with the use of opioids. The sedative effect of the drug is additive with that produced by anaesthetic agents.

Dantrolene

Uses Dantrolene is used in the treatment of:
1. malignant hyperthermia and the neuroleptic malignant syndrome
2. heat stroke and
3. muscle spasticity and may be of use
4. as an adjunct in the treatment of tetanus.

Chemical A phenyl hydantoin derivative.

Presentation As 25 or 100 mg capsules of dantrolene sodium as a lyophilised orange powder which contains 20 mg of dantrolene sodium and 3 g of mannitol (to improve the solubility), together with sodium hydroxide in each vial; this is reconstituted prior to use with 60 ml of water. A solution of pH 9.5 is produced.

Main Actions Muscular relaxation.

Mode of Action Dantrolene acts within skeletal muscle fibres to inhibit calcium ion release through inhibition of ryanodine receptors in the sarcoplasmic reticulum to cause a reduction in muscular contraction to a given electrical stimulus. Part of its action may be due to a marked GABA-ergic effect.

Routes of Administration/Doses For the treatment of acute hyperthermia, 1–10 mg/kg administered intravenously (either via a central vein or into a fast-running infusion) as required – an average of 2.5 mg/kg are required. For the prophylaxis of malignant hyperthermia, 4–8 mg/kg/day are given for 1–2 days prior to surgery in 3 to 4 divided doses; the role of this regime is controversial. The oral adult dose used for the prevention of spasticity is 25–100 mg 6-hourly. Therapeutic effects are observed within 15 minutes; the mean duration of action is 4–6 hours.

Effects
CVS No consistent effects have been reported from animal studies. Dantrolene may have antiarrhythmic effects in man. Dantrolene improves beta-adrenergic responsiveness in the failing human myocardium.
RS Negligible effects are produced by the drug in man.
CNS Dantrolene has marked central GABA-ergic effects; sedation may occur.
GU Dantrolene increases the effectiveness of voiding in many patients with neuromuscular disorders.
Metabolic/Other Dantrolene diminishes the force of electrically induced muscle twitches, whilst having no effect on action potentials in skeletal muscle.

Toxicity/Side Effects The drug is highly irritant if extravasated. With chronic use, muscular weakness, drowsiness and gastrointestinal disturbances may occur. Hepatic dysfunction occurs in up to 2% of patients which is reversible.

Kinetics

Absorption   20–70% of an oral dose is absorbed.

Distribution   Dantrolene is 80–90% protein-bound to albumin. The V_D is 0.6 l/kg.

Metabolism   Predominantly in the liver by hydroxylation (to an active metabolite) and by reduction and acetylation.

Excretion   15–25% is excreted in the urine, predominantly as the hydroxy metabolite. The clearance is 2.3 ml/kg/min and elimination half-life is 3–12 hours.

Special Points   There are no controlled trials of the effectiveness of dantrolene in the treatment of malignant hyperthermia or the malignant neuroleptic syndrome in man; however, more than 80% of patients with prodromal signs of the syndromes improve after receiving dantrolene. It has also been used successfully in the management of 'Ecstasy' toxicity.

Verapamil and dantrolene administered concurrently in animals may cause hyperkalaemia leading to ventricular fibrillation; these drugs are not recommended for use together in man.

Desflurane

Uses   Desflurane is used for the induction and maintenance of general anaesthesia.

Chemical   A halogenated ether.

Presentation   As a clear, colourless liquid that should be protected from light. The commercial preparation contains no additives and is flammable at a concentration of 17%. The molecular weight of desflurane is 168, the boiling point 23.5 °C and the saturated vapour pressure is 88.5 kPa at 20 °C. The MAC of desflurane is age-dependent and ranges from 5.75 to 10.65 (1.75–7.75 in the presence of 60% nitrous oxide), the oil/gas solubility coefficient 18.7 and the blood/gas solubility coefficient 0.42. Desflurane is stable in the presence of moist soda lime.

Main Action   General anaesthesia (reversible loss of both awareness and recall of noxious stimuli).

Mode of Action   The mechanism of general anaesthesia remains to be fully elucidated. General anaesthetics appear to disrupt synaptic transmission (especially in the area of the ventrobasal thalamus). This mechanism may include potentiation of the gamma-amino-butyric acid and glycine receptors and antagonism at NMDA receptors. Their mode of action at the molecular level appears to involve expansion of hydrophobic regions in the neuronal membrane, either within the lipid phase or within hydrophobic sites in cell membrane proteins.

Route of Administration/Dose   Desflurane is administered by inhalation. Because of the high saturated vapour pressure, desflurane must be administered by a specific pressurised and heated vaporiser The concentration used for the induction of anaesthesia is 4–11% and for maintenance, 2–6%.

Effects
CVS   Desflurane causes a decrease in myocardial contractility, but sympathetic tone is relatively well preserved. The cardiac index and left-ventricular ejection fraction are well maintained during desflurane anaesthesia in man. Desflurane causes a dose-dependent decrease in systemic vascular resistance and mean arterial pressure; the heart rate may increase via an indirect autonomic effect. The drug does not appear to cause the 'coronary steal' phenomenon in man. Desflurane does not sensitise the myocardium to the effects of catecholamines.

RS   Desflurane is a respiratory depressant, causing dose-dependent decreases in tidal volume and an increase in respiratory rate. The drug depresses the ventilatory response to CO_2. Desflurane is markedly irritant to the respiratory tract in concentrations greater than 6%.

CNS   The principal effect of desflurane is general anaesthesia. The drug causes cerebral vasodilation, leading to increased cerebral blood flow; the effects on intracranial pressure are unclear. Desflurane decreases cerebral oxygen consumption and is not associated with epileptiform activity. A centrally mediated decrease in skeletal muscle tone results from the use of desflurane.

AS   Desflurane does not decrease hepatic blood flow.

GU   Desflurane decreases renal cortical blood flow.

Metabolic/Other   Rapid alterations in desflurane concentration cause transient increases in catecholamine levels.

Toxicity/Side Effects   There is a high incidence of airway irritation and reactivity during the use of high concentrations of desflurane, making it unsuitable for use during gaseous induction. Desflurane is a trigger agent for the development of malignant hyperthermia.

Kinetics

Absorption   The major factors affecting the uptake of volatile anaesthetic agents are solubility, cardiac output and the concentration gradient between the alveoli and venous blood. Desflurane is exceptionally insoluble in blood; alveolar concentration therefore reaches inspired concentration very rapidly, resulting in a rapid induction of anaesthesia. An increase in the cardiac output increases the rate of alveolar uptake and slows the induction of anaesthesia. The concentration gradient between alveoli and venous blood approaches zero at equilibrium; a large concentration gradient favours the onset of anaesthesia.

Distribution   The drug is initially distributed to organs with a high blood flow (the brain, heart, liver and kidney) and later to less well-perfused organs (muscle, fat and bone).

Metabolism   0.02% of an administered dose is metabolised, predominantly to trifluoroacetic acid.

Excretion   Excretion is via the lungs, predominantly unchanged; trace quantities of trifluoroacetic acid are excreted in the urine. Elimination of desflurane is rapid due to its low solubility.

Special Points   Desflurane potentiates the action of co-administered depolarising and non-depolarising relaxants.

Dexmedetomidine

Uses Dexmedetomidine is used as a sedative for post-surgical patients requiring mechanical ventilation.

Chemical An imidazole derivative.

Presentation As a clear, colourless isotonic solution containing 100 µg/ml of dexmedetomidine base and 9 mg/ml of sodium chloride in water. The solution is preservative-free and contains no additives.

Main Actions Sedation, anxiolysis and analgesia.

Mode of Action Dexmedetomidine is a specific alpha-2 adrenoceptor agonist which acts via post-synaptic alpha-2 receptors to increase conductance through potassium ion channels.

Routes of Administration/Doses The drug is administered by intravenous infusion, commencing at 1 µg/kg for 10 minutes, then at 0.2–0.7 µg/kg/hour. The duration of use should not exceed 24 hours. Dexmedetomidine has also been administered transdermally and intramuscularly.

Effects
CVS The drug causes a predictable decrease in mean arterial pressure and heart rate.
RS Dexmedetomidine causes a slight increase in $PaCO_2$ and a decrease in minute ventilation with minimal change in respiratory rate – these effects are not clinically significant.
CNS The drug is sedative and anxiolytic – ventilated patients remain easily rousable and cooperative during treatment. Reversible memory impairment is an additional feature.

Metabolic/Other Dexmedetomidine causes a decrease in plasma epinephrine and norepinephrine concentrations. It does not impair adrenal steroidogenesis when used in the short term.

Toxicity/Side Effects Hypotension, bradycardia, nausea and a dry mouth are the most commonly reported side effects of the drug.

Kinetics

Distribution Dexmedetomidine is 94% protein-bound in the plasma; the V_D is 1.33 l/kg. The distribution half-life is 6 minutes.

Metabolism The drug undergoes extensive hepatic metabolism to methyl and glucuronide conjugates.

Excretion 95% of the metabolites are excreted in the urine. The elimination half-life is 2 hours and the clearance is 39 l/hour.

Special Points The drug shows a pharmacodynamic interaction with volatile agents and analgesic agents. The clearance is decreased in hepatic impairment, although renal impairment does not significantly alter its pharmacokinetics. Dexmedetomidine is currently licensed for use in the USA, but not Europe.

Dextran 40

Uses   Dextran 40 is used:
1. for plasma volume replacement in haemorrhage, burns or excessive fluid and electrolyte loss and
2. in the prophylaxis of post-operative thrombo-embolism.

Chemical   Dextran 40 is a polysaccharide derived from sucrose by the action of the bacterium *Leuconostoc mesenteroides*; the preparation is then further processed by hydrolysis and fractionation.

Presentation   As a clear, colourless 10% solution in either 5% dextrose or 0.9% saline. The preparation contains molecules with a weight average molecular weight of 40 000. 90% of molecules have a molecular weight within the range 10 000–75 000.

Main Actions   Plasma volume expansion and an antithrombotic effect.

Mode of Action   Each gram of dextran in the circulation will retain approximately 20 ml of water by its osmotic effect; a rapid infusion of 500 ml of Dextran 40 will maximally increase the circulating plasma volume by approximately 1000 ml. Molecules above 55 000 daltons are generally retained in the intra-vascular space, whereas those below 20 000 daltons have access to the interstitial space. Dextran 40 inhibits platelet adhesiveness and dilutes clotting factors, thereby improving peripheral perfusion. It is also adsorbed onto erythrocytes and interferes with fibrinogen binding, thereby interrupting the process of rouleaux formation.

Route of Administration/Dose   When used primarily as a plasma volume expander, Dextran 40 should be infused intravenously titrated against the clinical response. When used in the prophylaxis of post-operative thrombosis, the adult dose is 500 ml infused over 4–6 hours in the immediate peri-operative period, repeated on the next day. For high-risk cases, this may be continued on alternate days for up to two weeks.

Effects
CVS   The haemodyamic effects of Dextran 40 are proportional to the prevailing volaemic status; in the face of hypovolaemia, infusion of Dextran 40 restores cardiovascular parameters towards normal.
Metabolic/Other   Infusion of dextran reduces the serum lipid concentration and produces a reduction in the serum albumin.

Toxicity/Side Effects   Severe hypersensitivity reactions occur in 1 in 3300 – this is probably due to a cross-reaction with antibodies to a recent pneumococcal infection. Circulatory overload may occur with excessive administration. Increased capillary oozing due to improved perfusion pressure and capillary flow may be noted perioperatively. Acute renal failure may complicate the use of Dextran 40 when it is used in the management of profound hypovolaemia.

Kinetics   Data are incomplete.

Distribution   Dextran 40 is not significantly protein-bound; the V_D is 5.3–7.7 l. Chronic overdosage leads to storage of dextrans in the liver.

Metabolism   Occurs by the action of dextranases present in the lung, liver, kidney and spleen.

Excretion   The excretion of Dextran 40 is biphasic; 70% occurs by the renal excretion of small molecules, the remainder are metabolised and excreted as carbon dioxide and water. The plasma half-life is 4–9 hours.

Special Points   Dextran 40 does not interfere with cross-matching if enzymatic methods are used (although older preparations did).

If a dextran of molecular weight 1000 (not yet available in the UK) is infused prior to the administration of Dextran 40, the incidence of anaphylaxis is reduced 15–20-fold.

Dextran 70

Uses   Dextran 70 is used:
1. for plasma volume replacement in haemorrhage, burns or excessive fluid and electrolyte loss and
2. in the prophylaxis of post-operative thrombo-embolism.

Chemical   Dextran 70 is a polysaccharide derived from sucrose by the action of the bacterium *Leuconostoc mesenteroides*; the preparation is then further processed by hydrolysis and fractionation.

Presentation   As a clear, colourless 6% solution in either 5% dextrose or 0.9% saline. The preparation contains molecules with a weight average molecular weight of 70 000. 90% of molecules have a molecular weight within the range 20 000–115 000.

Main Actions   Plasma volume expansion and an antithrombotic effect.

Mode of Action   Each gram of dextran in the circulation will retain approximately 20 ml of water by its osmotic effect; an infusion of 500 ml of Dextran 70 will increase the circulating plasma volume by approximately 750 ml. Molecules above 55 000 daltons are generally retained in the intravascular space, whereas those below 20 000 daltons have access to the interstitial space. Dextran 70 exerts its antithrombotic action by reducing ADP-induced platelet aggregation and by reducing the activating effect of thrombin on platelets. The growth of white thrombus is impeded and the structure and stability of fibrin are altered by Dextran 70.

Route of Administration/Dose   When used primarily as a plasma volume expander, Dextran 70 should be infused intravenously titrated against the clinical response. When used in the prophylaxis of post-operative thrombosis, the adult dose is 500 ml infused over 4–6 hours in the immediate peri-operative period, repeated on the next day. For high-risk cases, this may be continued on alternate days for up to two weeks.

Effects
CVS   The haemodynamic effects of Dextran 70 are proportional to the prevailing volaemic status; in the face of hypovolaemia, infusion of Dextran 70 restores cardiovascular parameters towards normal. Modern dextrans, free of high molecular weight fractions, do not induce coagulation disturbances or interfere with normal platelet function.
RS   Dextran 70 appears to protect against the development of ARDS in patients with multiple trauma.
Metabolic/Other   Infusion of dextran reduces serum lipid levels and produces a reduction in the serum albumin concentration.

Toxicity/Side Effects Severe hypersensitivity reactions occur in 1 in 3300 – this is probably due to a cross-reaction with antibodies to a recent pneumococcal infection. Circulatory overload may occur with excessive administration of the colloid. Increased capillary oozing due to improved perfusion pressure and capillary flow may be noted per-operatively.

Kinetics Data are incomplete.

Distribution Chronic overdosage leads to storage of dextrans in the liver. There is no significant protein binding.

Metabolism 50% of an administered dose exceeds the renal threshold and is thus available for metabolism by dextranases present in the lung, liver, kidney and spleen to carbon dioxide and water.

Excretion The low molecular weight (<50 000) fraction is excreted unchanged in the urine. An elimination half-life of 23–25.5 hours has been postulated. 45–50% of a 500 ml infusion is excreted in 48 hours.

Special Points Dextran 70 does not interfere with cross-matching if enzymatic methods are used (although older preparations did).

If a dextran of molecular weight 1000 (not yet available in the UK) is infused prior to the administration of Dextran 70, the incidence of anaphylaxis is reduced 15–20-fold.

Dextrose

Uses Dextrose solutions are used:
1. to provide a source of water (5% solutions) and calories (10/20/50% solutions) and
2. in the treatment of hypoglycaemia.

Chemical Dextrose is D-glucopyranose D-glucose monohydrate, a monosaccharide obtained by the hydrolysis of cornstarch.

Presentation As a clear, colourless sterile solution containing 5/10/20/50% dextrose in water in ampoules or bags containing 500/1000 ml. The preparations are sterile and contain no buffers or bacteriostatic agents. The pH varies from 3.5–6.5, according to concentration. The 5% solution contains 170 kCal/l and has an osmolarity of 250 mOsm/l; the 10/20/50% solutions are appropriate multiples of these figures.

Main Actions An increase in the blood sugar concentration and glycogen deposition; ketosis and nitrogen loss are decreased.

Routes of Administration/Doses Dextrose solutions are administered intravenously; the 20% and 50% solutions should preferably be administered via a central vein. The dose depends upon the state of hydration, nutritional requirements and blood sugar concentration of the individual patient.

Effects
CVS The haemodyamic effects of dextrose solutions are proportional to the prevailing volaemic status; infusion of the crystalloid will temporarily restore cardiovascular parameters towards normal.
GU Renal perfusion is temporarily restored towards normal in hypovolaemic subjects transfused with the crystalloid.

Toxicity/Side Effects Overhydration leading to water intoxication, hyponatraemia, mental confusion and fits may occur with injudicious use of isotonic solutions. Hyperglycaemia and venous thrombosis may occur with the 10/20/50% solutions.

Kinetics Data are incomplete.

Absorption Dextrose is rapidly and completely absorbed when administered orally.

Distribution Dextrose solutions are initially distributed within the intravascular compartment and rapidly equilibrate within the intra- and extravascular space.

Metabolism Dextrose is completely metabolised to carbon dioxide and water.

Excretion   The metabolic products are excreted via the lungs and kidneys.

Special Points   Use of excessive quantities of dextrose solutions (especially in premenopausal women and prepubertal children) may result in cerebral oedema and respiratory arrest, a condition associated with poor neurological outcome.

Diamorphine

Uses Diamorphine is used:
1. for premedication
2. as an analgesic in the management of moderate to severe pain
3. in the treatment of left ventricular failure
4. as an antitussive agent and
5. to provide analgesia during terminal care.

Chemical A synthetic diacetylated morphine derivative.

Presentation As tablets containing 10 mg, and as a lyophilised white powder in ampoules containing 5/10/30/100/500 mg of diamorphine hydrochloride. A number of non-proprietary elixirs and suppositories are also available.

Main Actions Analgesia, euphoria and respiratory depression.

Mode of Action Diamorphine is a pro-drug; it does not possess an unsubstituted phenolic hydroxyl group at the 3-position and acts via active derivatives (6-o-acetylmorphine and morphine) which are mu-opioid receptor agonists. Opioids appear to exert their effects by increasing intracellular calcium concentration which, in turn, increases potassium conductance and hyperpolarisation of excitable cell membranes. The decrease in membrane excitability that results may decrease both pre-and post-synaptic responses.

Routes of Administration/Doses The average adult dose by the intravenous or intramuscular route is 5–10 mg. The corresponding intrathecal or epidural dose is 2.5–5 mg. Due to its higher lipid solubility, the drug has a more rapid onset of action than morphine and has a duration of action of 90 minutes after intramuscular administration.

Effects

CVS Diamorphine has little effect on the cardiovascular system when used in normal doses. In high doses, it may cause bradycardia due to a combination of increased vagal activity and decreased sympathetic activity; hypotension resulting from a decrease in systemic vascular resistance may occur.

RS The principal effect of the drug is respiratory depression in opioid-naive subjects, with a decreased ventilatory response to hypoxia and hypercapnia. Diamorphine also has a potent antitussive action. Bronchoconstriction may occur with the use of high doses of the drug.

CNS Diamorphine is 1.5–2 times as potent an analgesic agent as morphine. The drug tends to cause marked euphoria; there is a clinical impression that it causes less nausea and vomiting than morphine. Miosis is produced as a result of stimulation of the Edinger-Westphal nucleus. Seizures may occur with the use of high doses of the drug.

AS   Diamorphine decreases gastrointestinal motility and decreases gastric acid, biliary and pancreatic secretion; it also increases the common bile duct pressure by causing spasm of the sphincter of Oddi. There is a clinical impression that the drug causes less constipation than does an equipotent dose of morphine.

GU   The drug increases the tone of the ureters, bladder detrusor muscle and sphincter and may precipitate urinary retention.

Metabolic/Other   Mild diaphoresis and piloerection may occur with the use of diamorphine. Intrathecal diamorphine suppresses the metabolic response to surgery.

Toxicity/Side Effects   Respiratory depression, nausea and vomiting, hallucinations and dependence may complicate the use of diamorphine. Pruritus may occur after epidural or spinal administration of the drug.

Kinetics   Data are incomplete due to the instability of the drug *in vivo* and difficulties in assay methodology.

Absorption   Diamorphine is extensively absorbed when administered orally; the bioavailability appears to be low due to an extensive first-pass metabolism.

Distribution   The drug is 40% protein-bound in the plasma; the V_D is 350 l.

Metabolism   Diamorphine undergoes rapid enzymatic hydrolysis in the plasma and in association with red blood cells, probably via pseudocholinesterase and at least three esterases located within red blood cells. The initial metabolic product is 6-0-acetylmorphine (which is the active form of the drug) which is, in turn, further metabolised to morphine, with subsequent glucuronidation.

Excretion   50–60% of an administered dose appears in the urine as a morphine derivative; 0.13% is excreted unchanged. The elimination half-life of diamorphine is 3 minutes. The clearance of the morphine component is 3.1 ml/min/kg.

Special Points   Late respiratory depression has not been reported following the use of epidural diamorphine. The actions of the drug are all reversed by naloxone.

Diamorphine is not removed by dialysis.

Diazepam

Uses   Diazepam is used:
1. in the short-term treatment of anxiety and in the treatment of
2. status epilepticus
3. muscle spasm in tetanus and other spastic conditions
4. alcohol withdrawal and for
5. premedication
6. induction of anaesthesia and
7. sedation during endoscopy and procedures performed under local anaesthesia.

Chemical   A benzodiazepine.

Presentation   As tablets containing 2/5/10 mg, a syrup containing 0.4 mg/1 mg/ml, as 10 mg suppositories and as a solution for rectal administration containing 2/4 mg/ml of diazepam. The drug is also supplied as a clear yellow solution and as a white oil-in-water emulsion for injection containing 5 mg/ml.

Main Actions
1. hypnosis
2. sedation
3. anxiolysis
4. anterograde amnesia
5. anticonvulsant and
6. muscular relaxation.

Mode of Action   Benzodiazepines are thought to act via specific benzodiazepine receptors found at synapses throughout the central nervous system, but concentrated especially in the cortex and mid-brain. Benzodiazepine receptors are closely linked with GABA receptors, and appear to facilitate the activity of the latter. Activated GABA receptors open chloride ion channels which then either hyperpolarise or short-circuit the synaptic membrane.

Diazepam has Kappa-opioid agonist activity *in vitro*, which may explain the mechanism of benzodiazepine-induced spinal analgesia.

Routes of Administration/Doses   The adult oral dose is 2–60 mg/day in divided doses; the initial intravenous dose is 10–20 mg increasing according to clinical effect.

Effects
CVS A transient decrease in blood pressure and a slight decrease in cardiac output may occur following intravenous administration of diazepam. The coronary blood flow is increased secondary to coronary arterial vasodilation; a decrease in myocardial oxygen consumption has also been reported.

RS   Large doses cause respiratory depression; hypoxic drive is depressed to a greater degree than is hypercarbic drive.

CNS   Diazepam is anxiolytic and decreases aggression, although paradoxical excitement may occur. Sedation, hypnosis and anterograde amnesia occur after the administration of diazepam. The drug has anticonvulsant and analgesic properties and depresses spinal reflexes.

Toxicity/Side Effects   Depression of the central nervous system, including drowsiness, ataxia and headache, may complicate the use of diazepam. Rashes, gastrointestinal upsets and urinary retention have also been reported. Tolerance and dependence may occur with prolonged use of benzodiazepines; acute withdrawal of benzodiazepines in these circumstances may produce insomnia, anxiety, confusion, psychosis and perceptual disturbances. Intravenous diazepam is highly irritant to veins; the oil-in-water preparation is less so.

Kinetics

Absorption   Diazepam is rapidly absorbed after oral administration; the bioavailability is 86–100%. Absorption after intramuscular administration is slow and erratic.

Distribution   The drug is 99% protein-bound in the plasma; the V_D is 0.8–1.4 l/kg.

Metabolism   Diazepam is converted in the liver to active products; the major metabolite is desmethyldiazepam. Other metabolites are oxazepam (which is further metabolised by glucuronidation) and temazepam. These metabolites are active; desmethyldiazepam has a half-life of >100 hours.

Excretion   The metabolites are excreted in the urine as the oxidised and glucuronide derivatives; less than 1% is excreted unchanged. The clearance is 0.32–0.44 ml/min/kg (this is reduced by 42% by the concurrent administration of halothane) and the elimination half-life is 20–40 hours.

Special Points   Diazepam decreases the MAC of volatile agents and potentiates non-depolarising muscle relaxants. Cimetidine decreases the clearance of co-administered diazepam and thereby increases the plasma levels of the latter. Diazepam is adsorbed onto plastic.
   The drug is not removed by dialysis.

Diclofenac

Uses   Diclofenac is used in the treatment of:
1. rheumatoid and osteoarthritis
2. musculo-skeletal disorders
3. soft-tissue injuries
4. ankylosing spondylitis
5. acute gout
6. renal and biliary colic
7. dysmenorrhoea
8. minor post-surgical pain and as an adjunct to systemic opioid therapy and
9. as an antipyretic, and
10. to inhibit perioperative miosis and post-operative inflammation in cataract surgery.

Chemical   A phenylacetic acid derivative.

Presentation   As 25/50 mg tablets, 12.5/25/50/100 mg suppositories and in ampoules containing 25 mg/ml of diclofenac sodium for injection. An emulsified gel and eye drops for topical application are also available.

Main   Actions   Analgesic,   anti-inflammatory   and antipyretic.

Mode of Action   Diclofenac inhibits the enzyme cyclo-oxygenase which converts arachidonic acid to cyclic endoper-oxides, thus preventing the formation of prostaglandins and thromboxanes. Prostaglandins are involved in the sensitisation of peripheral pain receptors to noxious stimuli. The drug may also inhibit the lipo-oxygenase pathway by an action on hydroperoxy fatty acid peroxidase.
Diclofenac has no COX selectivity (COX-2:COX-1 ratio = 1:1).

Routes of Administration/Doses   The adult oral dose is 75–100 mg/day in divided doses; the rectal dose is 100 mg, usually administered as a single nocturnal dose. The intramuscular dose is 75 mg once or twice daily.

Effects
AS   Diclofenac causes less gastrointestinal damage than either indomethacin or aspirin. Dyspepsia, nausea, bleeding from gastric and duodenal vessels, mucosal ulceration, perforation and diarrhoea are expected COX-1 effects.
RS   Bronchoconstriction and pulmonary eosinophilia occur.
Metabolic/Other   Diclofenac interferes with neutrophil function. The plasma renin activity and aldosterone concentrations are reduced by 60–70%. The drug reversibly inhibits platelet aggregation, but has little effect on the bleeding time in man.

Toxicity/Side Effects Occur in 12% – complications are related to the duration of therapy and risks increase markedly after more than 5 days continuous therapy, especially in the elderly.

Disturbances of the gastrointestinal and central nervous system occur occasionally.

Rashes, hepatic, renal and haematological impairment have been reported.

Intramuscular injection may be painful and sterile abscesses have been reported.

Kinetics

Absorption The drug is well absorbed when administered by all routes. The oral bioavailability is 60%.

Distribution Diclofenac is 99.5% protein-bound in the plasma, predominantly to albumin. The V_D is 0.12–0.17 l/kg.

Metabolism Diclofenac undergoes significant first-pass metabolism, principally in the liver by hydroxylation with subsequent conjugation to inactive glucuronide and sulphate metabolites.

Excretion The drug is excreted in urine and bile, <1% unchanged. The clearance is 16 l/hr and the elimination half-life is 1.1–1.8 hours.

Special Points Renal impairment has little effect on the plasma concentration of diclofenac; the drug increases the plasma concentrations of co-administered digoxin and lithium.

Diclofenac may increase the effect of co-administered oral anticoagulants and sulphonylureas due to displacement from plasma proteins.

NSAIDs antagonise the antihypertensive effects of ACE inhibitors. The risk of renal impairment increases if NSAIDs & ACE inhibitors are co-administered.

Diclofenac should not be administered to aspirin-sensitive asthmatics.

Digoxin

Uses Digoxin is used in the treatment of:
1. atrial fibrillation and flutter
2. heart failure and may be of use
3. in the prevention of supraventricular dysrhythmias following thoracotomy.

Chemical A glycoside (sterol lactone + a sugar).

Presentation As 0.0625/0.125/0.25 mg tablets, an elixir containing 0.05 mg/ml and as a clear, colourless solution for injection containing 0.25 mg/ml of digoxin.

Main Actions Positive inotropism and slowing of the ventricular response.

Mode of Action Digoxin acts both directly and indirectly; its direct action is exerted by binding to and inhibiting the action of Na^+-K^+-ATPase within the sarcolemma cell membrane. This produces an increase in the intracellular sodium ion concentration and a decrease in intracellular potassium ion concentration. The increase in intracellular sodium ion concentration causes displacement of bound intracellular calcium ions. This increased availability of calcium ions results in a positive inotropic action. The decrease in intracellular potassium ion concentration leads to slowing of atrio-ventricular conduction and of the pacemaker cells. The drug also acts indirectly by modifying autonomic activity and increasing efferent vagal activity.

Routes of Administration/Doses The loading dose by both oral and parenteral routes is 10–20 μg/kg 6-hourly until the desired effect is achieved. Intravenous injection must be slow (at a rate not exceeding 0.025 mg/min) – the peak effects are observed 2 hours after intravenous administration. The maintenance dose is 10–20 μg/kg/day in divided doses; therapy should be adjusted according to response, guided (where appropriate) by measurement of serum levels of the drug. The therapeutic range 1–2 g/ml.

Effects
CVS The main action of digoxin is to increase the force of cardiac contraction; automaticity and contractility also increase. The heart rate is slowed due to a combination of improved haemodynamics, depression of sinus node discharge, slowing of atrio-ventricular nodal conduction, an increase in the atrio-ventricular nodal refractory period and an indirect vagotonic effect. Rapid intravenous administration of digoxin may cause vasoconstriction leading to hypertension and decreased coronary blood flow. The characteristic ECG changes produced by the drug include prolongation of the P-R

interval, S-T segment depression, T-wave flattening and short-ening of the Q-T interval.

GU   Digoxin has a mild intrinsic diuretic effect.

Toxicity/Side Effects   Side effects are common with digoxin, especially if the therapeutic range is exceeded. The gastrointestinal side effects include anorexia, nausea and vomiting, diarrhoea and abdominal pain. The neurological side effects of the drug include headache, drowsiness, confusion, visual disturbances, muscular weakness and coma. Digoxin may cause any form of dysrhythmia, especially junctional bradycardia, ventricular bigemini and second- or third-degree heart block. Rashes and gynaecomastia occur uncommonly. Digoxin-specific antibody fragments are available for the treatment of digoxin toxicity.

Kinetics

Absorption   Absorption from the gastrointestinal tract is highly variable and the bioavailability by this route varies from 60–90%. Absorption after intramuscular injection is erratic.

Distribution   Digoxin is 20–30% protein-bound in the plasma; the V_D is 5–11 l/kg. The concentrations achieved at steady-state in cardiac tissue are 15–30 times that of plasma.

Metabolism   Less than 10% of the dose undergoes hepatic metabolism via stepwise cleavage of the sugar moieties.

Excretion   50–70% of an administered dose of digoxin is excreted unchanged in the urine as a result of glomerular filtration and active tubular secretion. The clearance is dependent on renal function and may be calculated from the formula:
clearance = $(0.88 \times$ creatinine clearance $+ 0.33) \pm 52\%$; the elimination half-life is 1.6 days.

The dose interval should be increased in the presence of renal impairment.

Special Points   There is some controversy concerning DC cardioversion in digitalised patients.

Patients receiving suxamethonium, pancuronium or beta-adrenergic agonists concurrently with digoxin may exhibit an increased incidence of dysrhythmias.

The following states increase the likelihood of digoxin toxicity: hypokalaemia, hypernatraemia, hypercalcaemia, hypomagnesaemia, acid-base disturbances, hypoxaemia and renal failure. Co-administered verapamil, nifedipine, amiodarone and diazepam also increase plasma digoxin concentrations.

Digoxin is not appreciably removed by dialysis.

Diltiazem

Uses   Diltiazem is recommended for use:
1. in the treatment of stable and variant angina and may be of use in the treatment of:
2. hypertension
3. supraventricular tachycardias
4. Raynaud's phenomenon
5. migraine and
6. oesophageal motility disorders.

Chemical   A benzothiapine.

Presentation   As 60/90/120/180/240/300 mg tablets of diltiazem hydrochloride.

Main Actions   Diltiazem increases myocardial oxygen supply and decreases myocardial oxygen demand by coronary artery dilation, possibly aided by direct and indirect haemodynamic alterations.

Mode of Action   Diltiazem acts via dose-dependent inhibition of the slow inward calcium current in normal cardiac tissue.

Route of Administration/Dose   The adult oral dose is 30–120 mg 6–8 hourly.

Effects
CVS   Diltiazem is a potent peripheral and coronary arterial vasodilator, leading to a decrease in the systemic and pulmonary vascular resistances; the cardiac output increases due to a reduction in afterload. Little effect on the heart rate occurs in man; bradycardia tends to occur with chronic use. A-V nodal conduction is decreased by the drug; diltiazem is thus of use in the treatment of supraventricular tachycardias.
RS   The drug inhibits bronchoconstriction due to inhaled histamine in man.
AS   A significant reduction in lower oesophageal pressure is produced in patients with achalasia, although no effect is seen in normal subjects.
GU   Renal artery dilation leading to an increased renal plasma flow and subsequent diuresis occurs after the administration of diltiazem. Uterine activity is decreased *in vitro*.
Metabolic/Other   Platelet aggregation is decreased by diltiazem *in vitro*, although no significant effect on haemostasis can be demonstrated *in vivo*.

Toxicity/Side Effects   Occur in 2–10% and include headaches, flushing, peripheral oedema and bradycardia.

Kinetics

Absorption 90% of an oral dose is absorbed; the bioavailability by this route is 33–40% due to a significant first effect.

Distribution Diltiazem is 78–87% protein-bound in the plasma; the V_D is 5.3 l/kg.

Metabolism Occurs by deacetylation and demethylation in the liver with subsequent conjugation to glucuronide and sulphates – the metabolites are active.

Excretion 1–4% is excreted unchanged in the urine. The clearance is 11.5–21.3 ml/kg/min and the elimination half-life is 2–7 hours. Renal failure has no effect on the pharmacokinetics of diltiazem.

Special Points Caution should be used if the drug is administered concurrently with a beta-adrenergic antagonist as serious bradycardias may arise. All volatile agents in current use decrease calcium ion release from the sarcoplasmic reticulum and decrease calcium ion flux into cardiac cells; the negative inotropic effects of diltiazem are thus additive with those of the volatile agents. Experiments in animals have demonstrated an increased risk of sinus arrest if volatile agents and calcium antagonists are used concurrently. If withdrawn acutely (especially in the post-operative period) after chronic oral use, severe rebound hypertension may result. Calcium antagonists may also:
1. reduce the MAC of volatile agents by up to 20% and
2. increase the efficacy of neuromuscular blocking agents.
Diltiazem may increase the plasma concentration of co-administered digoxin by 20–60%. It also increases the toxicity of bupivacaine in animal models.

Disopyramide

Uses Disopyramide is used in the treatment of a wide variety of atrial and ventricular dysrhythmias, including the Wolff-Parkinson-White syndrome.

Chemical A tertiary amine.

Presentation As tablets containing 100/150/250 mg of disopyramide base or phosphate and as a solution for injection containing 10 mg/ml of disopyramide phosphate.

Main Action A class la antiarrhythmic agent.

Mode of Action Disopyramide acts by blockade of the fast inward sodium current, leading to prolongation of the duration of the action potential, effective refractory period and decreased membrane responsiveness and automaticity.

Routes of Administration/Doses The adult oral dose is 300–800 mg/day in divided doses. The intravenous loading dose is 2 mg/kg administered over not less than 5 minutes; if conversion to sinus rhythm occurs at any time, the injection should be curtailed. If a response is to occur, it will usually do so within 10–15 minutes of completion of the injection. The therapeutic range is 2–5 mg/ml.

Effects
CVS Disopyramide decreases sinus node automaticity, increases the effective refractory period of the atria and ventricles and slows conduction through the His-Purkinje system. The drug is a negative inotrope – following intravenous administration, the cardiac output decreases by 15% (i.e. to a greater degree than with equivalent doses of lignocaine). The effects on heart rate and blood pressure and variable and usually not significant. Disopyramide may widen the QRS complex and prolong the QT interval.
Metabolic/Other The drug may cause a decrease in fasting blood sugar levels.

Toxicity/Side Effects Disopyramide is usually well tolerated. Typical anticholinergic side effects may occur, as may allergic phenomena. Paraesthesiae and peripheral neuropathies may develop with continued use of the drug. Hypotension, an increase in the degree of any pre-existing block and serious ventricular dysrhythmias have been reported.

Kinetics

Absorption The drug is rapidly and completely absorbed when administered orally; due to a significant first-pass effect, the bioavailability of disopyramide by this route is 70–85%.

Distribution   The drug is protein-bound in the plasma to an extent that depends upon its concentration – values of 32–88% have been reported. The V_D is similarly concentration-dependent and varies from 0.51–1.2 l/kg.

Metabolism   The drug is dealkylated to a mono-N-dealkylated metabolite which has some antiarrhythmic activity.

Excretion   50–60% of the dose is excreted unchanged, mainly in the urine. The clearance is concentration-dependent and varies from 3.69–12.5 l/hr. The elimination half-life is 4.4–8.2 hours, which is increased in patients with renal or hepatic impairment.

Special Points   The drug should be used with caution in patients with impaired left ventricular function or in the presence of other negatively inotropic agents. Disopyramide is not removed by haemodialysis.

Dobutamine

Uses Dobutamine is used to provide inotropic support in patients with a low cardiac output secondary to:
1. myocardial infarction
2. cardiac surgery
3. cardiomyopathy
4. positive end expiratory pressure ventilation
5. in septic shock to increase oxygen transport to the tissues and
6. cardiac stress testing.

Chemical A synthetic isoprenaline derivative.

Presentation Dobutamine is presented in vials which hold a solution for injection containing 12.5/50 mg/ml of dobutamine hydrochloride, which needs to be diluted prior to infusion.

Main Action Positive inotrope.

Mode of Action Dobutamine acts directly on catecholamine receptors to activate adenyl cyclase, which catalyses the conversion of ATP to cAMP. This results in an increased cell membrane permeability to calcium ions which are necessary for depolarisation and completion of the contractile process.

Route of Administration/Doses Dobutamine is infused intravenously diluted in a suitable crystalloid to a volume of at least 50 ml. The dose range is 0.5–40 µg/kg/min, titrated against response; the drug acts within 1–2 minutes. Solutions should be used within 24 hours.

Effects
CVS The primary action of dobutamine is to increase cardiac contractility by a direct action on cardiac beta-1 adrenoceptors. Sino-atrial nodal automaticity is increased, leading to an increased heart rate; atrio-ventricular nodal conduction velocity is also increased by the drug. Dobutamine also has activity at alpha and beta-2 adrenoceptors and thus tends to have only moderate effect on the systemic vascular resistance. Myocardial perfusion may increase. The drug leads to a decrease in both the left ventricular end-diastolic pressure and the systemic vascular resistance and thus to an increase in cardiac index in patients with severe congestive cardiac failure.
CNS Stimulation occurs at high dose ranges.

GU The urine output increases secondary to an increase in cardiac output; dobutamine is devoid of any specific renal vasodilatory effect.

Metabolic/Other Dobutamine enhances natural killer cell activity. It decreases blood glucose and increases free fatty acid concentrations.

Toxicity/Side Effects Are uncommon at dose ranges below 10 µg/kg/min. Dysrhythmias, excessive tachycardia and hypertension, fatigue, nervousness, headache and chest pain may occur. Allergic phenomena have been reported.

Kinetics

Distribution Due to a half-life of 2 minutes, steady state concentrations occur within 8–10 minutes when the drug is given at a fixed rate. The V_D is 0.2 l/kg.

Metabolism The major route of metabolism is by methylation via catechol-O-methyl transferase to 3-O-methyldobutamine with subsequent conjugation to glucuronide.

Excretion The (inactive) 3-O-methyl derivative is excreted in the urine with 20% of the total dose appearing in the faeces. The clearance is 244 l/hour and the elimination half-life is 2 minutes.

Special Points Dobutamine should not be used in patients with cardiac outflow obstruction, e.g. cardiac tamponade or aortic stenosis. Tachyphylaxis may occur during prolonged infusion.

Dobutamine administration during anaesthesia leads to increased heat loss due to redistribution of blood flow to skin.

Domperidone

Uses Domperidone is used for the symptomatic treatment of nausea and vomiting from any cause.

Chemical A butyrophenone derivative.

Presentation As tablets containing 10 mg and a suspension containing 1 mg/ml of domperidone; 30 mg suppositories are also available.

Main Actions Increased gastrointestinal motility and tone, and a central antiemetic effect.

Mode of Action The effects of domperidone on gastro-intestinal mobility appear to be mediated by antagonism of peripheral dopaminergic (D_2-) receptors. Little else is known of the mechanism of action of the drug.

Routes of Administration/Doses The adult oral dose is 10–20 mg and the rectal dose 60 mg 4–8 hourly.

Effects
CVS Domperidone has no significant effects on cardiac output, heart rate, blood pressure or conduction.
CNS The drug does not readily cross the blood–brain barrier and is thus essentially devoid of central effects.
AS The drug increases lower oesophageal sphincter tone and the rate of gastric emptying. It has an antiemetic effect indistinguishable from that of metoclopramide in the prevention of post-operative vomiting, but appears to be more effective in the treatment of established post-operative vomiting.
Metabolic/Other The drug causes an increase in the serum prolactin concentration.

Toxicity/Side Effects Domperidone is generally very well tolerated; there are occasional reports of extra-pyramidal reactions occurring with the use of the drug. Galactorrhoea and gynaecomastia have also been reported.

Kinetics

Absorption The bioavailability is 13–17% when administered orally, due to first-pass metabolism in the gut wall and liver.

Distribution Domperidone is 92% protein-bound in the plasma; the V_D is 5.7 l/kg.

Metabolism 90% of the drug is metabolised by hydroxylation and oxidative N-dealkylation.

Excretion 30% appears in the urine and 60% in the faeces; the elimination half-life is 7.5 hours. Accumulation appears not to occur in the presence of renal impairment.

Special Points   Cardiac arrest has been reported after the rapid intravenous administration of domperidone. This preparation is no longer available.

Dopamine

Uses Dopamine is used in the management of:
1. low cardiac output states
2. septicaemic shock
3. impending renal failure to promote diuresis and
4. for the prevention of hepatorenal failure.

Chemical A naturally occurring catecholamine.

Presentation As a clear, colourless solution for injection containing 40/160 mg/ml of dopamine hydrochloride.

Main Actions Sympathomimetic and increased renal blood flow.

Mode of Action In low doses $(1–5 \, \mu g/kg/min)$, dopamine acts upon specific dopaminergic receptors, of which at least two types are recognised. D_1 receptors are a form of adenyl cyclase; D_2 receptors are not linked to adenyl cyclase and are involved in the central modulation of behaviour and movement. At higher dose ranges, the drug acts via direct and indirect stimulation of beta- and alpha-adrenergic receptors; at an infusion rate of $5–10 \, \mu g/kg/min$ beta-stimulation predominates, whereas at infusion rates exceeding $15 \, \mu g/kg/min$ alpha-effects predominate.

Route of Administration/Dose Dopamine is administered by intravenous infusion, diluted in dextrose/saline or Hartmann's solution. A dedicated central vein is preferred for the administration of the drug. A dose of $1–20 \, \mu g/kg/min$ may be used, titrated according to response. The drug acts within 5 minutes and has a duration of action of 10 minutes.

Effects

CVS The cardiovascular effects of dopamine depend upon the rate of infusion. At low doses $(<5 \, \mu g/kg/min)$, beta-adrenergic effects predominate leading to a positive inotropic effect, increased automaticity and an increase in cardiac output and coronary blood flow; the drug has little effect on heart rate. Systolic and diastolic blood pressure may decrease slightly due to a decrease in the systemic vascular resistance (a beta-2 effect). With the use of high doses $(>15 \, \mu g/kg/min)$ peripheral vasoconstriction (an alpha-adrenergic effect) occurs, leading to an increased venous return and systolic blood pressure. Dopamine has variable effects on the pulmonary vascular resistance.

RS Dopamine activates the carotid bodies and may decrease the ventilatory response to hypoxia.

CNS Dopamine is a central neurotransmitter involved in the modulation of movement; exogenous dopamine does not cross the blood–brain barrier except in its laevo-rotatory form. The drug causes marked nausea, due to a direct action on the chemosensitive trigger zone (which lies outside the blood–brain barrier). Increased intraocular pressure occurs with dopamine administration in critically ill patients.

AS   The drug causes vasodilation of the splanchnic circulation by an effect on dopaminergic receptors, and decreases gastroduodenal motility in the critically ill.

GU   In low doses (1–5 μg/kg/min) dopamine causes a marked decrease in the renal vascular resistance with a corresponding increase in renal blood flow. Dopamine produces diuresis via the D_1 receptors on the luminal and basal membranes of the proximal convoluted tubule. Natriuresis is produced by the inhibition of $Na^+ K^+$ ATPase. Creatinine clearance remains unaltered.

Metabolic/Other   Dopamine reduces the release of prolactin and aldosterone.

The drug appears to induce or aggravate the sick euthyroid syndrome and partial hypopituitarism and also depresses growth hormone secretion in the critically ill.

Toxicity/Side Effects   Tachycardia, dysrhythmias, angina, hypertension and nausea and vomiting may all follow the administration of the drug. Extravasation of dopamine may cause ischaemic tissue necrosis and skin sloughing.

Kinetics

Absorption   Dopamine is ineffective when administered orally.

Metabolism   Exogenous dopamine is metabolised in the plasma, liver and kidneys by monoamine oxidase and catechol-O-methyltransferase to homovanillic acid and 3,4-dihydroxyphenylacetic acid. 25% of an administered dose is converted to noradrenaline within adrenergic nerve terminals.

Excretion   Occurs principally in the urine as homovanillic acid and its sulphate and glucuronide derivatives; a small fraction is excreted unchanged. The clearance is 234–330 l/hr and the elimination half-life is 2 minutes.

Special Points   As with all inotropes, correction of hypovolaemia should be ensured before use of the drug. A reduced dose should be used in patients who have recently received MAOIs. Halogenated volatile anaesthetic agents may increase the likelihood of dysrhythmias occurring during the concurrent use of dopamine.

The drug is inactivated by alkaline solutions (e.g. sodium bicarbonate).

The dopaminergic stimulation is blocked by phenothiazines.

There is no evidence dopamine provides renal protection and it may worsen renal ischaemia.

Dopexamine hydrochloride

Uses Dopexamine is used in the treatment of:
1. low cardiac output states (including those complicating cardiac surgery)
2. acute heart failure
3. to increase splanchnic blood flow and
4. prevent renal shutdown.

Chemical A synthetic dopamine analogue.

Presentation As a clear solution containing 10 mg/ml of dopexamine hydrochloride; the solution should be discarded if it becomes discoloured.

Main Actions Arterial vasodilation, positive inotropism and renal arterial vasodilation.

Mode of Action Dopexamine is an agonist at dopaminergic D_1- and D_2-receptors and thus leads to relaxation of vascular smooth muscle in the renal, mesenteric, cerebral and coronary arterial beds (D_1-effects) and stimulation of sympathetic prejunctional receptors, thereby decreasing noradrenaline release (a D_2-effect). The drug also inhibits uptake-1 of noradrenaline and has potent beta-2 adrenergic agonist activity.

Routes of Administration/Doses Dopexamine should be diluted prior to administration in either dextrose or saline and administered via a central vein using a controlled infusion device. The initial dose is 0.5 μg/kg/min which may be increased as necessary to a maximum dose of 6 μg/kg/min.

Effects
CVS Dopexamine has positive inotropic and chronotropic effects, and thus increases cardiac output. The drug causes arteriolar vasodilation, leading to a mild decrease in diastolic blood pressure with a slight increase in systolic blood pressure; the left- and right-ventricular afterload, left ventricular end-diastolic pressure and pulmonary artery pressure decrease following the administration of the drug. Dopexamine also causes a slight increase in coronary artery blood flow with no attendant alteration in myocardial oxygen extraction. The drug has a low propensity to cause dysrhythmias.
RS Dopexamine causes measurable bronchodilatation.
CNS The drug increases the cerebral blood flow secondary to cerebral vasodilation. Nausea and vomiting may result from a weak D_2 effect at the chemoreceptor trigger zone.
AS Splanchnic blood flow may increase due to mesenteric vasodilation.
GU Dopexamine reduces renal vascular resistance, leading to an increase in renal plasma flow and an attendant diuresis and natriuresis.

Metabolic/Other   Beta-2 adrenergic stimulation may result in hypokalaemia and hyperglycaemia; the platelet count may also decrease due to temporary splenic sequestration of platelets.

Toxicity/Side Effects   The use of the drug may be complicated by headache, flushing, tremor, angina and dysrhythmias.

Kinetics   Data are incomplete.

Distribution   Dopexamine is 40% bound to red blood cells; the V_D is 317–446 ml/kg.

Metabolism   The drug is rapidly cleared from the blood by tissue uptake and is extensively metabolised by methylation and sulphate conjugation.

Excretion   Dopexamine is excreted as metabolites in the urine and faeces; the clearance is 30–35 ml/min/kg and the elimination half-life is 5–10 minutes.

Special Points   The use of dopexamine should be avoided in patients with uncorrected hypovolaemia, aortic stenosis, hypertrophic obstructive cardiomyopathy or a phaeochromocytoma.

Dopexamine has an unexplained antioxidant effect.

Doxacurium

Uses Doxacurium is used to facilitate intubation and controlled ventilation.

Chemical A benzylisoquinolinium which is a mixture of three *trans-trans* stereoisomers.

Presentation As a clear aqueous solution (with benzyl alcohol and hydrochloric acid) containing 1 mg/ml of doxacurium chloride presented in 5 ml vials.

Main Action Competitive neuromuscular blockade.

Mode of Action Doxacurium acts by competitive antagonism of acetylcholine at nicotinic (N2) receptors at the postsynaptic membrane of the neuromuscular junction.

Route of Administration/Dose Doxacurium is administered intravenously; the normal intubating dose is 0.05–0.08 mg/kg. Maintenance doses of 0.005–0.01 mg/kg are required at approximately 45 minute intervals. Satisfactory intubating conditions are produced within 4–9 minutes; a single dose will last 100 minutes. The mean recovery index is 54 minutes (range 14–184). The drug is non-cumulative with repeated administration.

Effects
CVS Doxacurium has no significant effect on mean arterial pressure, heart rate, cardiac index or pulmonary vascular resistance after rapid intravenous administration.
RS Neuromuscular blockade leads to apnoea.

Toxicity/Side Effects Transient cutaneous flushing is the most common side effect. Hypotension, bronchospasm and urticaria may all occur with an incidence of less than 1%.

Kinetics

Distribution The drug is 30% protein-bound in the plasma; the V_D is 0.13–0.3 l/kg.

Metabolism Doxacurium is not metabolised in man.

Excretion The unchanged drug is excreted in the bile and urine. The clearance is 1.21–5.7 ml/kg/min and the elimination half-life is 61–163 minutes. Renal failure increases the elimination half-life of doxacurium. There are no significant alterations of the pharmacokinetics of the drug in patients undergoing liver transplantation.

Special Points The duration of action of doxacurium is prolonged by isoflurane, enflurane and halothane by 25%. The following drugs may enhance the neuromuscular effects of doxacurium: aminoglycoside antibiotics, magnesium and lithium salts. Doxacurium does not act as a trigger agent for malignant hyperpyrexia in animal models. The drug is physically incompatible with alkaline solutions (e.g. barbiturates).

Doxapram

Uses Doxapram is used:
1. as a respiratory stimulant for the treatment of post-operative respiratory depression and acute-on-chronic respiratory failure and has been used
2. in the treatment of laryngospasm
3. to facilitate blind nasal intubation and
4. in the treatment of post-operative shivering.

Chemical A monohydrated pyrrolidinone derivative.

Presentation As a clear, colourless solution containing 20 mg/ml and as a solution for infusion containing 2 mg/ml in 5% dextrose of doxapram hydrochloride.

Main Action Respiratory stimulation.

Mode of Action Doxapram acts primarily by stimulating the peripheral chemoreceptors and secondarily by a direct action on the respiratory centre.

Routes of Administration/Doses The drug may be administered intravenously as a bolus of 1 mg/kg or as an infusion of 1.5–4 mg/kg. Given intravenously, doxapram acts in 20–40 seconds; its peak effect is seen at 1–2 minutes and the duration of action is 5–12 minutes, although pharmacological effects are detectable for two hours.

Effects
CVS Doxapram causes an increase in the cardiac output due primarily to an increase in the stroke volume. A slight increase in the blood pressure and heart rate may be produced by the drug.
RS The minute volume is increased by doxapram due to an increase in the tidal volume; at higher doses an increase in respiratory rate occurs. The carbon dioxide response curve is displaced to the left by the drug.
CNS The cerebral blood flow is increased following the administration of doxapram; the drug has less convulsant activity than other analeptic agents.
AS In animals, salivation and gastrointestinal tone and motility are increased by the drug.
GU In animal models, doxapram increases both the urine output and motility within the genito-urinary system.
Metabolic/Other Catecholamine and steroid secretion are increased in animal models. The metabolic rate may increase by up to 30% and may lead to hypoxia due to increased oxygen consumption.

Toxicity/Side Effects Restlessness, dizziness, hallucinations, excessive sweating and a sensation of perineal warmth have been described subsequent to the administration of doxapram.

Kinetics Data are incomplete.

Distribution The V_D is 1.5 l/kg.

Metabolism The metabolic pathway of doxapram in man is unknown.

Excretion 5% is excreted unchanged in the urine. The clearance is 370 ml/min and the half-life is 2–4 hours.

Special Points Doxapram has been shown:
1. possibly to decrease the incidence of post-operative chest infections
2. to lead to a more rapid return to consciousness after inhalational anaesthesia
3. to reverse opioid-induced respiratory depression without reversing analgesia and
4. to prevent the necessity for mechanical ventilation in some patients.

Droperidol

Uses Droperidol is used:
1. in premedication
2. in the technique of neuroleptanalgesia
3. in the treatment of nausea and vomiting occurring post-operatively or as a result of chemotherapy
4. in the treatment of psychosis and has been used
5. for the control of peri-operative hiccuping.

Chemical A butyrophenone derivative.

Presentation As 10 mg tablets, a syrup containing 1 mg/ml and as a clear solution for injection containing 5 mg/ml of droperidol.

Main Actions Antiemetic and neuroleptic.

Mode of Action The antiemetic and neuroleptic effects of the drug appear to be mediated by:
1. central dopaminergic (D_2) blockade leading to an increased threshold for vomiting at the chemoreceptor trigger zone and
2. post-synaptic GABA antagonism.

Routes of Administration/Doses The adult oral or intramuscular dose is 5–10 mg and the intravenous dose when used as a neuroleptic agent is 5–15 mg, although the drug appears to be an effective antiemetic in doses as low as 0.5 mg. The onset of action after intravenous administration is 3–20 minutes and the drug may act for up to 12 hours.

Effects
CVS Droperidol has minimal cardiovascular effects, but its antagonistic effects at alpha-adrenergic receptors may lead to hypotension in the presence of hypovolaemia.
RS The drug causes small decreases in minute volume, functional residual capacity and airways resistance.
CNS Droperidol induces neurolepsis; a state characterised by diminished motor activity, anxiolysis and indifference to the external environment. The seizure threshold is raised by the drug.
AS The drug has a powerful antiemetic effect via a central effect at the chemosensitive trigger zone.
Metabolic/Other Droperidol, in common with other dopamine antagonists, may cause hyperprolactinaemia. The drug reduces total body oxygen consumption.

Toxicity/Side Effects Extra-pyramidal effects occur in 1%. Gastrointestinal disturbances, abnormalities of liver function tests and allergic phenomena have been reported after the use of droperidol. Malignant neurolept syndrome may be precipitated by droperidol.

Kinetics

Absorption   The drug is well absorbed after intramuscular administration. The pharmacokinetics of droperidol after oral administration have not been elucidated.

Distribution   The drug is 85–90% protein-bound in the plasma; the V_D is 1.54–2.54 l/kg.

Metabolism   Droperidol is extensively metabolised in the liver (the major metabolic pathway in animals being oxidative N-dealkylation); the only metabolite that has been identified in man is 2-benzimidazolinone.

Excretion   75% of the dose is excreted in the urine (1% unchanged) and 22% in the faeces. The clearance is 9.7–18.5 ml/min/kg and the elimination half-life is 2–2.5 hours.

Special Points   Droperidol is pharmaceutically incompatible with thiopentone and methohexitone. The sedative effects of the drug are additive with those of other central nervous system depressants administered concurrently.

Edrophonium

Uses Edrophonium is used:
1. for the reversal of non-depolarising neuromuscular blockade
2. in the diagnosis of suspected phase II block
3. in the diagnosis of myasthenia gravis (the 'Tensilon test') and
4. in the differentiation of myasthenic and cholinergic crisis in myasthenic patients.

Chemical A synthetic quaternary ammonium compound.

Presentation As a clear, colourless solution for injection containing 10 mg/ml of edrophonium chloride.

Main Action Cholinergic.

Mode of Action Edrophonium is a prosthetic, reversible inhibitor of acetylcholinesterase; it competes with acetylcholine for the anionic site of the enzyme and reversibly binds to it. At least part of the effect of the drug appears to be exerted prejunctionally.

Route of Administration/Doses The drug is usually administered intravenously; it has a more rapid onset (its peak effect occurring at 0.8–2 minutes) and shorter duration of effect (10 minutes) than does neostigmine. The 'Tensilon test' for the diagnosis of myasthenia gravis consists of the slow administration of 2 mg of edrophonium, followed by a further 8 mg if clinical deterioration does not occur. When used in the differentiation of myasthenic and cholinergic crisis a dose of 2 mg of edrophonium is used – weakness will increase if the crisis is cholinergic (and improve if myasthenic) in nature. An anticholinergic agent (e.g. atropine) must be immediately available when these tests are performed. The dose for reversal of competitive neuromuscular blockade is 0.5–0.7 mg/kg by slow intravenous injection, preceded by an appropriate dose of an anticholinergic agent to counter the peripheral muscarinic side effects of the drug.

Effects
CVS The drug may cause bradycardia, leading to a fall in cardiac output; it decreases the effective refractory period of cardiac muscle and increases conduction time.
RS Edrophonium increases bronchial secretion and may cause bronchoconstriction.
CNS Agitation and dreaming may occur; the drug has a predictable miotic effect. Weakness leading to fasciculation and paralysis may occur when edrophonium is administered to normal subjects.

AS   The drug increases salivation, lower oesophageal and gastric tone, gastric acid output and lower gastrointestinal tract motility. Nausea and vomiting may occur.

GU   Edrophonium increases ureteric peristalsis and may lead to involuntary micturition.

Metabolic/Other   Sweating and lachrymation are increased by the drug.

Toxicity/Side Effects
The side effects are manifestations of its pharmacological actions as described above. Cardiac arrest has been reported after the use of edrophonium.

Kinetics
Data are incomplete.

Distribution
The V_D is 0.9–1.3 l/kg.

Metabolism
The metabolic fate of edrophonium is uncertain; it is not hydrolysed by anticholinesterases.

Excretion
Details of the excretory pathways of the drug are unknown. The clearance is 6.9–12.3 ml/min/kg and the elimination half-life is 110 minutes.

Special Points
The potency of edrophonium is 12–16 times less than that of neostigmine; the muscarinic effects of the drug are correspondingly easier to counteract than those of neostigmine. Edrophonium is less predictable than neostigmine when used to reverse profound competitive neuromuscular blockade.

Enalapril

Uses Enalapril is used for the treatment of:
1. essential and renovascular hypertension and
2. congestive heart failure.

Chemical An ester of enalaprilat.

Presentation As 2.5/5/10/20 mg tablets of enalapril maleate and in a fixed-dose combination with hydrochlorothiazide.

Main Action Antihypertensive.

Mode of Action Enalapril acts as an angiotensin-converting enzyme inhibitor and thus prevents the formation of angiotensin II from angiotensin I. Part of its action may also be exerted through modulation of sympathetic tone or of the kallikrein-kinin-prostaglandin system.

Route of Administration/Dose The adult oral dose is 5–40 mg daily according to response.

Effects
CVS Enalapril decreases the blood pressure by 15–20% after a single dose by reducing the systemic vascular resistance; it acts predominantly at arteries and arterioles. The cardiac output is little changed, except in the presence of heart failure, where it may increase by up to 25%. Little reflex tachycardia occurs.
GU The renal blood flow is increased following administration of the drug; the glomerular filtration rate remains unaltered. A natriuresis subsequently occurs but there is little overall effect on plasma volume.
Metabolic/Other Plasma renin activity is increased by the drug; the concentrations of aldosterone and angiotensin II are decreased and these changes are usually maintained during long-term treatment.

Toxicity/Side Effects Enalapril is usually well tolerated; hypotension, dizziness, fatigue, gastrointestinal upsets and rashes may occur. Renal function may deteriorate in patients with renovascular hypertension who receive the drug.

Kinetics

Absorption Enalapril is 60% absorbed when administered orally; the bioavailability by this route is 40%.

Distribution The drug is 50% protein-bound in the plasma.

Metabolism Enalapril is a pro-drug and is converted by hydrolysis in the liver to its active form, enalaprilat. No further metabolism occurs in man.

Excretion Unchanged enalapril and enalaprilat are excreted primarily in the urine; one-third is excreted in faeces. The clearance is 300 ml/min and the elimination half-life is 30–35 hours.

Special Points Enalapril has been shown to increase life expectancy in patients with congestive heart failure.

Accumulation may occur in patients with renal impairment – the drug is removed by dialysis.

The hypotensive effect of enalapril is additive with that of andesthetic agents; it may protect against the cardiovascular responses to laryngoscopy.

There is an increased incidence of renal failure with the co-administration of ACE inhibitors and NSAIDs in the presence of hypovolaemia.

Enflurane

Uses Enflurane is used for the induction and maintenance of general anaesthesia.

Chemical A halogenated methyl ethyl ether which is a geometric isomer of isoflurane.

Presentation As a clear, colourless liquid (that should be protected from light) with a characteristic sweet smell. The commercial preparation contains no stabilisers or preservatives; it is non-flammable in normal anaesthetic concentrations. The molecular weight of enflurane is 184.5, the boiling point 56.5°C and the saturated vapour pressure is 23.3 kPa at 20°C. The MAC of enflurane is 1.68 (0.57 in 70% nitrous oxide), the oil/water solubility coefficient 120 and the blood/gas solubility coefficient 1.91. The drug is readily soluble in rubber; it does not attack metals.

Main Action General anaesthesia (reversible loss of both awareness and recall of noxious stimuli).

Mode of Action The mechanism of general anaesthesia remains to be fully elucidated. General anaesthetics appear to disrupt synaptic transmission (especially in the area of the ventrobasal thalamus). This mechanism may include potentiation of the gamma-amino-butyric acid and glycine receptors and antagonism at NMDA receptors. Their mode of action at the molecular level appears to involve expansion of hydrophobic regions in the neuronal membrane, either within the lipid phase or within hydrophobic sites in cell membrane proteins.

Route of Administration/Dose Enflurane is administered by inhalation, conventionally via a calibrated vaporiser. The concentration used for the inhalational induction of anaesthesia is 1–10% and for maintenance, 0.6–3%.

Effects
CVS Enflurane is a negative inotrope; it also causes a decrease in the systemic vascular resistance and these two effects produce a decrease in mean arterial pressure. Unlike halothane, enflurane produces a slight reflex tachycardia. The drug decreases coronary vascular resistance; it also reduces the rate of phase IV depolarisation, increases the threshold potential and prolongs the effective refractory period. Enflurane is not markedly arrhythmogenic but does sensitise the myocardium to the effects of circulating catecholamines.
RS Enflurane is a powerful respiratory depressant, markedly decreasing tidal volume, although respiratory rate may increase during the administration of the drug. A slight increase in the P_aCO_2 may result in spontaneously breathing

subjects; the drug also decreases the ventilatory response to hypoxia and hypercapnia. Enflurane is non-irritant to the respiratory tract; it causes bronchodilatation and no increase in secretions. The drug inhibits pulmonary macrophage activity and mucociliary transport.

CNS The principal effect of enflurane is general anaesthesia; the drug has little analgesic effect. The drug increases cerebral blood flow, leading to an increase in intracranial pressure; it also decreases cerebral oxygen consumption. The drug may induce tonic/clonic muscle activity and may also produce epileptiform EEG traces, especially in the presence of hypocapnia. A marked decrease in skeletal muscle tone results from the use of enflurane, mediated by an effect on the post-junctional membrane.

AS Enflurane decreases splanchnic blood flow as a result of the hypotension it produces.

GU Enflurane decreases the renal blood flow and glomerular filtration rate; a small volume of concentrated urine results. The drug reduces the tone of the pregnant uterus.

Metabolic/Other Enflurane decreases the plasma noradrenaline concentration, and may increase blood sugar concentration. The drug causes a fall in body temperature predominantly by cutaneous vasodilation. Enflurane depresses white cell function for 24 hours post-operatively, but has no effect on platelet function.

Toxicity/Side Effects Enflurane is a recognised trigger agent for the development of malignant hyperthermia. The drug may also cause the appearance of myocardial dysrhythmias, particularly in the presence of hypoxia, hypercapnia or excessive catecholamine concentrations. Shivering ('the shakes') may occur post-operatively. There have been isolated reports of hepatotoxicity associated with the repeated use of enflurane; there is also the theoretical risk of fluoride ion toxicity occurring with the use of the drug, particularly in patients with renal failure.

Kinetics

Absorption The major factors affecting the uptake of volatile anaesthetic agents are solubility, cardiac output and the concentration gradient between the alveoli and venous blood. Enflurane is less soluble in blood than is halothane; alveolar concentration therefore reaches inspired concentration relatively rapidly, resulting in a rapid induction of anaesthesia. An increase in the cardiac output increases the rate of alveolar uptake and slows the induction of anaesthesia. The concentration gradient between alveoli and venous blood approaches zero at equilibrium; a large concentration gradient favours the onset of anaesthesia.

Distribution The drug is initially distributed to organs with a high blood flow (brain, heart, liver and kidney) and later to less well-perfused organs (muscles, fat and bone).

Enflurane

Metabolism 2.4% of an administered dose is slowly metabolised in the liver via cytochrome P-450 2El, principally by oxidation and dehalogenation; plasma fluoride ion concentrations may reach 10 times those observed after the use of halothane or isoflurane.

Excretion More than 80% is exhaled unchanged; 2.4% of an administered dose is excreted in the urine as non-volatile fluorinated compounds. The remainder is excreted via the skin, sweat and faeces.

Special Points Enflurane markedly potentiates the action of co-administered non-depolarising relaxants.

The dose of co-administered adrenaline should not exceed 10 ml of a 1:100 000 solution in a 10-minute period to guard against the development of ventricular dysrhythmias.

Enflurane is not recommended for use in epileptic patients.

Enoximone

Uses   Enoximone is used:
1. in the treatment of acute-on-chronic heart failure
2. during and after the withdrawal of cardiopulmonary bypass and
3. in the treatment of low-output states prior to cardiac transplantation.

Chemical   An imidazolone derivative.

Presentation   As a clear, yellow solution containing 5 mg/ml of enoximone.

Main Actions   Positive inotropism and vasodilation.

Mode of Action   Enoximone acts by inhibiting Type III phosphodiesterase, the enzyme responsible for the degradation of cAMP. The drug thus has a synergistic effect with those catecholamines which directly activate adenyl cyclase and leads to an increase in the intracellular concentration of cAMP.

Route of Administration/Doses   Enoximone is administered intravenously, diluted in a ratio of 1:1 with either water or saline, either by a slow bolus injection of 0.5–1 mg/kg to a maximum dose of 3 mg/kg every 3–6 hours, or by infusion at the rate of 90 µg/kg/min over 10–30 minutes and thereafter at the rate of 5–20 µg/kg/min. The drug acts within 10–30 minutes after intravenous administration; the mean duration of effect is 4–6 hours.

Effects
CVS   Enoximone has a positive inotropic action and leads to an increase in cardiac output; the left ventricular stroke work index and cardiac index increase by 40–55% in patients with heart failure. Similarly right atrial pressure, pulmonary capillary wedge pressure, pulmonary vascular resistance and systemic vascular resistance all decrease by 30%. The drug has little effect on myocardial oxygen consumption; myocardial efficiency and coronary blood flow increase in animal models. Enoximone usually has little effect on blood pressure or heart rate; dysrhythmias occur uncommonly.
Metabolic/Other   The drug has little effect on plasma renin activity or catecholamine concentrations. A decrease in the platelet count has been observed in a small percentage of patients receiving the drug.

Toxicity/Side Effects   Dysrhythmias, hypotension, central nervous system and gastrointestinal disturbances occur uncommonly with the use of enoximone.

Kinetics

Absorption   Enoximone is readily absorbed but undergoes extensive first-pass metabolism to an active sulphoxide form.

Distribution   The drug is 70% protein-bound in the plasma; the V_D is 2.1–8 l/kg.

Metabolism   Enoximone is primarily metabolised in the liver to an active sulphoxide form.

Excretion   The drug appears predominantly in the form of the suiphoxide in the urine; trace amounts are excreted unchanged. The clearance is 3.7–13 ml/min/kg and the elimination half-life is 6.2 hours. A decreased dose should be used in the presence of renal or hepatic impairment.

Enoximone appears to be partially removed by haemodialysis.

Ephedrine

Uses   Ephedrine is used in the treatment of:
1. hypotension occurring during general, spinal or epidural anaesthesia
2. nocturnal enuresis
3. narcolepsy
4. diabetic autonomic neuropathy
5. hiccups and
6. as a nasal decongestant.

Chemical   A naturally occurring sympathomimetic amine.

Presentation   As 15/30/60 mg tablets, an elixir containing 3 mg/ml, as 0.5/1% nasal drops, as a constituent of proprietary cold cures and as a clear, colourless solution for injection containing 30 mg/ml of ephedrine sulphate.

Main Action   Sympathomimetic.

Mode of Action   Ephedrine acts both indirectly (by causing release of noradrenaline from sympathetic nerve terminals) and directly by stimulation of alpha- and beta-adrenoreceptors.

Routes of Administration/Doses   The adult dose by the oral route is 30 mg 8-hourly; as a nasal decongestant 1–2 drops may be administered every 4 hours. The parenteral dose is 3–30 mg, titrated according to response. When administered orally, the drug acts within 60 minutes and has a duration of action of 3–5 hours. When administered intravenously, the onset of the drug's cardiovascular effects is rapid; the duration of action is about 1 hour.

Effects
CVS   The effects of ephedrine are similar to those of adrenaline, but are more prolonged as the drug is not metabolised by monoamine oxidase or catechol-O-methyltransferase. Ephedrine has positive inotropic and chronotropic actions, producing an increase in the cardiac output, cardiac work and myocardial oxygen consumption. Myocardial irritability is increased by the drug. Ephedrine increases the coronary blood flow, systolic and diastolic blood pressure and pulmonary artery pressure. An increase in the circulating volume may follow the use of the drug due to post-capillary vasoconstriction.
RS   Ephedrine is a respiratory stimulant and causes marked bronchodilatation.
CNS   Ephedrine has a stimulatory effect akin to that of amphetamine; the cerebral blood flow increases after the administration of the drug. Mydriasis occurs after topical use; ephedrine also has local anaesthetic properties.

AS The drug relaxes gastrointestinal smooth muscle and causes splanchnic vasoconstriction.

GU Ephedrine constricts renal blood vessels and may lead to a decrease in both the renal blood flow and glomerular filtration rate. The drug contracts the bladder sphincter and relaxes the detrusor muscle which may precipitate acute retention of urine. Ephedrine decreases uterine tone.

Metabolic/Other The drug increases the rate of hepatic glycogenolysis and may also increase basal metabolic rate and oxygen consumption secondary to central stimulation.

Toxicity/Side Effects Insomnia, anxiety, tremor, headache, dysrhythmias, nausea and vomiting and chest pain may complicate the use of the drug. Ephedrine is also irritant to mucous membranes.

Kinetics Data are incomplete.

Absorption Ephedrine is rapidly and completely absorbed when administered orally, intramuscularly or subcutaneously.

Distribution Ephedrine crosses the placental barrier.

Metabolism The drug is resistant to metabolism by monoamine oxidase and catechol-O-methyl transferase. Small amounts are metabolised in the liver by oxidative metabolism, demethylation and aromatic hydroxylation with subsequent conjugation.

Excretion 87–99% of an administered dose is excreted unchanged in the urine. The elimination half-life is 6.3 hours.

Special Points Tachyphylaxis occurs with prolonged use of the drug. Dysrhythmias occur with a greater frequency when ephedrine is used in the presence of halothane.

Clonidine premedication enhances the pressor effects of ephedrine.

Epinephrine

Uses Epinephrine is used in the treatment of:
1. anaphylactic and anaphylactoid shock
2. asystole
3. low cardiac output states
4. glaucoma and
5. as a local vasoconstrictor and
6. is added to local anaesthetic solutions to prolong their duration of action.

Chemical A catecholamine.

Presentation As a clear solution for injection containing 0.1/1 mg/ml of epinephrine hydrochloride, a 1% ophthalmic solution and as an aerosol spray delivering $280\,\mu g$ metered doses or epinephrine acid tartrate.

Main Actions Sympathomimetic.

Mode of Action Epinephrine is a directly acting sympathomimetic amine that is an agonist of alpha- and beta-adrenoreceptors; it has approximately equal activity at both alpha- and beta-receptors.

Routes of Administration/Doses The drug may be administered intravenously either as an intravenous bolus in doses of 0.1–1 mg for the treatment of asystole or as an infusion at the rate of $0.01–0.1\,\mu g/kg/min$, titrated according to response; low doses tend to produce predominantly beta-effects whilst higher doses tend to produce predominantly alpha-effects. The dose by the subcutaneous route is 0.1–0.5 mg. Epinephrine may be administered by inhalation; a maximum daily dose of 10–20 metered doses is recommended.

Effects
CVS Epinephrine is both a positive inotrope and a positive chronotrope and therefore causes an increase in cardiac output and myocardial oxygen consumption. The drug causes an increase in coronary blood flow. When administered as an intravenous bolus, epinephrine markedly increases peripheral vascular resistance producing an increase in systolic blood pressure, with a less marked increase in diastolic blood pressure. When administered as an intravenous infusion, the peripheral vascular resistance (a direct beta-2 effect) and diastolic blood pressure both tend to decrease. The heart rate initially increases and subsequently decreases due to a vagal reflex. The plasma volume decreases as a result of the loss of protein-free fluid into the extracellular fluid. Epinephrine increases platelet adhesiveness and blood coagulability (by increasing the activity of Factor V).

RS Epinephrine is a mild respiratory stimulant and causes an increase in both the tidal volume and respiratory rate. The drug is a potent bronchodilator but tends to increase the viscosity of bronchial secretions.

CNS Epinephrine only penetrates the central nervous system to a limited extent, but does have excitatory effects. The drug increases the cutaneous pain threshold and enhances neuromuscular transmission. Epinephrine has little overall effect on cerebral blood flow. It has weak mydriatic effects when applied topically to the eye.

AS The drug decreases intestinal tone and secretions; the splanchnic blood flow is increased.

GU Epinephrine decreases renal blood flow by up to 40%, although the glomerular filtration rate remains little altered. The bladder tone is decreased and the sphincteric tone increased by the drug, which may lead to difficulty with micturition. Epinephrine inhibits the contractions of the pregnant uterus.

Metabolic/Other The drug has profound metabolic effects; it decreases insulin secretion whilst increasing both glucagon secretion and the rate of glycogenolysis, resulting in elevation of the blood sugar concentration. The plasma renin activity is increased by the drug (a beta-1 effect) and the plasma concentration of free fatty acids is increased by the activation of triglyceride lipase. The serum potassium concentration transiently rises (due to release from the liver) following the administration of adrenaline; a more prolonged decrease in potassium concentration follows. Epinephrine administration increases the basal metabolic rate by 20–30%; in combination with the cutaneous vasoconstriction that the drug produces, pyrexia may result.

Toxicity/Side Effects Symptoms of central nervous system excitation, cerebral haemorrhage, tachycardia, dysrhythmias and myocardial ischaemia may result from the use of adrenaline.

Kinetics Data are incomplete.

Absorption The drug is inactivated when administered orally. Absorption is slower after subcutaneous than intramuscular administration. The drug is well absorbed from the tracheal mucosa.

Metabolism Exogenous adrenaline is predominantly first metabolised by catechol-O-methyl transferase predominantly in the liver to metadrenaline and normetadrenaline (uptake$_2$); some is metabolised by monoamine-oxidase within adrenergic neurones (uptake$_1$). The final common products of adrenaline metabolism are 3-methoxy 4-hydroxyphenylethylene and 3-methoxy 4-hydroxymandelic acid (which are inactive).

Excretion The inactive products appear predominantly in the urine.

Epinephrine

Special Points The dose of epinephrine should be limited to
1 μg/kg/30 minutes in the presence of halothane, and to
3 μg/kg/30 minutes in the presence of enflurane or isoflurane in
an attempt to prevent the appearance of serious ventricular dysrhythmias. Infiltration of epinephrine-containing solutions should
be avoided in regions of the body supplied by end arteries.

Epoeitin (recombinant human erythropoeitin)

Uses   Erythropoeitin is used for the treatment of anaemia associated with:
1.   chronic renal failure
2.   platinum-based chemotherapy
3.   low-birth-weight prematurity and is also used
4.   to increase the yield of autologous blood pre-operatively.

Chemical   A glycoprotein.

Presentation   Two forms (alpha and beta) of the drug are available, which are clinically indistinguishable. Epoietin alpha is presented as a solution for injection containing 2000/4000/10 000 units/ml. Epoietin beta is presented as a solution for injection containing 500/1000/5000/10 000 units/ml and as a powder for reconstitution prior to injection.

Main Action   Enhancement of erythropoeisis.

Mode of Action   Erythropoeitin specifically stimulates erythropoeisis by acting as a mitosis stimulating factor and differentiation hormone.

Routes of Administration/Doses   The drug is preferably administered subcutaneously initially as 50 units/kg three times a week, the dose is adjusted every four weeks in 25 units/kg increments. The maintenance dose is usually 25–100 units/kg three times weekly. The intravenous dose is usually 20–30% greater than the subcutaneous dose. For increasing the yield of autologous blood pre-operatively, the usual dose is 600 units/kg once or twice weekly for three weeks together with iron supplementation.

Effects
CVS   The drug causes a dose-dependent increase in blood pressure.
Metabolic/Other   Erythropoeitin's primary effect is to enhance erythropoeisis. It causes a dose-dependent increase in platelet count, but not thrombocytosis.

Toxicity/Side Effects   Hypertension, influenza-like symptoms and shunt thrombosis have been reported.

Kinetics   Data are incomplete and available only for patients with renal impairment.

Absorption   The bioavailability after subcutaneous administration is 23–42%.

Distribution   The V_D is 5 l.

Excretion   The elimination half-life is 8–15 hours.

Special Points   Epoeitin is not removed by haemofiltration or haemodialysis.

Epoprostenol

Uses   Epoprostenol is used:
1. as an anticoagulant during renal dialysis and cardiopulmonary bypass and may be of use in the treatment of
2. pre-eclampsia
3. Raynaud's disease
4. the haemolytic uraemic syndrome
5. septic shock and
6. pulmonary hypertension.

Chemical   A prostanoid (formerly called prostacyclin-PGI_2).

Presentation   As vials containing $500\,\mu g$ of freeze-dried epoprostenol sodium to be diluted before use in a mixture of sodium chloride and glycine.

Main Actions   Inhibition of platelet aggregation and vasodilation.

Mode of Action   Epoprostenol stimulates adenyl cyclase leading to an increase in the cAMP concentration within platelets; this, in turn, leads to inhibition of platelet phospholipase and cyclo-oxygenase and ultimately of platelet aggregation.

Routes of Administration/Doses   The drug may be administered intravenously or into the extracorporeal circulation; an infusion of 5 ng/kg/min should be started 15–30 minutes before dialysis is commenced and continued throughout the procedure. The effects of epoprostenol may persist for 30 minutes after cessation of an infusion.

Effects
CVS   The drug causes relaxation of vascular smooth muscle leading to a decrease in systemic vascular resistance, a slight tachycardia and a decrease in diastolic blood pressure.
RS   Epoprostenol causes a decrease in pulmonary vascular resistance and interferes with the mechanism of hypoxic pulmonary vasoconstriction.
CNS   The drug produces cerebral vasodilation leading to increased cerebral blood flow.
AS   Epoprostenol inhibits gastric acid secretion.
Metabolic/Other   Epoprostenol is the most powerful inhibitor of platelet aggregation known; the bleeding time may double with high doses. It also appears to have a fibrinolytic effect and increases red cell deformability. The drug stimulates renin secretion and may cause an increase in blood sugar concentrations.

Toxicity/Side Effects   Facial flushing and headache occur commonly after the administration of the drug. Gastro-intestinal upsets, chest, abdominal and jaw pain have also been reported.

Kinetics   Data are incomplete.

Metabolism   Epoprostenol is rapidly removed from the circulation by hydrolysis to 6-oxo-PGF$_{1alpha}$ in the blood, and by metabolism to a bicyclic 15-oxo derivative in the tissues.

Excretion   The plasma half-life is 30 second–3 minutes.

Special Points   Epoprostenol extends the life of filters during chronic renal replacement therapy and decreases the incidence of bleeding in these critically ill patients compared to heparin.

Erythromycin

Uses Erythromycin is used in the treatment of infections of:
1. the respiratory tract
2. skin, bone, joint and soft tissues and
3. oral/eye infections
4. sexually transmitted diseases and
5. for the prophylaxis of subacute bacterial endocarditis.

Chemical A macrolide.

Presentation As 250/500 mg tablets, a suspension containing 10/25/50 mg/ml and as 1 g vials of erythromycin lactobionate as a powder for reconstitution prior to intravenous infusion.

Main Actions Erythromycin is a bactericidal/bacteriostatic antibiotic that is active predominantly against Gram-positive organisms. Its spectrum of activity includes *Staphylococcus, Streptococcus, Neisseria, Clostridium, Bordetella, Bacteroides, Corynebacterium, Legionella, Treponema* sp., *Haemophilus influenzae* and *Mycoplasma* sp.

Mode of Action Erythromycin inhibits bacterial polypeptide synthesis by binding reversibly to the 50S subunit of bacterial ribosomes and inhibiting peptide translocase, thereby preventing the formation of polymerised peptides.

Route of Administration/Dose The adult oral dose is 1–4 g/day in divided doses.

Toxicity/Side Effects The estolate preparation may give rise to gastrointestinal disturbances, hepatitis, allergic phenomena and ototoxicity.

Kinetics

Absorption The bioavailability of erythromycin by the oral route is 10–60%.

Distribution Erythromycin is 81–87% protein-bound in the plasma; the V_D is 0.34–1.22 l/kg. The drug penetrates the central nervous system poorly.

Metabolism Occurs predominantly by demethylation in the liver.

Excretion 2–15% (according to the route of administration) of the dose is excreted unchanged in the urine. The clearance is 5–13.2 ml/min/kg and the elimination half-life is 1.6 hours.

Special Points Erythromycin is a prokinetic agent which enhances gastric motility. It may cause QT prolongation in the critically ill.

The drug is not removed by haemodialysis.

Erythromycin may potentiate the action of co-administered digoxin, midazolam, warfarin and theophylline due to inhibition of cytochrome P-450.

Esmolol

Uses   Esmolol is effective in the treatment of:
1. acute supraventricular dysrhythmias (atrial fibrillation or flutter)
2. peri-operative hypertension and
3. myocardial infarction.

Chemical   An aryloxypropanolamine.

Presentation   As a clear solution for injection containing 10/250 mg/ml of esmolol hydrochloride.

Main Actions   Negative inotropism and chronotropism.

Mode of Action   Esmolol acts by competitive blockade of beta-adrenoceptors; the drug is relatively selective for beta-1 receptors and has little or no intrinsic sympathomimetic activity.

Route of Administration/Dose   The drug is administered by intravenous infusion (preferably via a peripheral vein), diluted in any crystalloid with the exception of sodium bicarbonate, at a rate of 50–150 µg/kg/min according to response. Esmolol has a major advantage over other currently available beta-adrenergic antagonists in that its peak effects are observed within 6–10 minutes of administration, and are almost completely attenuated 20 minutes after cessation of the infusion. The advantages of this 'on–off' control are obvious.

Effects
CVS   Esmolol causes a fall in blood pressure and a dose-dependent fall in heart rate; the cardiac output falls by about 20% (i.e. to a similar extent as with propranolol). It slows atrioventricular conduction at doses that have no effect on other haemodynamic or electrocardiographic variables. The drug will obtund the cardiovascular responses to intubation and sternotomy, and protects against infarction in animal models of myocardial ischaemia.
RS   Esmolol appears to have little effect on airways resistance.

Toxicity/Side Effects   Hypotension, bradycardia, bronchospasm, nausea and vomiting, alteration of taste and central nervous system disturbances may occur with use of the drug.

Kinetics

Distribution   Esmolol is 56% protein-bound in the plasma; the V_D is 3.43 l/kg. Rapid but limited transplacental passage occurs in animal models.

Metabolism   Occurs primarily by hydrolysis by esterases located in red cells to methanol and a (major) primary acid metabolite which has weak beta-adrenergic antagonist activity but a long elimination half-life of 3.5 hours.

Excretion   70–80% appears in the urine as the major acid metabolite; <1% is excreted unchanged. The clearance is 285 ml/min/kg and the elimination half-life is 9.2 minutes. The drug should be used with caution in patients with renal impairment; hepatic disease has no effect.

Special Points   The drug has no effect on the pharmacokinetics of co-administered morphine or digoxin; it has been shown to increase the recovery time from suxamethonium from 5.6 to 8.3 minutes.

Ether

Uses   Ether is used for the induction and maintenance of general anaesthesia.

Chemical   Diethyl ether.

Presentation   As a clear, colourless liquid (that should be protected from light) with a characteristic sweet smell. Ether is flammable in air at concentrations of 1.83–48% and explosive in oxygen at concentrations of 2–82%. The molecular weight of ether is 74, the boiling point 35 °C and the saturated vapour pressure is 56.7 kPa at 20 °C. The MAC of ether is 1.92, the oil/water solubility coefficient 3.2 and the blood/gas solubility coefficient 12. Ether is relatively inert, but decomposes on exposure to air, heat and light to produce acetaldehyde and ether peroxide. Ether is no longer commercially available in the United Kingdom.

Main Actions   General anaesthesia (reversible loss of both awareness and recall of noxious stimuli) and analgesia.

Mode of Action   The mechanism of general anaesthesia remains to be fully elucidated. General anaesthetics appear to disrupt synaptic transmission (especially in the area of the ventrobasal thalamus), predominantly by inhibiting neuro-transmitter release and by interfering with the interaction of neurotransmitters with post-synaptic receptors. Their mode of action at the molecular level appears to involve expansion of hydrophobic regions in the neuronal membrane, either within the lipid phase or within hydrophobic sites in cell membrane proteins.

Route of Administration/Dose   Ether is administered by inhalation, conventionally via a calibrated vaporiser. The concentration used for the induction and maintenance of anaesthesia is 3–20%.

Effects
CVS   Ether is a negative inotrope *in vitro*; *in vivo*, sympathetic stimulation and catecholamine release and a vagolytic effect tend to offset this effect. The cardiac output is increased by 20%; the heart rate and systemic vascular resistance also increase and blood pressure is well maintained as a result. The drug causes dilatation of coronary arteries. Dysrhythmias are rare and the drug does not sensitise the myocardium to the effects of circulating catecholamines. Light ether anaesthesia produces peripheral vasoconstriction, whereas deeper anaesthesia results in vasodilation (due to an effect on the vasomotor centre) causing a decrease in both the cardiac output and blood pressure.

RS Ether is a respiratory stimulant; at light planes of anaesthesia the respiratory rate may exceed 30 breaths per minute; although the tidal volume decreases, the minute volume remains unaltered. The respiratory centre remains responsive to carbon dioxide at light planes and the P_aCO_2 remains constant. At deeper planes of anaesthesia, respiratory depression occurs and intubation becomes possible without the aid of muscle relaxants. Ether vapour is irritant and may cause breath-holding and coughing if the inspired concentration is increased too rapidly. The drug causes bronchodilatation with no increase in bronchial secretions.

CNS The principle effect of ether is general anaesthesia; the drug also has an analgesic effect. The drug causes cerebral vasodilation, leading to an increased cerebral blood flow and intracranial pressure. Ether decreases intraocular pressure and causes progressive pupillary dilatation. Clonus may occur at light planes due to increased stretch receptor reflexes. Skeletal muscle tone decreases as anaesthesia deepens as a result of both depression of spinal reflexes and a direct action on the neuromuscular junction. Depression of the medulla is a late event, occurring at very deep planes of anaesthesia.

AS The drug increases both salivation and lachrymation. Ether decreases gastrointestinal motility; hepatic function and biliary secretion are also transiently decreased. Splenic contraction may also occur, resulting in an elevated haematocrit and white cell count.

GU Ether causes renal arterial vasoconstriction and therefore decreases renal blood flow and the glomerular filtration rate; a small volume of concentrated urine results – albuminuria may also occur. The drug reduces the tone of the pregnant uterus.

Metabolic/Other Ether stimulates gluconeogenesis and may cause an increase in the blood sugar concentration. The drug occasionally causes metabolic acidosis in young children and patients unable to tolerate an increased lactate load.

Toxicity/Side Effects The predominant disadvantages of ether are its inflammability and the high incidence of postoperative nausea and vomiting (which occur in >50% of patients who receive the agent). The dramatic increase in salivation produced by the drug necessitates the use of antisialogogue premedication. Convulsions and post-operative shivering may complicate the use of ether.

Kinetics

Absorption The major factors affecting the uptake of volatile anaesthetic agents are solubility, cardiac output and the concentration gradient between the alveoli and venous blood. Ether is relatively soluble in blood; the alveolar concentration therefore reaches the inspired concentration relatively slowly, resulting in a slow induction of, and recovery from, anaesthesia. The irritant properties of the drug compound the slow induction. An increase in the cardiac output increases the rate of alveolar uptake and slows the induction of anaesthesia. The concentration gradient between alveoli and venous blood approaches zero at equilibrium; a large concentration gradient favours the onset of anaesthesia.

Distribution The drug is initially distributed to organs with a high blood flow (the brain, heart, liver and kidney) and later to less well-perfused organs (muscles and fat).

Metabolism 2–3% of an administered dose is metabolised in the liver, to yield acetaldehyde, alcohol, acetic acid and carbon dioxide.

Excretion 85–90% is exhaled unchanged; the metabolites are excreted in the urine.

Special Points Ether potentiates the action of co-administered non-depolarising relaxants. Diathermy should be used with extreme caution (if at all) in the presence of ether. Ether is cheap and has a wide safety margin; it therefore retains a useful role for anaesthesia in difficult circumstances.

Etomidate

Uses   Etomidate is used:
1. for the intravenous induction of general anaesthesia and for
2. treatment prior to surgery of Cushing's syndrome.

Chemical   A carboxylated imidazole derivative.

Presentation   As a clear, colourless solution for injection containing 2 mg/ml of etomidate in an aqueous vehicle of 35% propylene glycol and water. The pH of the aqueous solution is 8.1.

Main Action   Hypnotic.

Mode of Action   Etomidate appears to act upon GABA type A receptors to modulate fast inhibitory synaptic transmission within the CNS. Only the D-isomer demonstrates hypnotic activity.

Route of Administration/Dose   Etomidate is administered intravenously in a dose of 0.3 mg/kg; the drug acts in 10–65 seconds and its duration of action is 6–8 minutes. Etomidate is non-cumulative with repeated administration.

Effects
CVS   Etomidate is notable for its relative cardiovascular stability. Recommended doses of the drug may produce a slight decrease in cardiac output and systemic vascular resistance resulting in a mild degree of hypotension; tachycardia is produced only by high doses of the drug. Etomidate has little effect on myocardial oxygen delivery and consumption.
RS   The drug causes a dose-related decrease in respiratory rate and tidal volume; transient apnoea, coughing and hiccuping may occur.
CNS   Induction of anaesthesia with etomidate may be accompanied by the development of involuntary muscle movements, tremor and hypertonus. The drug decreases intracranial and intraocular pressure, the cerebral blood flow and cerebral metabolic rate. 20% of patients demonstrate generalised epileptiform EEG activity following the administration of etomidate.
AS   2–15% of patients who have received the drug experience nausea and vomiting post-operatively; this is increased to 40% if an opiate is co-administered.
Metabolic/Other   Etomidate is a potent inhibitor of steroidogenesis. Adrenal 11 beta-hydroxylase and cholesterol cleavage enzymes are inhibited by the drug, resulting in depression of cortisol and aldosterone synthesis for 24 hours after administration. This effect has been observed after both single doses and infusions. Etomidate has significant antiplatelet activities.

Toxicity/Side Effects   25–50% of patients who receive the drug experience pain on injection; the incidence of this is decreased by the addition of lignocaine. Venous thrombosis may also occur. Myoclonus may occur in unpremedicated patients. Histamine release and allergic phenomena are rare with the use of etomidate. The use of etomidate infusions for the sedation of critically ill patients is associated with an increased mortality. There is no conclusive evidence that anaesthetic doses of etomidate have any effect on morbidity or mortality.

Kinetics

Distribution   Etomidate is 76% protein-bound in the plasma; the V_D is 140–340 l. The relatively brief duration of effect of a bolus of the drug is due to redistribution to muscle and later to fat.

Metabolism   Occurs rapidly by plasma and hepatic esterases to yield inactive carboxylic metabolites.

Excretion   87% of an administered dose is excreted in the urine, 3% unchanged. The remainder is excreted in the bile. The clearance is 870–1700 ml/min (this is reduced by 31% in the presence of 67% nitrous oxide); the elimination half-life is 1–4.7 hours.

Special Points   Etomidate is porphyrinogenic in animal models and *in vitro*. The drug should not be mixed with pancuronium bromide.

Etomidate has been formulated as a lipid emulsion which appears to be less irritant on injection.

Fentanyl

Uses Fentanyl is used:
1. to provide the analgesic component of general anaesthesia
2. in combination with a major tranquilliser to produce neuroleptanalgesia
3. in premedication and has been used
4. for palliative care.

Chemical A tertiary amine which is a synthetic phenylpiperidine derivative.

Presentation As a clear, colourless solution for injection containing $50\,\mu g/ml$ of intranasal fentanyl citrate transdermal patches which deliver $25/50/75/100\,\mu g/hour$ over a 72-hour period and $200/400/600/800/1200/1600\,\mu g$ lozenges.

Main Actions Analgesia and respiratory depression.

Mode of Action Fentanyl is a highly selective mu agonist; the mu-opioid receptor appears to be specifically involved in the mediation of analgesia. Opioids appear to exert their effects by increasing intracellular calcium concentration, which in turn increases potassium conductance and hyperpolarisation of excitable cell membranes. The decrease in membrane excitability that results may decrease both pre- and post-synaptic responses.

Routes of Administration/Doses The adult dose for premedication by the intramuscular route is $50–100\,\mu g$. For the induction or supplementation of general anaesthesia, an intravenous dose of $1–100\,\mu g/kg$ may be used. Fentanyl may also be administered via the epidural route; a dose of $50–100\,\mu g$ is usually employed. The drug acts in 2–5 minutes when administered intravenously; a small dose has a duration of action of 30–60 minutes, whereas high ($>50\,\mu g/kg$) doses may be effective for 4–6 hours.

Effects
CVS The most significant cardiovascular effect that fentanyl demonstrates is bradycardia of vagal origin; cardiac output, mean arterial pressure, pulmonary and systemic vascular resistance and pulmonary capillary wedge pressure are unaffected by the administration of the drug. Fentanyl obtunds the cardiovascular responses to laryngoscopy and intubation.
RS Fentanyl is a potent respiratory depressant, causing a decrease in both the respiratory rate and tidal volume; it also diminishes the ventilatory response to hypoxia and hypercapnia. The drug is a potent antitussive agent. Chest wall rigidity (the 'wooden chest' phenomenon) may occur after the administration of fentanyl – this may be an effect of the drug on mu receptors located on GABA-ergic interneurones. Fentanyl

causes minimal release of histamine; bronchospasm is thus rarely precipitated by the drug.

CNS Fentanyl is 50–80 times more potent as an analgesic than morphine and has little hypnotic or sedative activity. Miosis is produced as a result of stimulation of the Edinger-Westphal nucleus. There have been several reports of seizure-like motor activity occurring in patients receiving fentanyl; however, no epileptic spike-wave patterns are demonstrable on the EEC (although beta-activity is initially decreased and alpha-activity is increased; subsequently alpha-activity disappears and delta-activity predominates).

AS Fentanyl decreases gastrointestinal motility and decreases gastric acid secretion; it also doubles the common bile duct pressure by causing spasm of the sphincter of Oddi.

GU The drug increases the tone of the ureters, bladder detrusor muscle and vesicular sphincter.

Metabolic/Other High doses of fentanyl will obtund the metabolic 'stress response' to surgery although the drug has no effect on white cell function. Unlike morphine, fentanyl does not increase the activity of antidiuretic hormone.

Toxicity/Side Effects Respiratory depression may occur post-operatively, possibly related to the appearance of a secondary peak in the plasma fentanyl concentration due to elution from muscle. Nausea, vomiting and dependence may also complicate the use of the drug.

Kinetics There is large interindividual variability in pharmacokinetics.

Absorption Fentanyl is absorbed orally and has a bioavailability by this route of 33%. Transdermal delivery produces 47% absorption at 24 hours, 88% at 48 hours and 94% by 72 hours.

Distribution The drug is 81–94% protein-bound in the plasma; the V_D is 0.88–4.41 l/kg. The short duration of action of a single dose of the drug is due to redistribution, rather than to metabolism (cf. thiopentone). Fentanyl is more lipid-soluble than morphine and thus crosses the blood–brain barrier more easily; it thus has a more rapid onset of action than morphine.

Metabolism Fentanyl appears to be metabolised primarily by N-dealkylation to norfentanyl with subsequent hydroxylation of this and the parent compound to hydroxypropionyl derivatives. The drug may also undergo hydroxylation and amide hydrolysis. Cytochrome P-450 3A4 plays the predominant role in fentanyl metabolism. As well as the liver, this is also found in human intestine. Some entero-systemic cycling of the drug may occur and first-pass metabolism occurs. The metabolites do not have appreciable analgesic activity.

Excretion 10% of an administered dose is excreted in the urine. The clearance is 0.4–1.5 l/min and the elimination half-life

Fentanyl

is 1.5–6 hours. Halothane decreases the clearance of fentanyl by 48%; a similar effect occurs with enflurane. The clearance of fentanyl is increased in surgical patients with renal impairment and decreased in patients with hepatic impairment.

Special Points   Fentanyl decreases the apparent MAC of co-administered volatile agents and increases the effect of non-depolarising muscle relaxants to a similar extent as does halothane. The drug is pharmaceutically incompatible with thiopentone and methohexitone.

It is unknown whether fentanyl is removed by haemodialysis.

Flecainide

Uses Flecainide is an antiarrhythmic agent used:
1. for the suppression of irritable foci, e.g. ventricular tachycardia and ventricular ectopics
2. in the treatment of re-entry dysrhythmias, e.g. the Wolff-Parkinson-White syndrome and
3. in the treatment of chronic pain syndromes.

Chemical An amide-type local anaesthetic.

Presentation As 50/100 mg tablets and as a 10 mg/ml solution of flecainide acetate for intravenous administration.

Main Action A class Ic antiarrhythmic.

Mode of Action Flecainide reduces the maximum rate of depolarisation in heart muscle and thereby stows conduction, particularly in the His-Purkinje system. It has a profound effect on conduction in accessory pathways, especially on retrograde conduction, and markedly suppresses ventricular ectopic foci. It is a local anaesthetic agent which depresses membrane responsiveness and conduction velocity with no effect on the duration of the action potential.

Route of Administration/Doses The adult oral dose is 100–200 mg 12-hourly. Intravenously, flecainide may be administered as a bolus dose of 2 mg/kg over 10 minutes followed by an infusion of 1.5 mg/kg/hr for 1 hour, reducing to 0.25 mg/kg/hr.

Effects
CVS Flecainide is generally well tolerated; the blood pressure and heart rate usually remain unchanged. The drug has negative inotropic potential.
CNS Visual disturbances may occur, and are probably a central effect of the drug.

Toxicity/Side Effects Reversible liver damage, dizziness, paraesthesiae, headaches and nausea may complicate the use of the drug.

Kinetics

Absorption Flecainide is rapidly and completely absorbed after oral administration; the bioavailability is 85–90%.

Distribution Flecainide is 37–58% protein-bound in the plasma; the V_D is 5.8–10 l/kg.

Metabolism Occurs in the liver to two major metabolites – meta-O-dealkylated flecainide and its lactam.

Excretion   10–50% of the dose is excreted unchanged in the urine. The clearance is 10 ml/min/kg and the elimination half-life is 7–15 hours after intravenous administration and 12–27 hours after oral administration.

Special Points   Flecainide increases plasma digoxin levels by 15% when the two drugs are administered concurrently. Hypokalaemia reduces the effectiveness of the drug; a reduced dose should be used in renal or hepatic failure.

Flecainide is not removed by haemodialysis.

Flucloxacillin

Uses Flucloxacillin is used in the treatment of:
1. respiratory tract infections
2. skin and soft tissue infections
3. osteomyelitis and for
4. prophylaxis during surgery.

Chemical A semi-synthetic isoxazolyl penicillin.

Presentation As 250/500 mg capsules and in vials containing 250/500/1000 mg of flucloxacillin sodium and as a syrup containing 25/50 mg/ml of flucloxacillin magnesium.

Main Actions Flucloxacillin is an acid-stable, penicillinase-resistant, narrow spectrum bactericidal antibiotic active against *Staphylococcus aureus*, Group A beta-haemolytic streptococci and pneumococci.

Mode of Action Flucloxacillin acts in the manner typical of penicillins; by binding to a cell wall penicillin-binding protein and thereby interfering with the activity of the enzymes which are involved in the cross-linking of bacterial cell wall peptidoglycans.

Routes of Administration/Doses The adult oral and intramuscular dose is 250–500 mg 6-hourly; the corresponding intravenous dose is 250 mg–2 g 6-hourly.

Toxicity/Side Effects Gastrointestinal and central nervous system disturbances, rashes, sore throat and glossitis may complicate the use of the drug. Flucloxacillin may cause both pseudomembranous colitis and jaundice in the critically ill.

Kinetics

Absorption Flucloxacillin is 50–70% absorbed when administered orally.

Distribution The drug is 95% protein-bound in the plasma; the V_D is 6.8–9.4 l.

Metabolism 8–13% is metabolised to an active form, 5-hydroxymethyl-flucloxacillin and 4% is hydrolysed in the liver to penicilloic acid, which is inactive.

Excretion Excretion of the drug occurs by glomerular filtration and tubular secretion, 35–75% of the dose appearing in the urine according to the dose and route of administration. The clearance is 3 ml/min/kg and the elimination half-life is 46 min.

Special Points Reduction of the dose of flucloxacillin should be considered if the creatinine clearance is <10 ml/min; the drug is not significantly removed by haemodialysis. Precipitation may occur if flucloxacillin is co-administered with an aminoglycoside.

Flumazenil

Uses Flumazenil is used:
1. as an aid to weaning and neurological assessment of ventilated patients who have received benzodiazepine sedation during intensive care
2. as part of the 'wake-up' test during scoliosis surgery
3. to reverse oversedation after endoscopy
4. to facilitate gastric lavage in patients after benzodiazepine overdose and
5. has also been used in the treatment of hepatic encephalopathy and
6. alcohol intoxication.

Chemical An imidazobenzodiazepine.

Presentation As a clear, colourless solution containing 100 µg/ml of flumazenil.

Main Action Reversal of the actions of benzodiazepines.

Mode of Action Flumazenil is a competitive antagonist at central benzodiazepine receptors.

Routes of Administration/Doses Flumazenil is administered intravenously, titrated in 100 µg increments to a total maximum adult dose of 1 mg. It acts in 30–60 seconds and lasts 15–140 minutes. It may also be infused intravenously at 100–400 µg/hour.

Effects Flumazenil appears to have no intrinsic effects other than a slight intrinsic anticonvulsant effect.

Toxicity/Side Effects Hypertension, dysrhythmias, dizziness, nausea and vomiting, facial flushing, anxiety and headache have been described. Resedation after prior administration of a benzodiazepine and convulsions in epileptics have also been reported.

Kinetics

Absorption Flumazenil is well absorbed when administered orally, but undergoes significant first-pass hepatic metabolism.

Distribution The drug is 50% protein-bound in the plasma; the V_D is 0.9 l/kg.

Metabolism Flumazenil is extensively metabolised in the liver to a carboxylic acid and glucuronide, both of which are inert.

Excretion   95% is excreted in the urine, <0.1% unchanged. The clearance is 700–1100 ml/min and the elimination half-life is 53 minutes.

Special Points   Flumazenil improves the quality of emergence from anaesthesia and reduces post-operative shivering.

Fluoxetine

Uses   Fluoxetine is used for the treatment of:
1. depression
2. bulimia
3. obsessive–compulsive disorders.

Chemical   A propylamine derivative.

Presentation   As 20/60 mg tablets and a suspension containing 4 mg/ml of fluoxetine hydrochloride.

Main Action   Antidepressant.

Mode of Action   Fluoxetine selectively inhibits the neuronal re-uptake of serotonin by the pre-synaptic serotonin re-uptake pump. *In vitro* it exhibits very weak anticholinergic and antihistaminergic activity.

Routes of Administration/Doses   Fluoxetine is administered as a single daily dose of 20–60 mg.

Effects
CVS   The drug has no effects.
AS   Fluoxetine decreases dietary intake in animal models.
Metabolic/Other   Fluoxetine decreases plasma sodium concentration, possibly by causing inappropriate ADH secretion. It also elevates serum corticosterone concentrations.

Toxicity/Side Effects   The drug causes dose-related gastrointestinal effects (nausea, abdominal pain, diarrhoea). Hypersensitivity reactions of all types may occur.

Kinetics

Absorption   The drug is well absorbed orally; the bioavailability is 72%.

Distribution   Fluoxetine is 94% protein-bound in the plasma; the V_D is 31 l/kg.

Metabolism   The drug undergoes extensive first-pass hepatic metabolism, in part to an active desmethyl-metabolite.

Excretion   60% of an administered dose is excreted in the urine. The clearance is 43 l/hr and the elimination half-life is 1–4 days.

Special Points   The pharmocokinetics are altered by hepatic, but not renal, impairment. Pentazocine co-administration can result in severe CNS excitatory responses.

Furosemide

Uses   Furosemide is used in the treatment of:
1. oedema of cardiac, renal or hepatic origin
2. chronic renal insufficiency
3. hypertension
4. raised intracranial pressure
5. symptomatic hypercalcaemia and
6. conversion of oliguric to polyuric renal failure.

Chemical   An anthranilic acid (sulphonamide) derivative.

Presentation   As a clear solution (which must be protected from light) for injection containing 10 mg/ml and as 20/40/500 mg tablets of furosemide. A number of fixed-dose combinations with amiloride, triamterene, spironolactone and potassium chloride are also available.

Main Action   Diuresis.

Mode of Action   Furosemide acts by inhibition of active chloride ion reabsorption in the proximal tubule and ascending limb of the loop of Henle – by reducing the tonicity of the renal medulla, a hypotonic or isotonic urine is produced. The mechanism of action at a cellular level may be exerted via inhibition of Na^+-K^+-ATPase or by inhibition of glycolysis.

Routes of Administration/Doses   The adult oral dose is 20–2000 mg daily, the intramuscular dose is 20–50 mg. Intravenous administration is titrated according to response – a range of 10–1000 mg is recommended. The infusion rate should not exceed 4 mg/min as ototoxicity may result.

Effects
CVS/RS   Pulmonary and systemic vasodilation occur leading to symptomatic relief of breathlessness prior to diuresis.
GU   A diuresis occurs within a few minutes and lasts 2 hours when frusemide is administered intravenously; correspondingly, diuresis starts one hour after oral administration and lasts 4–6 hours. Free water clearance is increased by the drug. The renal blood flow is increased and redistributed in favour of inner cortico-medullary flow. Oxygen consumption in the loop of Henle is reduced to basal levels and may protect the kidney from is ischaemia.
Metabolic/Other   The drug causes a metabolic alkalosis and may be diabetogenic; the serum urate concentrations are increased.

Toxicity/Side Effects   Hypokalaemia, hypocalcaemia, hypomagnesaemia and metabolic alkalosis may occur after the administration of furosemide. Transient auditory nerve damage, pancreatitis, skin rashes and bone marrow depression have been reported. Furosemide causes interstitial nephritis in high doses; this is a common cause of acute renal failure when co-administered with an aminoglycoside – the two drugs are synergistic in this respect. Deafness is also more likely to result when furosemide and an aminoglycoside are co-administered.

Kinetics

Absorption   Furosemide is 60–70% absorbed after oral administration; the bioavailability by this route is 43–71%.

Distribution   The drug is 96% protein-bound in the plasma, almost exclusively to albumin. The V_D is 0.11–0.13 l/kg.

Metabolism   Furosemide appears to be metabolised primarily in the kidney to a glucuronide.

Excretion   80% is excreted in the urine as unchanged and glucuronidated furosemide, the rest appears in the faeces. The clearance is 2.2 ml/min/kg and the elimination half-life is 45–92 minutes.

Special Points   The effects of curariform muscle relaxants may be enhanced by furosemide, probably due to hypokalaemia. The response to concurrently administered vasopressors may be diminished and that to vasodilators enhanced, both phenomena being manifestations of a contracted circulating blood volume.

The drug is not removed by haemodialysis.

Gabapentin

Uses Gabapentin is used in the treatment of:
1. post-herpetic neuralgia
2. painful diabetic neuropathy
3. partial seizures and
4. neuropathic pain.

Chemical An acetic acid derivative which is a structural analogue of GABA.

Presentation As 600/800 mg tablets, 100/300/400 mg capsules and an oral solution containing 50 mg/ml of gabapentin.

Main Actions Anticonvulsant and analgesic.

Mode of Action Gabapentin is structurally related to GABA but does not interact with GABA receptors. It interacts instead with a unique binding site at voltage-dependent Ca^{++} channels. It may also:
1. stimulate glutamate decarboxylase (the enzyme which converts glutamate to GABA)
2. increase the synaptic release of GABA and
3. modulate neuronal transmission at NMDA receptors.

Routes of Administration/Doses The drug is administered orally in an adult dose of up to 1800 mg/day in three divided doses. The dose needs to be reduced in patients with renal impairment.

Effect

CNS Gabapentin has analgesic and anticonvulsant properties and improves sleep in patients with neuropathic pain.

Toxicity/Side Effects Dizziness, ataxia, nystagmus, headache, tremor, diplopia, nausea and vomiting occur with a frequency >5%.

Kinetics

Absorption Gabapentin is well absorbed orally and has a bioavailability of 60%.

Distribution The drug is 3% protein-bound in the plasma; the V_D is 0.85 l/kg.

Metabolism Gabapentin is not metabolised in man.

Excretion The drug is excreted uncharged, predominantly in the urine. The elimination half-life is 5–7 hours. The clearance is related to the creatinine clearance.

Special Point Gabapentin enhances the analgesic effect of co-administered morphine. It is removed by haemodialysis.

Gentamicin

Uses   Gentamicin is used in the treatment of:
1.   urinary tract infections
2.   severe respiratory tract infections
3.   severe neonatal infections and
4.   septicaemia.

Chemical   An aminoglycoside.

Presentation   As a clear solution for injection containing 10/40 mg/ml of gentamicin sulphate and as creams/drops/ointments for topical application. Gentamicin is also available as a constituent of bone cement and as beads. It can be administered intrathecally.

Main Actions   Gentamicin is active against a wide range of Gram-positive and Gram-negative organisms including *Escherichia coli, Klebsiella, Proteus, Pseudomonas aeruginosa* and *Staphyloccus* sp. Gentamicin is inactive against *Streptococcus* sp. and anaerobes. Acquired resistance is common due to plasmid transmission.

Mode of Action   Gentamicin binds irreversibly to specific bacterial ribosomal proteins and inhibits protein synthesis by interfering with initiation of the polypeptide chain and by inducing misreading of mRNA. Gentamicin exhibits a post-antibiotic effect.

Routes of Administration/Doses   The initial adult intravenous and intramuscular dose is 60–80 mg 8-hourly; subsequent therapy should be guided by measurements of the plasma concentration of the drug. A single daily infusion of 5 mg/kg achieves levels above MIC; Subsequent dosing needs to be adjusted using drug levels and creatinine measurements.

Toxicity/Side Effects   Ototoxicity (with vestibular and auditory components) and nephrotoxicity (a form of acute tubular necrosis occurring 5–7 days after exposure) are the most serious side effects of the drug and both are correlated with high trough concentrations of gentamicin. Headaches, nausea and vomiting, rashes and abnormalities of liver function tests have also been reported in association with the use of the drug.

Kinetics

Absorption   Gentamicin is not significantly absorbed ($>1\%$ of dose) when administered orally and is not inactivated in the gastrointestinal tract.

Distribution   Gentamicin is $<10\%$ protein-bound in the plasma; the V_D is 0.14–0.7 l/kg (which is increased in the presence

of renal impairment). High concentrations are found in the renal cortex.

Metabolism   No metabolism of the drug occurs in man.

Excretion   The drug is excreted unchanged almost completely by glomerular filtration. The clearance is 1.18–1.32 ml/min/kg and the elimination half-life is 1–3 hours (which markedly increases as renal function deteriorates).

Special Points   Monitoring of plasma concentrations should commence after 3–5 doses of gentamicin and 24 hours after any change in dose. Trough samples are taken immediately before a dose and peak samples should be taken 1 hour after intramuscular and 10 minutes after intravenous administration. The optimum peak concentrations are 4–12 mg/l and the corresponding trough concentration is <2 mg/ml. Fever reduces the peak serum concentrations. The dosage and dose interval will require adjustment if the creatinine clearance is <70 ml/min.

The drug is removed by haemodialysis and haemofiltration.

Aminoglycosides prolong the action of non-depolarising muscle relaxants by inhibiting pre-synapric acetylcholine release and by stabilisation of the post-synaptic membrane at the neuromuscular junction. This effect may be reversed by the administration of intravenous calcium.

Glibenclamide

Uses   Glibenclamide is used in the treatment of non-insulin-dependent (type II) diabetes mellitus.

Chemical   A sulphonylurea.

Presentation   As 2.5/5 mg tablets of glibenclamide.

Main Action   Hypoglycaemia.

Mode of Action   Glibenclamide acts by liberating insulin from pancreatic beta-cells; it appears to act by binding to the plasma membrane of the beta-cell and producing prolonged depolarisation, reducing the permeability of the membrane to potassium. This in turn leads to opening of calcium channels; the resulting influx of calcium causes triggering of insulin release. Sulphonylureas may also act by altering peripheral insulin receptor number and sensitivity.

Route of Administration/Dose   The adult oral dose is 2.5–15 mg daily. The peak effect occurs 2 hours after administration and the duration of action is 12 hours.

Effects

Metabolic/Other   The main effect of glibenclamide is to decrease the blood sugar concentration; healthy subjects show a smaller decrease than do diabetic subjects. Sulphonylureas are ineffective in pancreatectomised patients and insulin-dependent diabetics. The drug also causes a decrease in the plasma triglyceride, cholesterol and free fatty acid concentration.

Toxicity/Side Effects   Gastrointestinal disturbances, cholestatic jaundice and alterations in liver function tests may complicate the use of glibenclamide. Hypoglycaemia, rashes, reversible leucopenia and thrombocytopenia have also been reported.

Kinetics

Absorption   The drug is completely absorbed when administered orally, bioavailability is 100%.

Distribution   Glibenclamide is 97% protein-bound in the plasma, predominantly to albumin; the V_D is 0.15 l/kg.

Metabolism   The drug is extensively (95%) metabolised in the liver by hydroxylation to three major inactive metabolites.

Excretion   30–50% of the dose is excreted in the urine, the remainder in the faeces. The clearance is 78 ml/min/kg and the elimination half-life is 1–2 hours. The elimination of the drug is impaired in the presence of severe renal impairment.

Special Points   It is generally recommended that treatment with glibenclamide be discontinued 24 hours prior to elective surgery.

The following drugs may potentiate the effect of sulphonylureas either by displacement from plasma proteins or by inhibition of their hepatic metabolism and result in hypoglycaemia: NSAIDs, salicylates, sulphonamides, oral anticoagulants, MAOIs and beta-adrenergic antagonists. Conversely, the following drugs tend to counteract the effect of sulphonylureas and result in loss of diabetic control: thiazide and other diuretics, steroids, phenothiazines, phenytoin, sympathomimetic agents and calcium antagonists.

Glucagon

Uses Glucagon is recommended for use:
1. in the treatment of hypoglycaemia and
2. to facilitate radiological investigation of the gastrointestinal tract and has been used in the management of
3. cardiogenic shock
4. renal colic
5. acute diverticulitis and
6. propranolol overdose.

Chemical A polypeptide hormone extracted from the alpha-cells of the pancreatic islets of Langerhans.

Presentation As vials containing 1/10 mg of lyophilised glucagon hydrochloride with lactose – this is reconstituted in glycerol and water prior to use.

Main Actions Elevation of blood sugar concentration, positive inotropism and chronotropism and relaxation of smooth muscle.

Mode of Action Glucagon acts via cell membrane receptors which stimulate adenylate cyclase activity, leading to an increase in the intracellular concentrations of cAMP. The final effects of the hormone are mediated via a cascade of protein kinases.

Routes of Administration/Doses Glucagon may be administered intravenously, intramuscularly or subcutaneously in a dose of 1–5 mg for an adult. The drug may also be infused intravenously (diluted in 5% dextrose) at a rate of 1–20 mg/hr. Glucagon acts within 1 minute when administered intravenously and in 8–10 minutes when administered intramuscularly or subcutaneously – the ensuing increase in the blood sugar concentration lasts 10–30 minutes.

Effects
CVS Glucagon has marked positive inotropic, and some-what less marked positive chronotropic effects and acts synergistically with beta-adrenergic agonist drugs in this respect. The drug does not increase myocardial irritability.
AS The drug reduces tone throughout the entire gastrointestinal tract, including the common bile duct; gastric and pancreatic secretion are simultaneously inhibited.
GU Glucagon decreases the ureteric tone and has an effect similar to (but less potent than) 'low-dose' dopamine in improving the renal blood flow and urine output.
Metabolic/Other Glucagon increases gluconeogenesis, glycogenolysis, lipolysis, proteolysis and ketogenesis leading to an increase in the blood sugar concentration. It also stimulates the release of endogenous catecholamines and may cause

hypokalaemia secondary to an increase in the rate of insulin secretion.

Toxicity/Side Effects   The drug is usually well tolerated; nausea and vomiting, hypo- or hyperglycaemia, diarrhoea and allergic phenomena may complicate the use of glucagon.

Kinetics

Absorption   Glucagon is inactive when administered orally. The bioavailability appears to be similar when administered intramuscularly or subcutaneously.

Metabolism   The drug is degraded by proteolysis in approximately equal quantities by splanchnic, hepatic and renal routes. The precise metabolic pathways are unknown.

Excretion   The clearance is 8–12 ml/min/kg and the elimination half-life is 3–6 minutes.

Special Points   The clearance of glucagon is halved in patients with renal failure; the drug is not removed by haemodialysis. Glucagon potentiates the anticoagulant effect of warfarin but not that of heparin.

Glyceryl trinitrate

(Nitroglycerin)

Uses   Glyceryl trinitrate is used in the treatment of:
1. stable, unstable and variant angina
2. left ventricular failure secondary to myocardial infarction and
3. in the peri-operative control of blood pressure and
4. for the prophylaxis of phlebitis associated with venous cannulation and may be of use in
5. decreasing infarct size in patients with acute myocardial infarction and used.
6. to promote venodilation when administering peripheral total parenteral nutrition.

Chemical   An organic nitrate which is an ester of nitric acid.

Presentation   As 300/500/600 µg tablets for sublingual administration, 1/2/3/5 mg tablets for buccal administration, an oral spray delivering 400 µg per metered dose, a slow-release transdermal patch delivering 5/10 mg per 24 hours and as a clear solution for injection (which must be protected from light) containing 0.5/1/5 mg/ml of glyceryl trinitrate.

Main Actions   Vasodilation of both arteries and veins.

Mode of Action   The precise mode of action of glyceryl trinitrate is unknown. It may act by:
1. causing efflux of calcium ions from smooth and cardiac muscle cells
2. affecting prostaglandin synthesis
3. blockade of alpha-adrenoreceptors in the pulmonary circulation or
4. by increasing cGMP synthesis, leading to activation of a cGMP-dependent protein kinase and dephosphorylation of the light chain of myosin within muscle cells.

Routes of Administration/Doses   The adult dose is 0.3 mg by the sublingual route, 0.4–0.8 mg when delivered by buccal spray, 1–5 mg when delivered by the buccal route in tablet form, 5–10 mg/24 hours when administered transdermally and (diluted in dextrose or saline) at the rate of 10–400 µg/min when administered intravenously. The maximum effect occurs in 15–30 minutes when administered buccally or sublingually, and 90–120 seconds after intravenous administration.

Effects
CVS   At low dose ranges, glyceryl trinitrate causes venodilation, and at higher concentrations venous and arterial vasodilation. The systolic blood pressure decreases more than does the diastolic blood pressure; the central venous pressure, pulmonary

artery pressure, left ventricular end-diastolic pressure and myocardial oxygen consumption all decrease with the use of glyceryl trinitrate. The cardiac output is usually unaltered or decreased slightly by administration of the drug; it may increase in patients with heart failure who have a high systemic vascular resistance. The coronary blood flow may decrease or remain unchanged. A reflex tachycardia occurs in normal subjects; no effect is observed on the heart rate in patients with heart failure. Glyceryl trinitrate is thought to relieve angina primarily by reducing myocardial oxygen demand (secondarily to a fall in left ventricular end-diastolic pressure and myocardial wall tension): myocardial oxygen supply is simultaneously increased by redistribution of the coronary blood flow to the subendocardium.

RS The drug causes bronchodilatation; intrapulmonary shunting may increase but the mechanism of hypoxic pulmonary vasoconstriction appears to be unaffected in man.

CNS The intracranial pressure may increase due to cerebral vasodilation.

AS Glyceryl trinitrate relaxes the smooth muscle of the gastrointestinal and biliary tracts.

GU The renal blood flow may decrease in patients with congestive cardiac failure secondary to a fall in blood pressure with no accompanying change in renal vascular resistance.

Toxicity/Side Effects Hypotension, sinus tachycardia and occasionally bradycardia, nausea and vomiting may result from administration of the drug. Headaches occur more commonly with oral or sublingual than with intravenous administration.

Kinetics The data vary widely.

Absorption Absorption is rapid and efficient after sublingual administration but slow after oral or transdermal administration; the bioavailability is 3% after oral administration due to a significant first-pass effect.

Distribution Glyceryl trinitrate is 60% protein-bound in the plasma in animal models; the V_D is 0.04–2.9 l/kg.

Metabolism The drug is rapidly metabolised in the liver and red blood cells by reduction to dinitrates, mononitrates and nitrites, all of which are less active than the parent compound.

Excretion 80% is excreted in the urine; trace amounts are exhaled as carbon dioxide. The clearance after intravenous administration is 0.3–1 l/min/kg and the elimination half-life is 1–3 minutes.

Special Points 40–80% of the dose of intravenous glyceryl trinitrate is adsorbed onto plastic giving sets. The drug has been shown to increase the duration of pancuronium-induced neuromuscular blockade and may also slow the catabolism of opioids. Clinically important tolerance does not occur with continued intravenous administration of the drug.

The drug is not removed by dialysis.

Excess cardiovascular mortality has been noticed with the use of nitrates and sildenafil.

Glycopyrronium

Uses Glycopyrronium is used:
1. in premedication where an antisialogogue action is desired
2. to protect against the peripheral muscarinic effects of anticholinesterases
3. for the treatment of bradycardias in anaesthetised patients and
4. for the treatment of hyperhydrosis (via topical administration).

Chemical A quaternary ammonium compound.

Presentation As a clear solution for injection containing 0.2 mg/ml of glycopyrronium and as a powder for topical application. It is also supplied in a fixed-dose combination containing 0.5 mg of glycopyrronium and 2.5 mg of neostigmine per ml.

Main Actions Anticholinergic; glycopyrronium has a particularly profound anti-secretory action.

Mode of Action Glycopyrronium acts by competitive antagonism of acetylcholine at peripheral muscarinic receptors.

Routes of Administration/Doses The adult intravenous and intramuscular dose is 0.2–0.4 mg; the paediatric dose is 4–10 μg/kg. The peak effect occurs 3 minutes after intravenous injection.

Effects
CVS Glycopyrronium has little effect on the blood pressure when used in normal doses and causes less dysrhythmias than atropine. Tachycardia occurs when the drug is administered intravenously in doses greater than 0.2 mg to anaesthetised patients. Glycopyrronium is protective against bradycardias due to the oculocardiac reflex or suxamethonium when administered intravenously. The vagolytic effects of the drug last approximately 2–3 hours.
RS The drug has a significant and long-lasting bronchodilator effect and causes an increase in the physiological dead space.
CNS Glycopyrronium is unable to cross the blood–brain barrier and is theoretically devoid of any central effects; however, headache and drowsiness are well-recognised sequelae of the drug. Post-anaesthetic recovery appears to be significantly more rapid with glycopyrronium than with atropine. Glycopyrronium has no effect on pupil size or accommodation.
AS The drug has a powerful antisialogogue effect that lasts approximately 8 hours after intravenous or intramuscular injection – the drug is five times as potent as atropine in this

respect. Glycopyrronium reduces gastric volume by 90% for 4 hours after administration and reduces antral motility. The drug reduces lower oesophageal sphincter tone.

Metabolic/Other   The drug inhibits sweat gland activity, but little effect is produced on body temperature. Glycopyrronium has a weak local anaesthetic action.

Toxicity/Side Effects   Typical anticholinergic side-effects are produced by the drug; dry mouth, difficulty in micturition, and inhibition of sweating.

Kinetics   Data are incomplete.

Absorption   Oral absorption is poor and erratic; bioavailability by this route is 5%. The drug seems to be absorbed in comparable amounts when administered by either the intramuscular or intravenous route.

Distribution   Redistribution of the drug occurs rapidly – 90% disappears from the plasma in 5 minutes. The drug crosses the placenta and may cause a fetal tachycardia. The V_D is 0.2–0.64 l/kg.

Metabolism   In animals, glycopyrronium occurs by hydroxylation and oxidation in the liver; very little biotransformation of the drug occurs in man.

Excretion   Excretion occurs in the urine (85%) and bile (15%), 80% unchanged. The clearance of glycopyrronium is 0.89 l/min and the elimination half-life is 0.6–1.1 hours.

Special Points   When used in combination with neostigmine to reverse non-depolarising neuromuscular blockade, glycopyrronium causes less initial tachycardia and less anticholinesterase-induced late bradycardia than atropine (and control of secretions is superior) due to the fact that the time course of action of neostigmine and glycopyrronium are better matched.

The drug is physically incompatible with thiopentone, methohexitone and diazepam.

Haloperidol

Uses   Haloperidol is used in the treatment of:
1. schizophrenia and related psychoses
2. nausea and vomiting
3. motor tics and hiccuping and
4. for premedication.

Chemical   A butyrophenone derivative.

Presentation   As 0.5/1.5/5/10/20 mg tablets, a syrup containing 2/10 mg/ml and as a clear solution for injection containing 5 mg/ml of haloperidol. A depot preparation containing 50/100 mg/ml of haloperidol decanoate is also available.

Main Actions   Antiemetic and neuroleptic.

Mode of Action   The antiemetic and neuroleptic effects of the drug appear to be mediated by:
1. central dopaminergic (D_2-) blockade leading to an increased threshold for vomiting at the chemoreceptor trigger zone and
2. post-synaptic GABA antagonism.

Routes of Administration/Doses   The adult oral dose is 1–15 mg daily in divided doses. The initial intramuscular dose is 2–30 mg, with additional doses of 5 mg until the symptoms are controlled. The intravenous dose is 1–5 mg. The drug has a longer duration of action than droperidol.

Effects
CVS   Haloperidol has minimal cardiovascular effects, but its antagonistic effects at alpha-adrenergic receptors may lead to hypotension in the presence of hypovolaemia.
RS   The drug has minimal effect on respiration.
CNS   Haloperidol induces neurolepsis; a state characterised by diminished motor activity anxiolysis and indifference to the external environment. The seizure threshold is raised by the drug.
AS   The drug has a powerful antiemetic effect via a central effect at the chemosensitive trigger zone.
Metabolic/Other   Haloperidol, in common with other dopamine antagonists, may cause hyperprolactinaemia.

Toxicity/Side Effects   Extra-pyramidal effects occur relatively commonly during the use of haloperidol; these include the neuroleptic malignant syndrome (a complex of symptoms that include catatonia, cardiovascular lability, hyperthermia and myoglobinaemia) which has a mortality in excess of 10%. Gastrointestinal and haemopoietic disturbances, abnormalities of liver function tests and allergic phenomena have been reported after the use of the drug.

Kinetics

Absorption   The drug is well absorbed after oral administration; the bioavailability by this route is 50–88%.

Distribution   The drug is 92% protein-bound in the plasma; the V_D is 18–30 l/kg.

Metabolism   Haloperidol is extensively metabolised in the liver; a reduced metabolite may be active.

Excretion   The clearance is 11.3 ml/min/kg and the elimination half-life is 10–38 hours, dependent upon the route of administration.

Special Points   Haloperidol is the preferred agent for the treatment of delirium in the critically ill adult. The sedative effects of the drug are additive with those of other central nervous system depressants administered concurrently. Hypotension resulting from the administration of the drug should not be treated using epinephrine, as a further decrease in the blood pressure may result.

Haloperidol is not removed by dialysis.

Halothane

Uses   Halothane is used for the induction and maintenance of general anaesthesia.

Chemical   A halogenated hydrocarbon containing bromine, chlorine and fluorine.

Presentation   As a clear, colourless liquid (that should be protected from light) with a characteristic sweet smell. The commercial preparation contains 0.01% thymol which prevents decomposition on exposure to light; it is non-flammable in normal anaesthetic concentrations. The molecular weight of halothane is 197.4, the boiling point 50.2 °C and the saturated vapour pressure is 32 kPa at 20 °C. The MAC of halothane is 0.75 (0.29 in the presence of 70% nitrous oxide), the oil/water solubility coefficient 220 and the blood/gas solubility coefficient 2.5. The drug is readily soluble in rubber; it does not attack metals in the absence of water vapour, but will attack brass, aluminium and lead in the presence of water vapour.

Main Action   General anaesthesia (reversible loss of both awareness and recall of noxious stimuli).

Mode of Action   The mechanism of general anaesthesia remains to be fully elucidated. General anaesthetics appear to disrupt synaptic transmission (especially in the area of the ventrobasal thalamus). The mechanism may include potentiation of gamma-amino-butyric acid and glycine receptors and antagonism at NMDA receptors. Their mode of action at the molecular level appears to involve expansion of hydrophobic regions in the neuronal membrane, either within the lipid phase or within hydrophobic sites in cell membrane proteins.

Route of Administration/Dose   Halothane is administered by inhalation, conventionally via a calibrated vaporiser. The concentration used for the inhalational induction of anaesthesia is 2–4% and for maintenance, 0.5–2%.

Effects
CVS   Halothane causes a dose-related decrease in myocardial contractility and cardiac output, with an attendant decrease in cardiac work and myocardial oxygen consumption, possibly by inhibition of calcium ion flux within myocardial cells and of the interaction between calcium ions and the contractile proteins. The heart rate decreases as a result of vagal stimulation; the systemic vascular resistance is decreased by 15–18% leading to a decrease in systolic and diastolic blood pressure; halothane also obtunds the baroreceptor reflexes. The drug has little effect on coronary vascular resistance. The threshold potential and refractory period of myocardial cells are increased; the drug also decreases the rate of phase IV repolarisation. Halothane causes marked sensitisation of the myocardium to

catecholamines, although it does not itself increase the concentration of circulating catecholamines.

RS Halothane is a respiratory depressant, markedly decreasing the tidal volume, although the respiratory rate may increase. A slight increase in P_aCO_2 may result in spontaneously breathing subjects; the drug also decreases the ventilatory response to hypoxia and hypercapnia and inhibits the mechanism of hypoxic pulmonary vasoconstriction. Halothane is non-irritant to the respiratory tract; it causes bronchodilatation by a direct effect on the bronchial smooth muscle and also inhibits histamine-induced bronchoconstriction. Bronchial secretions are reduced by the drug.

CNS The principal effect of halothane is general anaesthesia; the drug has little, if any, analgesic effect. The drug causes cerebral vasodilation, leading to an increase in both the cerebral blood flow and intracranial pressure; it also decreases cerebral oxygen consumption. A centrally mediated decrease in skeletal muscle tone results from the use of halothane.

AS The drug decreases salivation and gastric motility; splanchnic blood flow decreases as a result of the hypotension the drug produces.

GU Halothane decreases renal blood flow by 40% and the glomerular filtration rate by 50%; a small volume of concentrated urine results. The drug reduces the tone of the pregnant uterus.

Metabolic/Other Halothane decrease plasma noradrenaline concentration, whilst increasing the concentrations of thyroxine and growth hormone. It also inhibits leucocyte phagocytosis. The drug causes a fall in body temperature, predominantly by cutaneous vasodilation. Halothane causes a significant decrease in nitric oxide synthase activity.

Toxicity Side/Effects Halothane is a potent trigger agent for the development of malignant hyperthermia. The drug may also cause the appearance of myocardial dysrhythmias, particularly in the presence of hypoxia, hypercapnia or excessive catecholamine concentrations. Shivering ('halothane shakes') may occur post-operatively. The most serious side effect, halothane hepatitis, occurs (rarely) after the repeated use of the drug in the same individual. Halothane hepatitis is thought to be the result of an immune reaction to a metabolite formed by a reductive metabolic pathway. The risk of this complication is increased by obesity, peri-operative hypoxaemia and a short interval between consecutive exposures. It has been recommended that a period of at least 6 months should elapse prior to repeated administration of the drug to any individual.

Kinetics

Absorption The major factors affecting the uptake of volatile anaesthetic agents are solubility, cardiac output and the concentration gradient between the alveoli and venous blood. Halothane is relatively insoluble in blood; alveolar concentration therefore reaches inspired concentration relatively rapidly, resulting in a rapid induction of anaesthesia. An increase in the cardiac output increases the rate of alveolar uptake and slows the induction of anaesthesia. The concentration gradient between alveoli and venous blood approaches zero at equilibrium; a large concentration gradient favours the onset of anaesthesia.

Distribution The drug is initially distributed to organs with a high blood flow (the brain, heart, liver and kidney) and later to less well-perfused organs (muscles, fat and bone).

Metabolism 20% of an administered dose is metabolised in the liver via cytochrome P-450 2El, principally by oxidation and dehalogenation to yield trifluorocetic acid, trifluorocetylethanolamide, chlorobromodifluorethylene and chloride and bromide radicals.

Excretion 60–80% is exhaled unchanged; the metabolites are excreted in the urine. Excretion of metabolites may continue for up to 3 weeks after the administration of halothane.

Special Points Halothane potentiates the action of co-administered non-depolarising relaxants. The dose of co-administered adrenaline should not exceed 10 ml of a 1:100 000 solution in a 10-minute period to guard against the development of ventricular dysrhythmias.

Hartmann's solution

Uses Hartmann's solution is used:
1. in the treatment of dehydration
2. for the acute expansion of intravascular volume and
3. to provide maintenance fluid and electrolyte requirements in the peri-operative period.

Chemical Compound sodium lactate.

Presentation As a clear, colourless sterile solution in 500/1000 ml bags containing 131 mmol of sodium ions, 111 mmol of chloride ions, 2 mmol of calcium ions, 5 mmol of potassium ions and 29 mmol of lactate ions (which are converted to bicarbonate ions in the liver) per litre. The pH of the solution is 6–7.3.

Main– Action Intravascular volume expansion.

Route of Administration/Dose Hartmann's solution is administered intravenously at a rate titrated against the patient's clinical status.

Effects
CVS The haemodynamic effects of Hartmann's solution are proportional to the prevailing circulating volume and are short-lived.
GU Renal perfusion is temporarily restored towards normal in hypovolaemic patients transfused with the crystalloid.
Metabolic/Other 1 litre of one-sixth molar sodium lactate is potentially equivalent to 290 ml of 5% sodium bicarbonate in its acid-neutralising effect and to 600 ml of 5% dextrose in its antiketogenic effect.

Toxicity/Side Effects The predominant hazard is that of overtransfusion, leading to hypernatraemia, pulmonary oedema and metabolic alkalosis.

Kinetics Data are incomplete.

Distribution Hartmann's solution is initially distributed into the plasma but later equilibrates with the extracellular fluid.

Metabolism The lactate component is oxidised in the liver to bicarbonate and glycogen over a period of about 2 hours. This is dependent on cellular oxidative activity and the mechanism may be depressed by hypoxia and liver dysfunction.

Excretion Via the urine.

Heparin

Uses Heparin is used for:
1. the prevention of venous thromboembolic disease
2. the priming of haemodialysis and cardiopulmonary bypass machines and for maintaining the patency of indwelling lines and the treatment of
3. disseminated intravascular coagulation and
4. fat embolism.

Chemical Commercial heparin is a mixture of acid mucopolysaccharides (of molecular weight 3000–60 000 daltons) extracted from bovine lung or porcine intestinal mucosa.

Presentation As a clear solution of heparin sodium, containing 1000/5000/25 000 IU/ml and as heparin calcium, containing 25 000 IU/ml.

Main Action Anticoagulant.

Mode of Action The drug acts by binding reversibly to antithrombin III and enhancing its ability to inhibit certain proteases in the coagulation cascade (XIII, XII, XI, X, IX, plasmin and thrombin). It also binds directly to several coagulation proteases and thereby facilitates their reaction with antithrombin III.

Routes of Administration/Doses The intravenous dose of heparin is titrated (at approximately 1000 IU/hour) to maintain activated partial thromboplastin time at 1.5–2 times the control value. The subcutaneous dose is 5000 IU 8–12 hourly. 1 IU of heparin will prevent 1 ml of citrated sheep plasma from clotting for 1 hour after the addition of 0.2 ml 1:100 calcium chloride solution. Heparin sodium contains at least 120 IU/mg.

Effects
Metabolic/Other In addition to its anticoagulant effects, heparin inhibits platelet aggregation by fibrin. Heparin increases hepatic triglyceride and other lipase activities in plasma, leading to an increase in plasma free fatty acid concentration.

Toxicity/Side Effects Excessive bleeding is the most commonly reported side effect; osteoporosis and aldosterone suppression have also been reported. Thrombocytopenia occurs in approximately 5% of patients who receive the drug and occurs more commonly when bovine heparin is used. This may be asymptomatic or be associated with life-threatening arterial and venous thromboses, a condition which carries a mortality of 30%.

Kinetics

Absorption There are no data concerning oral administration. The bioavailability appears to be the same for intravenous or subcutaneous administration.

Distribution One-third is bound in the plasma to antithrombin III and the rest to albumin, fibrinogen and proteases. The V_D is 40–100 ml/kg.

Metabolism Heparin appears to be desulphated and depolymerised (by heparinases) in the liver, kidneys and reticuloendothelial system.

Excretion Small amounts are excreted unchanged in the urine; renal impairment has little effect on the pharmacokinetics of heparin. The clearance is 0.5–2 ml/kg/min and the elimination half-life is 0.5–2.5 hours. Heparin elimination is markedly decreased during hypothermia, e.g. during cardiopulmonary bypass.

Special Points It is controversial whether low-dose heparin therapy contraindicates epidural or spinal anaesthesia; most authorities would agree that full heparinisation does.

During heparin therapy, the thrombin time, whole-blood clotting time and activated partial thromboplastin time (kaolin cephalin time) are all prolonged. The bleeding time is unaffected by heparin and the drug has no fibrinolytic activity. Specific antagonism of the effects of heparin may be achieved by the use of protamine (qv).

Low-molecular-weight heparin acts via antithrombin III to inhibit factor Xa. It is effective and has the apparent advantages of once-daily administration, safety during pregnancy and causing thrombocytopenia less frequently.

Heparin is not removed by haemodialysis.

Hetastarch

Uses   Hetastarch is used:
1. for plasma volume replacement in haemorrhage, burns or excessive fluid and electrolyte loss
2. for the priming of extracorporeal circuits and
3. for leucapheresis.

Chemical   Hetastarch is a synthetic polymer derived from amylopectin. The hydroxyethyl groups are substituted into the glucose units to retard degradation by serum amylase.

Presentation   As a clear, pale yellow 6% solution of hetastarch in 0.9% saline. The preparation contains molecules with a weight average molecular weight of 450 000 and a number average molecular weight of 69 000. 90% of molecules have a molecular weight within the range 10 000–1 000 000. The solution contains 154 mmol of sodium and 154 mmol of chloride per litre; the osmolarity is 310 mOsm/litre.

Main Action   Plasma volume expansion.

Mode of Action   The colloidal properties of hetastarch are akin to those of human albumin, although the former exerts a greater colloid osmotic effect and the plasma volume thus increases slightly more than by the volume of hetastarch infused.

Route of Administration/Dose   Hetastarch is administered intravenously as required to restore the circulating volume: it should not be normally used in a volume exceeding 20 ml/kg/day. The increase in plasma volume lasts 24–36 hours.

Effects
CVS   The haemodynamic effects of hetastarch are proportional to the prevailing volaemic status; in the face of hypovolaemia, hetastarch infusion restores cardiovascular parameters towards normal. Hetastarch may interfere with platelet function and prolong the prothrombin, partial thromboplastin and bleeding times to a degree which is usually clinically insignificant.
GU   Renal perfusion is restored towards normal in hypovolaemic subjects transfused with the colloid.
Metabolic/Other   Hetastarch has no effect on the blood sugar concentration. The serum amylase concentration may become elevated.

Toxicity/Side Effects   The use of hetastarch may be complicated by circulatory overload, pyrexia, itching, salivary gland enlargement, headache and vomiting. Anaphylactoid reactions occur at a frequency of 0.0004–0.0006%.

Kinetics

Distribution   Tissues such as the spleen which have a high macrophage activity take up a small fraction of the administered dose and retain it for prolonged periods.

Metabolism   Molecules with a molecular weight >50 000 are sequentially hydrolysed by serum amylase to fragments which are subsequently excreted renally or removed by the reticulo-endothelial system.

Excretion   Molecules with a molecular weight <50 000 are rapidly excreted by glomerular filtration. 90% is excreted with an elimination half-life of 17 days.

Special Points   Hetastarch does not interfere with blood cross-matching, although it may lead to rouleaux formation when administered in large volumes.

It inhibits endothelial activation, thus preventing neutrophil adhesion during sepsis syndrome. Starches appear to be more effective than albumin in maintaining intravascular volume in capillary leak syndromes.

Renal failure and clotting abnormalities are relative contraindications to the use of starches.

Human albumin solution (HAS)

Uses   HAS is used:
1. for plasma volume replacement in haemorrhage, burns or excessive fluid and electrolyte loss
2. for the priming of extracorporeal circuits
3. in the treatment of hypoalbuminaemic states and
4. as a replacement fluid during therapeutic plasma exchange.

Chemical   A protein solution

Presentation   As a clear, straw-coloured fluid for infusion containing 4.5/5/20/25% of protein (of which 96% is albumin); the solutions contain sodium carbonate, sodium bicarbonate and/or acetic acid to adjust the pH to 6.4–7.4 and stabilisers but no preservatives. The solutions are prepared from pooled venous plasma from healthy subjects who are HepBsAg and HIV negative; the solutions are pasteurised at 60 °C for 10 hours. The sodium content of HAS is 130–160 mmol/l.

Main Actions   Plasma volume expansion and reversal of hypoalbuminaemia.

Mode of Action   Albumin is intimately involved in the regulation of plasma volume due to its colloid oncotic pressure; 5% HAS is iso-oncotic, but 20/25% HAS will draw 3/3.5 times the administered volume into the circulation from the tissues within 15 minutes.

Routes of Administration/Doses   HAS is administered by intravenous infusion according to clinical requirements; the haematocrit should be monitored and maintained above 25% – circulatory overload must be avoided.

Effects
CVS   The haemodynamic effects of HAS are proportional to the prevailing volaemic status; in the face of hypovolaemia, HAS infusion restores cardiovascular parameters towards normal. Myocardial depression has been reported with HAS. Although it contains no clotting factors, HAS does not interfere with the mechanism of blood clotting.
GU   Renal perfusion is restored towards normal in hypovolaemic subjects transfused with the colloid.

Toxicity/Side Effects   The major concern with the use of HAS is circulatory overload. Allergic reactions and aluminium toxicity occur infrequently.

Kinetics   Data are incomplete.

Metabolism   Exogenous albumin enters the amino acid pool and undergoes biotransformation within the liver.

Excretion   The elimination half-life is 16–18 days.

Special Points   HAS does not inhibit endothelial activation in sepsis. There is little evidence to support the use of albumin to improve outcome in the critically ill. Its effects on plasma volume are not predictable, especially in pathological states associated with leaky capillary membranes.

Hydralazine

Uses Hydralazine is used in the treatment of:
1. chronic moderate to severe hypertension
2. acute, severe hypertension
3. pre-eclampsia and
4. congestive heart failure.

Chemical A pthalazine derivative.

Presentation As 25/50 mg tablets of hydralazine hydrochloride and in ampoules containing 20 mg of hydralazine hydrochloride as a white lyophilised powder which is reconstituted prior to use in water.

Main Action Peripheral vasodilation.

Mode of Action Hydralazine appears to act directly on vascular smooth muscle by interfering either with calcium entry into the cell or the release of calcium from intracellular stores; this leads to electromechanical decoupling and inhibition of contraction.

Routes of Administration/Doses The adult oral dose is 50–200 mg/day in divided doses; the intravenous dose is 20–40 mg administered slowly. The drug takes 15–20 minutes to act when administered intravenously and has a duration of action of 2–6 hours.

Effects
CVS Hydralazine causes predominantly arteriolar vasodilation leading to a decrease in the systemic vascular resistance; a compensatory tachycardia develops and the cardiac output increases.
CNS Cerebral blood flow increases after the administration of hydralazine.
GU The renal blood flow increases secondarily to the increased cardiac output; however, hydralazine usually produces sodium retention and a decrease in urine volume.
Metabolic/Other Plasma renin activity is increased by the drug.

Toxicity/Side Effects Minor side effects, such as headache, flushing, sweating, nausea and vomiting, are common. The drug may precipitate angina in patients with myocardial ischaemia. A lupus-like syndrome may occur when high doses are used. Peripheral neuropathies and blood dyscrasias occur rarely with the use of hydralazine.

Kinetics

Absorption The bioavailability of oral hydralazine is dependent on acetylator status (v.i.) and thus the extent of first-pass metabolism – average values are 16–35%.

Distribution   Hydralazine is 87% protein-bound in the plasma; the V_D is 4.2 l/kg.

Metabolism   The drug is primarily metabolised by acetylation and oxidation with subsequent conjugation. Phenotypically determined populations of fast and slow acetylators exist.

Excretion   50–90% is excreted in the urine, 1–2% unchanged. Up to 10% may appear in the faeces. The clearance is 1.4 l/kg/hr and the elimination half-life is 0.67–3.6 hours.

Special Points   The drug is commonly used in combination with a beta-adrenergic antagonist to obtund the compensatory tachycardia and increased plasma renin activity caused by hydralazine.

The hypotensive effects of volatile agents and hydralazine are additive. A dose of 0.4 mg/kg has been recommended 10 minutes prior to induction in order to obtund the pressor response to intubation.

The drug crosses the placenta and may produce a fetal tachycardia when used in pregnancy or labour.

The addition of hydralazine to dextrose solutions is not recommended.

Hydralazine is not removed by haemodialysis.

Hydrocortisone

Uses Hydrocortisone is used:
1. as replacement therapy in adrenocortical deficiency states and in the treatment of
2. allergy and anaphylaxis
3. asthma
4. a panoply of autoimmune disorders
5. eczema and contact sensitivity syndromes and
6. in leukaemia chemotherapy regimes and
7. for immunosuppression after organ transplantation.

Chemical A glucocorticosteroid.

Presentation As 10/20 mg tablets of hydrocortisone, in vials containing a white lyophilised powder which is diluted in water to yield a solution containing 100 mg of hydrocortisone sodium succinate and as a variety of topical creams and retention enemas, some of which are fixed dose combinations.

Main Action Anti-inflammatory.

Mode of Action Corticosteroids act by controlling the rate of protein synthesis; they react with cytoplasmic receptors to form a complex which directly influences the rate of RNA transcription. This directs the synthesis of lipocortins.

Routes of Administration/Doses The adult dose by the intravenous route is 100–500 mg 6–8 hourly; the drug acts within 2–4 hours and has duration of action of 8 hours when administered intravenously. The corresponding oral dose is 10–20 mg/day, using the lowest dose that is effective and on alternate days if possible to limit the development of side effects. The intra-articular dose is 5–50 mg daily.

Effects
CVS In the absence of corticosteroids vascular permeability increases, small blood vessels demonstrate an inadequate motor response and cardiac output decreases. Steroids have a positive effect on myocardial contractivity and cause vasoconstriction by increasing the number of alpha-1 adrenoreceptors and beta-adrenoreceptors and stimulating their function.
CNS Corticosteroids increase the excitability of the central nervous system; the absence of glucorticoids leads to apathy, depression and irritability.
AS Hydrocortisone increases the likelihood of peptic ulcer disease; it also decreases the gastrointestinal absorption of calcium.
GU Hydrocortisone has weak mineralocorticoid effects and produces sodium retention and increased potassium excretion; the urinary excretion of calcium is also increased by the drug. The drug increases the glomerular filtration rate and stimulates tubular secretory activity.

Metabolic/Other   Hydrocortisone exerts profound effects on carbohydrate, protein and lipid metabolism. Glucocorticoids stimulate gluconeogenesis and inhibit the peripheral utilisation of glucose; they cause a redistribution of body fat, enhance lipolysis and also reduce the conversion of amino acids to protein. Hydrocortisone is a potent anti-inflammatory agent which inhibits all stages of the inflammatory process by inhibiting neutrophil and macrophage recruitment, blocking the effect of lymphokines and inhibiting the formation of plasminogen activator. Corticosteroids increase red blood cell, neutrophil and haemoglobin concentrations, whilst depressing other white cell lines and the activity of lymphoid tissue.

Toxicity/Side Effects   Consist of an acute withdrawal syndrome and a syndrome (Cushing's) produced by prolonged use of excessive quantities of the drug. Cushing's syndrome is characterised by growth arrest, a characteristic appearance consisting of central obesity, a moon face and buffalo hump, striae, acne, hirsutism, skin and capillary fragility together with the following metabolic derangements: altered glucose tolerance, fluid retention, a hypokalaemic alkalosis and osteoporosis. A proximal myopathy, cataracts and an increased susceptibility to peptic ulcer disease may also complicate the use of the drug.

Kinetics

Absorption   Hydrocortisone is well absorbed when administered orally or rectally; the oral bioavailability is 54% and the rectal bioavailability is 30–90%.

Distribution   The drug is reversibly bound in the plasma to albumin (20%) and a specific corticosteroid-binding globulin (70%); the drug is >90% protein-bound at low concentrations but only 60–70% protein-bound at higher concentrations. The V_D is 0.3–0.5 l/kg according to the dose.

Metabolism   Occurs in the liver to tetrahydrocortisone.

Excretion   The clearance of hydrocortisone is dose-dependent and ranges from 167–283 ml/min; the elimination half-life is 1.2–1.8 hours.

Special Points   Cortisone and hydrocortisone (cortisol) are metabolically interconvertible; only the latter is active. The conversion of cortisone to hydrocortisone is rapid and extensive and occurs as a first-pass effect in the liver. Hydrocortisone is one-quarter as potent as an anti-inflammatory agent as prednisolone. It has been recommended that peri-operative steroid cover be given:
1. to patients who have received high-dose steroid replacement therapy for >2 weeks in the preceding year prior to surgery

Hydrocortisone

2. to patients undergoing pituitary or adrenal surgery.

Glucocorticoids antagonise the effects of anticholinesterase drugs.

Relative adrenal insufficiency is reported in the critically ill and low-dose hydrocortisone replacement has been shown to decrease the time to 'shock' reversal and may decrease mortality.

Hyoscine

Uses   Hyoscine is used:
1.   in premedication
2.   in the prophylaxis of motion sickness and
3.   as an antispasmodic.

Chemical   Hyoscine is an alkaloid derived from *Scopolia carniolica* and is an ester of tropic acid and scopine. Scopolamine is 1-hyoscine.

Presentation   Hyoscine hydrobromide is presented as a clear solution for injection containing 0.4 mg/ml and as a fixed-dose combination with papaveretum. Hyoscine butylbromide is presented as a clear solution containing 20 mg/ml and in 10 mg tablet form. A transdermal preparation delivering 0.5 mg of hyoscine is also available.

Main Actions   Anticholinergic, with marked sedative effects.

Mode of Action   The drug acts by competitive antagonism of acetylcholine at muscarinic receptors (hyoscine has little effect at nicotinic receptors).

Routes of Administration/Doses   Hyoscine may be administered intramuscularly, intravenously, subcutaneously, transdermally or orally. The intramuscular dose for premedication is 0.008 mg/kg. The adult oral dose is 20 mg 6-hourly.

Effects
CVS   Hyoscine has less effect than atropine on cardiovascular parameters. When administered intravenously, an initial tachycardia may be followed by a bradycardia.
RS   The drug causes a marked decrease in bronchial secretions, mild bronchodilatation and mild stimulation of respiration.
CNS   Hyoscine is a central nervous system depressant, causing 'twilight sleep' and amnesia. It has antanalgesic, antiemetic and anti-Parkinsonian properties. Hyoscine may also cause the central anticholinergic syndrome.
AS   A marked antisialogogue, hyoscine is also antispasmodic throughout the gut and biliary tree.
GU   The tone of the bladder and ureters is reduced following administration of the drug.
Metabolic/Other   Hyoscine has a more marked effect on the eye and sweat gland activity than atropine.

Toxicity/Side Effects   The central anticholinergic syndrome is the main side effect and may be prolonged, especially in the elderly; peripheral anticholinergic side effects may also occur following the use of hyoscine.

Kinetics

Absorption   Hyoscine is poorly absorbed after oral administration; the bioavailability is 10% by this route. The drug is well absorbed following subcutaneous or intramuscular administration.

Distribution   Hyoscine is 11% protein-bound in the plasma; the V_D is 2.0 l/kg.

Metabolism   The drug is extensively metabolised in liver and tissues to scopine and scopic acid.

Excretion   2% of an oral dose is excreted unchanged in the urine and 5% in the bile. The clearance is 45 l/hour and the elimination half-life is 2.5 hours.

Special Points   The drug may induce acute clinical and biochemical manifestations in patients with porphyria.

Imipenem

Uses Imipenem is a broad spectrum antibiotic used in the treatment of:
1. urinary and respiratory tract infections
2. intra-abdominal sepsis
3. bone and joint infections and
4. bacteraemia.

Chemical A semi-synthetic thienamycin antibiotic presented in a fixed dose combination with cilastatin, a renal peptidase inhibitor which decreases renal metabolism of imipenem to increase the concentration of active circulating imipenem. Cilastatin otherwise has no effect on the bactericidal activity of imipenem.

Presentation In vials containing 500 mg of imipenem monohydrate with 500 mg of cilastatin sodium or twice the quantities of both.

Main Actions Imipenem has a remarkably wide spectrum of activity – the broadest of any currently available. It is active against Gram-positive and Gram-negative aerobes and anaerobes, including most staphylococcal (including MRSA) and streptococcal species, *Pseudomonas aeruginosa, Haemophilus influenzae, Neisseria gonorrhoeae, Escherichia coli, Proteus, Klebsiella, Salmonella* and *Shigella* sp. It is very active against most beta-lactamase-producing bacteria.

Mode of Action Imipenem inhibits cell wall synthesis by binding covalently to penicillin-binding proteins in the bacterial cell membrane and inhibiting transpeptidases involved in cell wall synthesis. Imipenem may have a post-antibiotic effect.

Route of Administration/Doses The drug is administered by intravenous infusion over 20–30 minutes; the adult dose is 1–2 g daily in 3–4 divided doses. The maximum recommended dose is 50 mg/kg/day.

Effects
CVS Hypotension may occur with rapid intravenous injection.

Toxicity/Side Effects Imipenem is usually well tolerated; gastrointestinal upsets (including pseudomembranous colitis), rashes, eosinophilia and abnormalities of liver function tests may occur. Seizures have been reported in up to 2% of patients receiving imipenem. The drug is highly irritant to veins.

Kinetics

Distribution Imipenem is 20% protein-bound in the plasma; the V_D is 0.23–0.31 l/kg.

Metabolism   The drug undergoes partial post-excretory metabolism in the renal proximal tubules via dehydropeptidase-1 (a dipeptidase that is inhibited by cilastatin).

Excretion   60–75% of the dose is excreted unchanged in the urine; the drug is non-cumulative in patients with normal renal function. The clearance is 3–3.67 ml/min/kg and the elimination half-life is approximately 1 hour.

Special Points   The dosage should be reduced in renal failure; both drugs are removed by haemodialysis.

Imipenem has low endotoxin-releasing potential; the clinical significance of this is unknown.

Imipramine

Uses   Imipramine is used for the treatment of:
1. depression and
2. nocturnal enuresis.

Chemical   A dibenzazepine derivative.

Presentation   As 10/25 mg tablets and a syrup containing 5 mg/ml of imipramine hydrochloride.

Main Action   Antidepressant.

Mode of Action   Tricyclic antidepressants may potentiate the action of biogenic amines within the central nervous system by preventing their re-uptake at nerve terminals. They also antagonise muscarinic cholinergic, alpha-1 adrenergic and H_1 and H_2 histaminergic receptors.

Route of Administration/Doses   The adult oral dose is 25–50 mg 6–8 hourly.

Effects
CVS   Imipramine causes postural hypotension as a result of peripheral alpha-adrenergic blockade; a compensatory tachycardia may develop. The tricyclic antidepressants are also negatively inotropic; they also have characteristic effects on ECG morphology, including T-wave flattening and inversion.
RS   Imipramine has little effect on respiratory function when normal doses are used.
CNS   The predominant effect of the drug is an antidepressant action, which may take several weeks to develop; sedation, weakness and fatigue are also commonly produced.
AS   High doses of imipramine increase the gastric emptying time.
Metabolic/Other   The drug may produce excessive sweating by an unknown mechanism.

Toxicity/Side Effects   Occur in 5% and include palpitations, dysrhythmias, tremor, confusion, mania and hepatic dysfunction. Anticholinergic side effects (blurred vision, dryness of the mouth, constipation and urinary retention) may also occur. Overdose of the drug may result in fits, coma and fatal dysrhythmias.

Kinetics

Absorption   The drug is well absorbed when administered orally; the bioavailability is 19–35%.

Distribution   Imipramine is 95% protein-bound in the plasma; the V_D is 15–31 l/kg.

Metabolism   The drug is demethylated to an active form, desimipramine; this is inactivated by hydroxylation with subsequent conjugation to glucuronide.

Excretion   The glucuronide conjugates are excreted in the urine. The clearance is 11–19 ml/min/kg and the elimination half-life is 11–25 hours.

Special Points   Scopolamine and the phenothiazines displace tricyclic antidepressants from their binding sites on plasma proteins and thus increase the activity of the latter; barbiturates increase the rate of hepatic metabolism of tricyclic antidepressants and decrease their activity.

Imipramine accentuates the cardiovascular effects of adrenaline; care should be exercised when local anaesthetic agents containing adrenaline are used in patients receiving the drug. Imipramine also increases the likelihood of dysrhythmias occurring during general anaesthesia.

Imipramine is not removed by haemodialysis.

Indometacin

Uses Indometacin is used in the treatment of:
1. rheumatoid and osteoarthritis
2. gout
3. ankylosing spondylitis
4. acute musculoskeletal disorders
5. dysmenorrhoea and has been used
6. to promote the closure of a patent ductus arteriosus.

Chemical An indoleacetic acid derivative.

Presentation As capsules containing 25/50 mg, as slow-release preparations containing 25/50/75 mg, as 100 mg suppositories and as a suspension containing 5 mg/ml of indometacin.

Main Actions Analgesic, anti-inflammatory and antipyretic.

Mode of Action Indometacin acts by inhibiting prostaglandin production (by 60–95% according to dose) by causing reversible blockade of the conversion of arachidonic acid to PGG_2, a reaction catalysed by COX. Indometacin does not exhibit COX selectivity.

Routes of Administration/Doses The adult oral or rectal dose is 50–200 mg/day in divided doses.

Effects
CVS The drug may cause hypertension, dysrhythmias and salt and water retention leading to the development of peripheral oedema. It promotes the closure of the ductus arteriosus in neonates.
AS Indometacin causes hyperaemia of the gastric mucosa and may cause ulceration at high doses. Reversible abnormalities of liver function tests may also occur.
GU Interstitial nephritis leading to an impairment of renal function and hyperkalaemia occurs infrequently.
Metabolic/Other Indometacin is a more potent anti-inflammatory agent than aspirin or hydrocortisone and a more potent analgesic and antipyretic agent than aspirin in animal models. It also inhibits platelet aggregation and prolongs the bleeding time (which remains within the normal range).

Toxicity/Side Effects Occur frequently (in 35–50%) – the list of reported side effects is legion. The most common side effects are gastrointestinal and central nervous system disturbances (headache, dizziness and depression). Hypersensitivity reactions and haemopoietic disturbances may also occur.

Kinetics

Absorption Indometacin is rapidly and well absorbed after oral administration. The bioavailability is 80% via the oral route and 80% when administered rectally.

Distribution The drug is 99% protein-bound in the plasma, predominantly to albumin. The V_D is 0.5–0.8 l/kg.

Metabolism Occurs in the liver by demethylation and deacylation with subsequent conjugation to glucuronide. Enterohepatic cycling of the conjugates occurs.

Excretion One-third is excreted in the faeces and the rest in the urine; 10% of this is excreted unchanged. The clearance is 1–2.5 ml/min/kg and the elimination half-life is 2.6–11.2 hours.

Special Points The drug should be taken with food or milk to decrease the incidence of gastrointestinal upsets. Indometacin may increase the effect of co-administered oral anticoagulants and sulphonylureas due to displacement from plasma proteins.

The drug is not removed by haemodialysis.

Insulin

Uses Insulin is used in the management of:
1. type I diabetes mellitus
2. diabetic emergencies
3. the peri-operative control of blood sugar concentration
4. hyperkalaemia and
5. to improve glucose utilisation during total parenteral nutrition and
6. in provocation tests for growth hormone.

Chemical A polypeptide hormone. Human insulin is produced commercially by recombinant DNA techniques; bovine insulin differs by three, and porcine insulin by one amino acid from human insulin.

Presentation A wide variety of insulin preparations is available; the standard preparations contain 100 units/ml. The source may be human recombinant, bovine or porcine and each may be modified by the addition of zinc or protamine to retard absorption.

Main Actions Stimulation of carbohydrate metabolism, protein synthesis and lipogenesis.

Mode of Action Insulin binds to and activates a specific membrane-bound receptor; the effects of this may be mediated by alterations in the intracellular concentrations of cyclic nucleotides. Insulin exerts a direct effect on lipoprotein lipase, increases the rate of transcriptional and translational events during protein synthesis and controls membrane polarisation and ion transport by activating Na^+-K^+-ATPase.

Routes of Administration Insulin may be administered intravenously, intramuscularly and subcutaneously in a dose titrated according to the blood sugar estimations. It may be diluted for intravenous infusion in saline/dextrose, but has an improved stability in gelatin solutions. The apparent dose requirement is increased by 20% when bovine or porcine insulin is used in place of human insulin.

Rapidly acting insulins act within 1 hour and have a duration of action of 5–7 hours; slow-acting preparations act within 4 hours and have a duration of action of 18–36 hours.

Effects

Metabolic/Other Insulin has profound effects upon carbohydrate, fat and protein metabolism. The drug increases the rate of diffusion of glucose into all cells, and specifically into hepatocytes by enhancing the activity of glucokinase (which causes the initial phosphorylation of glucose, thereby 'trapping' glucose intracellularly). The drug increases the rate of glycogen synthesis by enhancing the activity of phosphofructokinase (which is involved in glucose phosphorylation) and glycogen synthetase (which polymerises monosaccharides to form glycogen). Insulin simultaneously inhibits glycogenolysis by an action on phosphorylase and inhibits gluconeogenesis. It also facilitates diffusion of glucose into muscle cells.

Insulin causes fat deposition in adipose tissue by increasing the hepatic synthesis of fatty acids; these are utilised within the liver to form triglycerides which are released into the bloodstream; insulin simultaneously activates lipoprotein lipase in adipose tissue which splits triglycerides into fatty acids, enabling them to be absorbed into adipose tissue where they are stored. The drug also inhibits a hormone-sensitive lipase thereby preventing hydrolysis of triglycerides and facilitates glucose transport into fat cells, leading to an increased supply of glycerol which is used in the manufacture of storage triglycerides.

Insulin causes active transport of amino acids into cells, and increases mRNA translation and DNA transcription; in addition, it inhibits the catabolism of proteins.

The drug also causes an increase in the rate of potassium and magnesium transport into cells.

Toxicity/Side Effects   The commonest acute side effect of insulin is hypoglycaemia. Chronic use may be complicated by localised allergic reactions, lipodystrophy and insulin resistance due to antibody formation.

Kinetics

Absorption   Insulin is inactive when administered orally, since it is destroyed by gastrointestinal proteases.

Distribution   The drug exhibits little protein-binding; the V_D is 0.075 l/kg (0.146 l/kg in the diabetic subject).

Metabolism   Insulin is rapidly metabolised in liver, muscle and kidney by glutathione insulin transhydrogenase.

Excretion   The metabolites appear in the urine. The clearance is 33.3 ml/mm/kg (18.5 ml/min/kg in the diabetic subject) and the elimination half-life is 1.6–3.4 minutes (5.3–7.8 minutes in the diabetic subject).

Special Points   The co-administration of steroids, thyroxine, thiazide diuretics and sympathomimetic agents tend to counteract the effects of insulin on carbohydrate metabolism. Many regimes of insulin administration have been described for the peri-operative management of diabetic patients.

Insulin is not removed by dialysis.

Tight blood sugar control in critical illness has been shown to decrease mortality, especially in surgical patients.

Ipratropium

Uses Ipratropium is used in the treatment of asthma and chronic obstructive airways disease.

Chemical A synthetic quaternary ammonium compound which is a derivative of atropine.

Presentation As an isotonic solution of ipratropium bromide containing 0.25 mg/ml for nebulisation or as a metered-dose aerosol delivering 200 µg/dose (18 µg of which is available to the patient).

Main Actions Bronchodilatation.

Mode of Action Ipratropium acts by competitive inhibition of cholinergic receptors on bronchial smooth muscle, thereby blocking the bronchoconstrictor action of vagal efferent impulses. It may also inhibit acetylcholine enhancement of mediator release by blocking cholinergic receptors on the surface of mast cells.

Routes of Administration/Doses The drug is administered by inhalation of a nebulised solution or aerosol in an adult dose of 100–500 µg 6-hourly or 1–2 puffs 6-hourly respectively. The maximum effect is achieved in 1.5–2 hours and lasts 4–6 hours.

Effects
CVS No effect on cardiovascular function is observed after administration by inhalation. When administered intravenously, tachycardia with an increase in blood pressure and cardiac output and a fall in central venous pressure may result.
RS Bronchodilatation is the principal effect of the drug. No effect is seen on the viscosity or volume of secretions or the effectiveness of mucociliary clearance. The oxygen saturation remains unaltered following the administration of ipratropium.
CNS The drug has no effect, since ipratropium is unable to cross the blood–brain barrier.
AS When given orally in large doses, gastric secretion and salivation are decreased by the drug.

Toxicity/Side Effects None of the typical anticholinergic side effects is observed if ipratropium is administered by inhalation. 20–30% of patients receiving the drug experience transient local effects – dryness or unpleasant taste in the mouth. Local deposition of the nebulised drug on the eye may cause mydriasis and difficulty with accommodation.

Kinetics

Absorption The bioavailability of the drug when administered orally is 3–30% and 5% by the inhaled route.

Distribution   The V_D is 0.4 l/kg.

Metabolism   Ipratropium is metabolised to 8 inactive metabolites.

Excretion   Occurs in approximately equal proportions in the urine and faeces. The clearance is 11.8 l/hour and the elimination half-life is 3.2–3.8 hours.

Special Points   Ipratropium is less effective than beta-adrenergic agonists in the treatment of asthma, although its effectiveness in the treatment of bronchitis appears to be equal to that of the beta-adrenergic agonists. An additive effect with the latter drugs is difficult to prove.

Isoflurane

Uses Isoflurane is used:
1. for the induction and maintenance of general anaesthesia and has been used
2. for sedation during intensive care.

Chemical A halogenated methyl ether which is a structural isomer of enflurane.

Presentation As a clear, colourless liquid with a pungent smell. The commercial preparation contains no stabilisers or preservatives; it is non-flammable in normal anesthetic concentrations. The molecular weight of isoflurane is 184.5, the boiling point 48.5 °C and the saturated vapour pressure is 32 kPa at 20 °C. The MAC of isoflurane is 1.15 (0.50 in 70% nitrous oxide), the oil/water solubility coefficient 174 and the blood/gas solubility coefficient 1.4. The drug is readily soluble in rubber; it does not attack metals.

Main Action General anaesthesia (reversible loss of both awareness and recall of noxious stimuli).

Mode of Action The mechanism of general anaesthesia remains to be fully elucidated. General anaesthetics appear to disrupt synaptic transmission (especially in the area of the ventro-basal thalamus). The mechanism may include potentiation of gamma-amino-butyric acid and glycine receptors and antagonism at NMDA receptors. Their mode of action at the molecular level appears to involve expansion of hydrophobic regions in the neuronal membrane, either within the lipid phase or within hydrophobic sites in cell membrane proteins.

Routes of Administration/Dose Isoflurane is administered by inhalation, conventionally via a calibrated vaporiser. The concentration used for the inhalational induction of anaesthesia is 1–4% and for maintenance, 0.5–3%.

Effects
CVS Isoflurane is a mild negative inotrope; it also causes a marked decrease in the systemic vascular resistance and these two effects produce a decrease in mean arterial pressure. Unlike halothane, isoflurane produces a reflex tachycardia. The drug reduces the rate of phase IV depolarisation, increases the threshold potential and prolongs the effective refractory period. Isoflurane causes coronary vasodilation, which in the presence of fixed coronary arterial stenotic lesions, may lead to redistribution of coronary blood flow from the endo- to epicardium ('coronary steal' effect). Isoflurane is not markedly arrhythmogenic and causes little

sensitisation of the myocardium to the effects of circulating catecholamines.

RS Isoflurane is a respiratory depressant, decreasing the tidal volume with little effect on respiratory rate. A slight increase in P_aCO_2 may occur in spontaneously breathing subjects; the drug also decreases the ventilatory response to hypoxia and hypercapnia. Isoflurane is irritant to the respiratory tract and may cause coughing, breath-holding and an increase in bronchial secretions; it also causes bronchodilatation.

CNS The principal effect of isoflurane is general anaesthesia; the drug has little analgesic effect. The drug increases cerebral blood flow when used in normocapnic patients in a concentration exceeding $1 \times MAC$, leading to an increase in intracranial pressure; it also decreases cerebral oxygen consumption. A decrease in skeletal muscle tone results from the use of isoflurane, mediated by an effect on the post-junctional membrane.

AS Hepatic blood flow is well maintained during the administration of isoflurane.

GU The drug reduces the tone of the pregnant uterus.

Toxicity/Side Effects Isoflurane appears to be a trigger agent for the development of malignant hyperthermia (three reported cases). There have been isolated reports of hepatotoxicity associated with the repeated use of isoflurane; nephrotoxicity does not occur with the use of the drug as the fluoride ion concentrations it produces are insignificant.

Kinetics

Absorption The major factors affecting the uptake of volatile anaesthetic agents are solubility, cardiac output and the concentration gradient between the alveoli and venous blood.

Isoflurane is less soluble in blood than is enflurane; alveolar concentration should therefore reach inspired concentration relatively rapidly, resulting in a rapid induction of anaesthesia (although the irritant nature of the drug tends to offset this effect). An increase in the cardiac output increases the rate of alveolar uptake and slows the induction of anaesthesia. The concentration gradient between alveoli and venous blood approaches zero at equilibrium; a large concentration gradient favours the onset of anaesthesia.

Distribution The drug is initially distributed to organs with a high blood flow (the brain, heart, liver and kidney) and later to less well-perfused organs (muscles, fat and bone).

Metabolism 0.2% of an administered dose is slowly metabolised in the liver, principally by oxidation and dehalogenation.

Excretion Isoflurane is principally exhaled unchanged; 0.2% of an administered dose is excreted in the urine as non-volatile fluorinated compounds.

Special Points Isoflurane potentiates the action of co-administered non-depolarising relaxants. It is suitable for use in epileptic patients.

Isoprenaline

Uses   Isoprenaline is used in the treatment of:
1. complete heart block (whilst awaiting transvenous pacing)
2. asthma
3. torsade de pointes and is used to provide
4. inotropic support.

Chemical   A synthetic catecholamine.

Presentation   As 30 mg tablets and as clear solutions for injection containing 0.02/1 mg/ml of isoprenaline hydrochloride. An aerosol delivering 80/400 µg of isoprenaline sulphate per metered dose is also available.

Main Actions   Positive inotropism, positive chronotropism and bronchodilatation.

Mode of Action   Isoprenaline is a beta-adrenergic agonist; its actions are mediated by membrane-bound adenylate cyclase and the subsequent formation of cAMP.

Routes of Administration/Doses   The initial adult oral dose is 30 mg 8-hourly; the dose may be increased as required to a maximum of 840 mg/day. The aerosol may be used essentially as required. Isoprenaline may also be administered as an infusion, diluted in water or 5% dextrose, at the rate of 0.5–8 µg/min, according to response. The positive chronotropic effect becomes apparent after 20 minutes.

Effects
CVS   Isoprenaline is a powerful positive inotrope and chronotrope and thus causes an increase in the cardiac output and systolic blood pressure. The drug causes a decrease in the peripheral vascular resistance (a beta-2 effect); as a result, the diastolic blood pressure tends to decrease. The drug increases automaticity and enhances atrioventricular nodal conduction; it also increases coronary blood flow which tends to offset the increase in myocardial oxygen consumption that it produces.
RS   The drug is a potent bronchodilator and increases anatomical dead space and ventilation/perfusion mismatching, which may lead to hypoxia.
CNS   Isoprenaline is a central nervous system stimulant.
AS   Isoprenaline decreases gastrointestinal tone and motility; the mesenteric blood supply is increased by the drug.
GU   The administration of isoprenaline reduces renal blood flow in normotensive subjects, but may increase renal perfusion in shock states. The drug also reduces uterine tone.
Metabolic/Other   In common with adrenaline, isoprenaline increases the plasma concentration of free fatty acids and may cause hyperglycaemia. Isoprenaline inhibits antigen-induced histamine release and the formation of Slow-Releasing Substance of Anaphylaxis.

Toxicity/Side Effects The use of isoprenaline may be complicated by excessive tachycardia, palpitations, angina, dysrhythmias, hypotension and sweating. The use of iso-prenaline inhalers by asthmatic patients has been associated with an excess mortality.

Kinetics Quantitative data are lacking.

Absorption The drug is well absorbed when administered orally, but is subject to an extensive first-pass metabolism in the intestinal mucosa and liver.

Distribution Isoprenaline is 65% protein-bound in the plasma.

Metabolism Isoprenaline is a relatively poor substrate for the action of monoamine oxidase; the drug is predominantly metabolised by catechol-O-methyltransferase in the liver to sulphated conjugates.

Excretion 15–75% of an administered dose of isoprenaline is excreted unchanged in the urine, the remainder, as sulphated conjugates. The plasma half-life is 1–7 minutes.

Special Points Hypoxia, hypercapnia and the co-administration of halothane, trilene or cyclopropane increase the likelihood of the development of dysrhythmias during the use of isoprenaline. Tachyphylaxis may occur with prolonged use.

Ketamine

Uses   Ketamine is used:
1. for the induction of anaesthesia, especially in poor-risk patients with hypotension or asthma
2. as a sole agent for short procedures, such as intraocular examinations, burns dressings and radiological and radiotherapy procedures in children
3. as an agent for mass casualties in the field
4. for analgesia both post-operatively and in patients receiving intensive care
5. for pain relief in patients with chronic pain and
6. for the reversal of severe unresponsive asthma.

Chemical   A phencyclidine derivative.

Presentation   As a colourless solution containing 10/50/100 mg/ml of racemic ketamine hydrochloride. The 50 and 100 mg/ml preparations contain 1 in 10 000 benzethonium chloride as a preservative.

Main Actions   Dissociative anaesthesia (a combination of profound analgesia with superficial sleep).

Mode of Action   Ketamine is a non-competitive antagonist of the NMDA receptor Ca^{2+} channel pore and also inhibits NMDA receptor activity by interaction with the phencyclidine binding site. It may also modulate opioid and muscarinic receptor activity.

Routes of Administrati'on/Doses   The intramuscular dose is 10 mg/kg; the onset of action is 2–8 minutes and the duration of action is 10–20 minutes. The corresponding intravenous dose is 1.5–2 mg/kg administered over a period of 60 seconds; the onset of action occurs within 30 seconds and the duration of action is 5–10 minutes. Ketamine may be infused intravenously at the rate of 50 µg/kg/min. The drug is also effective when administered orally, extradurally (in an adult dose of 10 mg), intrathecally, rectally or nasally.

Effects
CVS   Ketamine causes tachycardia, an increase in the blood pressure, central venous pressure and cardiac output secondary to an increase in sympathetic tone. Baroreceptor function is well maintained and dysrhythmias are uncommon.
RS   Ketamine causes mild stimulation of respiration with relative preservation of airway reflexes. Bronchodilatation is a feature of the action of the drug.
CNS   The state of dissociative anaesthesia is produced by the drug. The cerebral blood flow, cerebral metabolic rate and intraocular pressure are increased; amnesia is a marked feature. Visceral pain is poorly obtunded by ketamine. The EEG

demonstrates dominant theta activity and loss of the alpha rhythm. At high doses, ketamine exhibits local anaesthetic properties.

AS Post-operative nausea and vomiting are common; salivation is increased following the administration of the drug. Ketamine has no effect on gastrointestinal motility.

GU Ketamine increases uterine tone.

Metabolic/Other The levels of circulating adrenaline and noradrenaline are increased following the administration of ketamine. The tone and activity of striated muscle may also increase.

Toxicity Transient rashes occur in 15% of patients receiving the drug. Emergence delirium, unpleasant dreams and hallucinations are notable complications of the use of ketamine (vi). The hypertonus produced by ketamine may require positioning of the patient prior to induction. Pain on injection (especially intramuscularly) may be alleviated by combination with lignocaine.

Kinetics

Absorption Ketamine is well absorbed after oral or intramuscular administration; the oral bioavailability is 20%.

Distribution Ketamine is 20–50% protein-bound in the plasma; the V_D is 3 l/kg. The distribution half-life is 11 minutes; recovery is thus primarily due to redistribution from brain to peripheral tissues.

Metabolism Ketamine is converted in the liver by N-demethylation and hydroxylation of the cyclohexylamine ring. Some of the metabolites are pharmacologically active.

Excretion The conjugated metabolites are excreted in the urine. The clearance is 17 ml/kg/min and the elimination half-life is 2.5 hours.

Special Points Antisialogogue premedication is recommended prior to the use of ketamine. Emergence phenomena are less frequent in the young and elderly. These may be reduced in incidence if the patient is left undisturbed during the recovery period or by premedication with opioid–hyoscine or opioid–hyoscine–droperidol. The incidence of unpleasant dreams is reduced by premedication with lorazepam or diazepam.

Ketamine, in low dose, reduces tourniquet hypertension under general anaesthesia.

Ketamine reduces the requirement for inotropic support in septic patients. In animal models of endotoxic shock, ketamine reduces pulmonary damage by enhancing haemodynamic stability and reducing pulmonary hypertension and extravasation.

Ketamine and thiopentone are pharmaceutically incompatible.

Incidents of abuse have been reported.

Labetalol

Uses   Labetalol is used in the treatment of:
1. all grades of hypertension
2. hypertensive emergencies and has been used
3. to produce controlled hypotension during anaesthesia
4. for the control of the reflex cardiovascular responses to intubation and
5. in the management of acute myocardial infarction.

Chemical   A synthetic salicylamide derivative.

Presentation   As a clear solution for injection containing 5 mg/ml, and as 50/100/200/400 mg tablets of labetalol hydrochloride.

Main Action   Antihypertensive.

Mode of Action   Labetalol acts by selective antagonism of alpha-1, beta-1 and beta-2 adrenoceptors (the ratio of alpha: beta effects is 1:3 when administered orally and 1:7 when administered intravenously). The drug has some intrinsic sympathomimetic activity at beta-2 adrenoceptors and may cause some vasodilation directly by stimulation of beta-2 receptors in vascular smooth muscle.

Routes of Administration/Doses   The adult oral dose is 100–800 mg 12-hourly. The drug may also be administered intravenously as a 5–20 mg bolus injected over 2 minutes, with subsequent increments to a maximum adult dose of 200 mg, or by infusion (diluted in dextrose or dextrose saline) at the rate of 20–160 mg/hour. When administered intravenously, labetalol acts in 5–30 minutes and has a mean duration of action of 50 minutes.

Patients should remain supine whilst receiving the drug via the intravenous route and subsequently assume the upright position cautiously, as profound postural hypotension may occur.

Effects

CVS   Intravenous labetalol causes a 20% (greater in hypertensive patients) decrease in the systolic and diastolic blood pressure; the heart rate and cardiac output may decrease by 10%. The drug reduces the systemic vascular resistance by 14%; limb blood flow increases and coronary vascular resistance may decrease. Labetalol inhibits platelet aggregation *in vitro*.

RS   With single doses, the drug has no effect on FEV_1, FVC or specific airways resistance in patients with obstructive airways disease. Chronic use of the drug has no clinically significant effect on respiratory function.

CNS   Labetalol has no effect on cerebral blood flow; autoregulation is well maintained.

GU Labetalol decreases renal vascular resistance by 20%, leading to an increase in renal blood flow. The glomerular filtration rate, however, remains unchanged.

Metabolic/Other The concentrations of adrenaline, nora-drenaline and prolactin increase acutely in hypertensive patients given labetalol intravenously. The drug may also decrease plasma renin activity and the concentration of angiotensin II. The ESR and serum transaminase concentration may increase following the administration of the drug; labetalol has no effect on plasma lipid concentration.

Toxicity/Side Effects
The side effects of beta-blockade (asthma, Raynaud's phenomenon, heart failure, cramps, night-mares etc.) occur less frequently during the use of labetalol than do the side effects of alpha-blockade (dizziness, formica-tion, nasal congestion etc.). Gastrointestinal disturbances may also complicate the use of labetalol.

Kinetics

Absorption
Labetalol is rapidly absorbed when adminis-tered orally but, due to a significant first-pass metabolism, the bioavailability shows an eight-fold variation (11–86%).

Distribution
The drug is 50% protein-bound in the plasma; the V_D is 2.5–15.7 l/kg.

Metabolism
Labetalol is extensively metabolised in the liver (and possibly in the gut-wall) to several inactive conjugates.

Excretion
Occurs predominantly as inactive conjugates in the urine (5% is excreted unchanged) with some appearing in the faeces. The clearance is 13–31 ml/min/kg) and the elimina-tion half-life is 3–8 hours. Renal impairment has no effect on the kinetics of labetalol; the dose should be reduced in the pres-ence of hepatic impairment.

Special Points
In the presence of concentrations of halothane >3%, labetalol causes a significant decrease in car-diac output, stroke volume, mean arterial pressure and central venous pressure.

Haemodialysis will remove <1% of a dose of labetalol.

Levo thyroxine/ Triiodothyronine

Uses   Thyroid hormones are used in the treatment of:
1. hypothyroidism
2. myxoedema coma and
3. goitre.

Chemical   Both hormones are iodine-containing amino acid derivatives of thyronine.

Presentation   Levo thyroxine is presented as tablets containing $50/100\,\mu g$ of levo thyroxine sodium. Triiodothyronine is presented as $20\,\mu g$ tablets and a white lyophilised powder for reconstitution in water containing $20\,\mu g$ of triiodothyronine.

Main Actions   Modulation of growth and metabolism.

Mode of Action   The thyroid hormones, probably predominantly triiodothyronine, combine with a 'receptor protein' within the cell nucleus and thereby activate the DNA transcription process leading to an increase in the rate of RNA synthesis and a generalised increase in protein synthesis.

Routes of Administration/Doses   The adult oral dose of levo thyroxine is 25–$300\,\mu g$ daily in divided doses, titrated according to the clinical response and results of thyroid function tests. The corresponding dose of triiodothyronine is 10–$60\,\mu g$ daily; the dose by the intravenous route is 5–$20\,\mu g$ 4–12 hourly; close monitoring is essential during intravenous administration. There is a 24-hour latency period before the effects of levo thyroxine are manifested; the peak effect occurs in 6–7 days. Triiodothyronine acts in 6 hours and the peak effect is observed within 24 hours.

Effects
CVS   The thyroid hormones are positively inotropic and chronotropic; these effects may be mediated by an increase in the number of myocardial beta-adrenergic receptors. The systolic blood pressure is increased by 10–$20\,\text{mmHg}$; the diastolic blood pressure decreases and mean arterial pressure remains unchanged. Vasodilation results from the increase in peripheral oxygen consumption; the circulating blood volume also increases slightly.
RS   The thyroid hormones increase the rate and depth of respiration secondary to the increase in the basal metabolic rate.
CNS   The hormones have a stimulatory effect on central nervous system function; tremor and hyperreflexia may result. Their physiological function also includes mediation of negative feedback on the release of thyroid-stimulating hormone from the pituitary.

AS   Appetite is increased following the administration of levo thyroxine or triiodothyronine; the secretory activity and motility of the gastrointestinal tract are also increased.

GU   The thyroid hormones are involved in the control of sexual function and menstruation.

Metabolic/Other   Thyroid hormones promote gluconeogenesis and increase the mobilisation of glycogen stores. Lipolysis is stimulated leading to an increase in the concentration of free fatty acids; hypercholesterolaemia may result from increased cholesterol turnover. The rate of protein synthesis is enhanced.

Toxicity/Side Effects   Excessive administration of the thyroid hormones results in the clinical state of thyrotoxicosis.

Kinetics

Absorption   Both levo thyroxine and triiodothyronine are completely absorbed when administered orally.

Distribution   Both hormones are bound to thyroid-binding globulin and thyroid-binding pre-albumin in the plasma; levo thyroxine is 99.97% bound and triiodothyronine is 99.5% bound. The V_D of levo thyroxine is 0.2 l/kg and that of triiodothyronine is 0.5 l/kg.

Metabolism   35% of levo thyroxine is converted to triiodothyronine in the periphery (predominantly in the liver and kidney) and some to inactive reverse T3. Both levo thyroxine and triiodothyronine undergo conjugation to glucuronide and sulphate and are excreted in the bile; some enterohepatic circulation occurs.

Excretion   20–40% of an administered dose is excreted in the faeces unchanged. The clearance of levo thyroxine is 1.7 ml/min and the elimination half-life is 6–7 days; the clearance of triiodothyronine is 17 ml/min and the elimination half-life is 2 days.

Special Points   The thyroid hormones increase the anticoagulant activity of co-administered warfarin. Beta-adrenergic antagonists interfere with the conversion of levo thyroxine to triiodothyronine and lead to a relative increase in the inactive reverse T3 fraction.

A 'sick' euthyroid state has been described in critical illness.

Lidocaine

Uses Lidocaine is used:
1. as a local anaesthetic and
2. in the treatment of ventricular dysrhythmias.

Chemical A tertiary amine which is an amide derivative of diethylaminoacetic acid.

Presentation As a clear, colourless 0.5/1/1.5/2% solution for injection of lidocaine hydrochloride (with or without 1:200 000 adrenaline); a gel containing 21.4 mg/ml of lidocaine hydrochloride (with or without chlorhexidine gluconate); a 5% ointment, a 10% spray and a 4% aqueous solution for topical application and as a cream/suppositories (in combination with hydrocortisone) for rectal administration.

Main Actions Reversible neural blockade and class Ib antiarrhythmic actions.

Mode of Action Local anaesthetics diffuse in their uncharged base form through neural sheaths and the axonal membrane to the internal surface of cell membrane sodium ion channels; here they combine with hydrogen ions to form a cationic species which enters the internal opening of the sodium ion channel and combines with a receptor. This produces blockade of the sodium ion channel, thereby decreasing sodium ion conductance and preventing depolarisation of the cell membrane.

Routes of Administration/Doses Lidocaine may be administered topically, by infiltration, intrathecally or epidurally; the toxic dose of lidocaine is 3 mg/kg (7 mg/kg with adrenaline). The adult intravenous dose for the treatment of acute ventricular dysrhythmias is a bolus injection of 1 mg/kg, administered over 2 minutes. This is normally followed by an infusion which begins at the rate of 4 mg/min for the first hour, 2 mg/min for the next hour and subsequently of 1 mg/min. Lidocaine acts in 2–20 minutes, dependent on the rate of administration and has a duration of action of 200–400 minutes (dependent upon the presence of vasoconstrictors and the concentration used).

Effects
CVS In low concentrations, lidocaine decreases the rate of phase IV depolarisation, the duration of the action potential, the effective refractory period and conduction velocity. It has few haemodynamic effects when used in low doses, except to cause a slight increase in the systemic vascular resistance leading to a mild increase in the blood pressure. In toxic concentrations, the drug decreases peripheral vascular resistance and myocardial contractility, producing hypotension and possibly cardiovascular collapse.

RS The drug causes bronchodilatation at subtoxic concentrations. Respiratory depression occurs in the toxic dose range.
CNS The principal effect of lidocaine is reversible neural blockade; this leads to a characteristically biphasic effect in the central nervous system. Initially, excitation (lightheadedness, dizziness, visual and auditory disturbances and fitting) occurs, due to the blockade of inhibitory pathways in the cortex; with increasing doses, depression of both facilitatory and inhibitory pathways occur, leading to central nervous system depression (drowsiness, disorientation and coma). Local anaesthetic agents block neuromuscular transmission when administered intra-arterially; it is thought that a complex of neuro-transmitter, receptor and local anaesthetic is formed which has negligible conductance.
AS Local anaesthetics depress contraction of the intact bowel.
Metabolic/Other Lidocaine may have some anticholinergic and antihistaminergic activity.

Toxicity/Side Effects Allergic reactions to the amide-type local anaesthetic agents are extremely rare. The side effects are predominantly correlated with excessive plasma concentrations of the drug, as described above. Lidocaine has a relatively narrow therapeutic index; its toxicity is related to the cardiac output (and therefore to the hepatic blood flow).

Kinetics

Absorption The absorption of local anaesthetic agents is related to:
1. the site of injection (intercostal > epidural > brachial plexus > subcutaneous)
2. the dose – a linear relationship exists between the total dose and the peak blood concentrations achieved and
3. the presence of vasoconstrictors, which delay absorption.
The bioavailability of lidocaine by the oral route is 24–46%, due to a high extraction and first-pass metabolism by the liver.

Distribution Lidocaine is 64% protein-bound in the plasma, predominantly to alpha-1 acid glycoprotein; the V_D is 0.7–1.5 l/kg.

Metabolism 70% of the dose is metabolised in the liver by N-dealkylation with subsequent hydrolysis to mono-ethyl-glycine and xylidide; the latter is further metabolised prior to excretion in the urine.

Excretion Less than 10% of an administered dose is excreted unchanged in the urine. The clearance is 6.8–11.6 ml/min/kg and the elimination half-life is 90–110 minutes. The clearance is reduced in the presence of cardiac and hepatic failure.

Lidocaine

Special Points The onset and duration of conduction blockade is related to the pKa, lipid solubility and extent of protein binding of the drug. A low pKa and a high lipid solubility are associated with a rapid onset time; a high degree of protein binding is associated with a long duration of action. The pKa of lidocaine is 7.7 and the heptane:buffer partition coefficient is 2.9.

Due to lidocaine's narrow therapeutic index, plasma concentrations of the drug need to be monitored in patients with cardiac and hepatic impairment.

Lidocaine is not removed by haemodialysis.

Intravenous administration of lidocaine decreases nitrous oxide and halothane requirements by 10% and 28%, respectively. Local anaesthetic agents significantly increase the duration of action of both depolarising and non-depolarising relaxants.

EMLA (Eutectic Mixture of Local Anaesthetics) is a white cream used to provide topical anaesthesia prior to venepuncture, and has also been used to provide anaesthesia for split-skin grafting. It contains 2.5% lidocaine and 2.5% prilocaine in an oil–water emulsion. When applied topically under an occlusive dressing, local anaesthesia is achieved after 1–2 hours and lasts for up to 5 hours. The preparation causes temporary blanching and oedema of the skin; detectable methaemoglobinaemia may also occur.

Linezolid

Uses Linezolid is used in the treatment of:
1. nosocomial and community-acquired pneumonia
2. complex skin and soft tissue infections and
3. MRSA infection.

Chemical An oxazolidinone.

Presentation As 600 mg tablets and a solution for intravenous administration containing 2 mg/ml of linelozid.

Main Action Antibacterial vs. a wide range of Gram-positive organisms, particularly *Enterococcus, Streptococcus* and *Staphylococcal* sp., and Gram-positive anaerobes including *Clostridium perfringens.*

Mode of Action Linezolid inhibits bacterial protein synthesis by binding specifically to the 50S ribisomal subunit, thereby preventing initiation complex formation.

Routes of Administration/Doses The adult oral and intravenous dose is 600 mg 12-hourly.

Toxicity/Side Effects Headache, abnormalities of liver function tests, taste alteration and gastrointestinal disturbances are common. Fertility may be affected reversibly. Skin and bleeding disorders, phlebitis and pancreatitis may also occur.

Kinetics

Absorption Linezolid is rapidly absorbed after oral administration and has an oral bioavailability approaching 100%.

Distribution The drug is 31% protein-bound in the plasma; the V_D is 0.64 l/kg.

Metabolism Linezolid is metabolised by oxidation to two inactive carboxylic acid metabolites.

Elimination 30% is excreted unchanged in the urine, the metabolites are excreted in the urine and faeces. The elimination half-life is 5 hours and the clearance 120 ml/min.

Special Points Linezolid is a reversible nonselective MAOI. It enhances the effects of ephedrine on the blood pressure.

Lithium

Uses Lithium is used in the treatment of:
1. mania and hypomania and in the prophylaxis of
2. recurrent bipolar depression
3. recurrent affective disorders and
4. as an adjunct in the treatment of chronic pain of non-malignant origin.

Chemical An alkali metal.

Presentation As tablets containing 200/250/400/450 mg of lithium carbonate.

Main Action Antipsychotic.

Mode of Action The precise mode of action of lithium is unknown; it may act by stabilisation of membranes or by alteration of central neurotransmitter function.

Route of Administration/Dose The adult oral dose is 0.4–1.2 g/day; serum levels should be monitored within one week of starting lithium and regularly thereafter, as the drug has a narrow therapeutic index. The therapeutic level is 0.5–1.5 mmol/l.

Effects
CVS Prolonged lithium therapy may lead to reversible ECG changes, especially T-wave depression.
CNS The drug has no effect on central nervous system function in normal subjects, although an increase in muscle tone occurs commonly. Lithium appears to lower the seizure threshold in epileptics.
GU Over one-third of patients receiving lithium develop polyuria and polydipsia due to antagonism of the effects of ADH.
Metabolic/Other With prolonged use of lithium, retention of sodium (secondary to an increase in aldosterone secretion) may occur, as may hypercalcaemia and hypermagnesaemia. The drug has mild insulin-like effects on carbohydrate metabolism.

Toxicity/Side Effects At therapeutic serum levels, disturbances of thyroid function, weight gain, tremor, pretibial oedema and allergic phenomena may occur. Excessive serum concentrations may result in nausea and vomiting, abdominal pain, diarrhoea, ataxia, convulsions, coma, dysrhythmias and death. Nephrogenic diabetes insipidus occurs in 5–20% of patients on long-term lithium treatment.

Kinetics

Absorption The drug is rapidly absorbed when administered orally; the bioavailability is 100%.

Distribution Lithium exhibits no demonstrable protein-binding in the plasma; the V_D is 0.45–1.13 l/kg.

Excretion 95% of a dose of lithium is excreted in the urine; the remainder in sweat. The clearance is 0.24–0.46 ml/min/kg and the elimination half-life is 14–30 hours.

Special Points Renal, cardiac and thyroid function should be monitored regularly during lithium therapy. Co-administration of lithium and diazepam has been reported to lead to hypothermia; the drug may also increase the duration of action of both depolarising and non-depolarising relaxants.

The drug is removed by haemodialysis.

Lorazepam

Uses   Lorazepam is used:
1. in the short-term treatment of anxiety
2. as a hypnotic
3. in premedication and
4. for the treatment of status epilepticus.

Chemical   A hydroxybenzodiazepine.

Presentation   As 1/2.5 mg tablets and as a clear, colourless solution for injection containing 4 mg/ml of lorazepam.

Main Actions
1. hypnosis
2. sedation
3. anxiolysis
4. anterograde amnesia
5. anticonvulsant and
6. muscular relaxation.

Mode of Action   Benzodiazepines are thought to act via specific benzodiazepine receptors found at synapses throughout the central nervous system, but concentrated especially in the cortex and mid-brain. Benzodiazepine receptors are closely linked with GABA receptors, and appear to facilitate the activity of the latter. Activated GABA receptors open chloride ion channels which then either hyperpolarise or short-circuit the synaptic membrane.

Routes of Administration/Doses   The adult oral or sublingual dose is 1–4 mg/day in divided doses. The intravenous or intramuscular dose is 0.025–0.05 mg/kg; intramuscular injection is painful.

Effects
CVS   Lorazepam appears to have no direct cardiac effects.
RS   Mild respiratory depression occurs following the administration of the drug, which is of clinical significance only in patients with lung disease.
CNS   The drug produces sedation, anterograde amnesia and an anticonvulsant effect.
AS   Lorazepam has no effect on basal gastric acid secretion, but decreases pentagastrin-stimulated gastric acid secretion by 25%.
Metabolic/Other   Circulating cortisol and glucose levels fall when lorazepam is used in premedication, probably secondarily to its anxiolytic effect.

Toxicity/Side Effects   Drowsiness, sedation, confusion and impaired coordination occur in a dose-dependent fashion. Paradoxical stimulation has been reported and occurs more frequently when hyoscine is administered concurrently.

Tolerance and dependence may occur with prolonged use of benzodiazepines; acute withdrawal of benzodiazepines in these circumstances may produce insomnia, anxiety, confusion, psychosis and perceptual disturbances.

Kinetics

Absorption   Lorazepam has a bioavailability of 90% when administered by the oral or intramuscular route.

Distribution   The drug is 88–92% protein-bound in the plasma; the V_D is 1 l/kg. Lorazepam is less extensively distributed than diazepam and thus has a longer duration of action, despite the shorter elimination half-life of lorazepam.

Metabolism   Lorazepam is conjugated directly in the liver to glucuronide to form an inactive water-soluble metabolite.

Excretion   80% of an orally-administered dose appears in the urine as the glucuronide. The clearance is 1 ml/min/kg and the elimination half-life is 8–25 hours – this is unaffected by renal disease.

Special Points   The co-administration of cimetidine does not impair the metabolic clearance of lorazepam.

The drug is not removed by haemodialysis.

Magnesium sulphate

Uses   Magnesium has been used in the management of:
1. pre-eclampsia and eclampsia
2. hypomagnesaemia associated with malabsorption syndromes (especially chronic alcoholism) and critical illness
3. premature labour (as a tocolytic)
4. acute myocardial infarction
5. torsade de pointes and other ventricular dysrhythmias
6. barium poisoning
7. asthma
8. cerebral oedema
9. spasms occurring with tetanus
10. autonomic hyperreflexia secondary to chronic spinal cord injury and is
11. a component of cardioplegic solutions.

Chemical   An inorganic sulphate.

Presentation   A clear, colourless solution of magnesium sulphate containing 2.03 mmol/ml of ionic magnesium.

Main Actions   Magnesium is an essential co-factor in over 300 enzyme systems. It is also essential for the production of ATP, DNA, RNA and protein function.

Mode of Action   The precise mechanism of magnesium's anticonvulsant activity remains unknown; it produces a dose-dependent pre-synaptic inhibition of acetylcholine release at the neuromuscular junction.

Routes of Administration/Doses   Magnesium sulphate may be administered intravenously or intramuscularly. A number of dose regimes have been described for the use of magnesium sulphate in the management of pre-eclampsia, e.g. 16 mmol administered intravenously over 20 minutes followed by an infusion of 4–8 mmol/hour. Serum concentrations should be monitored repeatedly and the dose adjusted correspondingly. Loss of deep tendon reflexes is a useful clinical sign of impending toxicity.

Effects
CVS   Magnesium acts peripherally to cause vasodilation and may cause hypotension when used in high doses. The drug slows the rate of SA node impulse formation and prolongs SA conduction time, the PR interval and AV nodal effective refractory period. Magnesium attenuates both the vasoconstrictor and arrhythmogenic actions of adrenaline.
RS   Magnesium is an effective bronchodilator and attenuates hypoxic pulmonary vasoconstriction.
CNS   The drug is a CNS depressant and exhibits anticonvulsant properties. High concentrations inhibit catechol release from adrenergic nerve terminals and the adrenal medulla.

AS Magnesium sulphate acts as an osmotic laxative when administered orally.

GU The drug exerts a renal vasodilator and diuretic effect. It decreases uterine tone and contractility; placental perfusion may increase secondary to a decrease in uterine vascular resistance. Magnesium crosses the placenta and may cause neonatal hypotonia and neonatal depression.

Metabolic/Other Magnesium prolongs the clotting time of whole blood, decreases thromboxane B_2 synthesis and inhibits thrombin-induced platelet aggregation.

Toxicity/Side Effects Minor side effects include warmth, flushing, nausea, headache and dizziness. Dose-related side effects include somnolence, areflexia, AV and intraventricular conduction disorders, progressive muscular weakness and cardiac arrest. The toxic effects can be reversed by the administration of calcium. Intramuscular injection of magnesium sulphate is painful.

Kinetics

Absorption 25–65% of ingested magnesium is absorbed.

Distribution Magnesium is 30% protein-bound in the plasma.

Excretion More than 50% of an exogenous magnesium load is excreted in the urine, even in the presence of significant magnesium deficiency.

Special Points Magnesium enhances the effects of other CNS depressants and neuromuscular blocking agents; 30–50% of the normal dose of non-depolarising relaxants should be used to maintain neuromuscular blockade in the presence of magnesium sulphate. Acute administration of magnesium sulphate prior to the use of suxamethonium appears to prevent potassium release and may reduce the incidence and severity of muscle pains.

Magnesium deficiency is present in 20–65% of patients receiving intensive care.

Mannitol

Uses   Mannitol is used:
1. to reduce the pressure and volume of cerebrospinal fluid
2. to preserve renal function during the peri-operative period in jaundiced patients and in those undergoing major vascular surgery
3. in the short-term management of patients with acute glaucoma
4. for bowel preparation prior to colorectal procedures
5. to initiate a diuresis in transplanted kidneys and
6. in the treatment of rhabdomyolysis.

Chemical   An alcohol, derived from Dahlia tubers.

Presentation   As sterile, pyrogen-free solutions of 10% and 20% mannitol in water; crystallisation may occur at low temperatures.

Main Action   Osmotic diuresis and antioxidant.

Mode of Action   Mannitol is a low-molecular-weight (182 daltons) compound and is thus freely filtered at the glomerulus and not reabsorbed; neither does it cross the intact blood–brain barrier. Its action as a diuretic rests upon the fact that it increases the osmolality of the glomerular filtrate and tubular fluid, increasing urinary volume by an osmotic effect. Mannitol decreases CSF volume and pressure by:
1. decreasing the rate of CSF formation and
2. by withdrawing brain extracellular water across the blood–brain barrier into the plasma; if the barker is disrupted, mannitol passes into the brain extravascular space and is ineffective.
Mannitol also acts as a hydroxyl radical scavenger.

Routes of Administration/Doses   For the reduction of elevated intracranial pressure, a dose of 1 g/kg is infused intravenously over 15 minutes prior to operative treatment. Subsequently, intermittent doses of 0.25–0.5 g/kg may be used for the treatment of persistently elevated intracranial pressure. The diuretic dose is 0.5–1 g/kg. Mannitol acts within a few minutes and lasts 1–4 hours.

The oral dose for bowel preparation is 100 ml of the 20% solution – care should be taken to maintain adequate hydration.

Effects
CVS   The acute administration of mannitol increases the cardiac output; blood pressure increases by 5–10 mmHg.
CNS   Mannitol induces a significant reduction in intracranial pressure with preservation of cerebral blood flow in patients with intact autoregulation; in patients with defective autoregulation,

a minimal reduction in intracranial pressure with an increase in cerebral blood flow occurs.

GU   Renal blood flow is increased and the rate of renin secretion decreases; mannitol washes out the medullary interstitial gradient, leading to a decreased ability to produce concentrated urine. Diuresis occurs 1–3 hours after administration.

Metabolic/Other   The plasma sodium and potassium concentrations may fall and urea increase with the use of high doses of mannitol.

Toxicity/Side Effects   Circulatory overload and rebound increases in intracranial pressure may occur following the use of mannitol. Allergic responses are rare; the drug is irritant to tissues and veins. Mannitol may have toxic effects on distal convoluted tubule and collecting duct cells, causing vacuolisation.

Kinetics

Absorption   After oral administration, approximately 17.5% is absorbed in the small bowel.

Distribution   The drug shows a biphasic distribution to plasma and extracellular water; complex fluid shifts occur in response to this. The V_D is 0.47 l/kg.

Metabolism   Mannitol is not metabolised in man.

Excretion   The drug is excreted unchanged in the urine: the clearance is 7 ml/min/kg and the elimination half-life is 72 minutes.

Special Points   Blood should not be co-administered with mannitol. A total dose exceeding 3 g/kg/day may produce a serum osmolality greater than 320 mOsm/l. Rebound increases in intracranial pressure may occur after the cessation of mannitol therapy.

Metaraminol

Uses   Metaraminol is used as an adjunct in the treatment of:
1. hypotension occurring during general or spinal anaesthesia and
2. for the management of hypotension occurring during cardiopulmonary bypass.

Chemical   A synthetic sympathomimetic amine.

Presentation   As a clear solution containing 10 mg/ml of metaraminol tartrate.

Main Action   Peripheral vasoconstriction.

Mode of Action   Metaraminol is a direct- and indirect-acting sympathomimetic agent that has agonist effects at both alpha- and beta-adrenoceptors, although alpha-agonist activity predominates.

Routes of Administration/Doses   The adult dose by intravenous infusion of metaraminol diluted in saline or dextrose should be titrated according to response; bolus doses of 0.5–5 mg may be administered intravenously with extreme caution. The corresponding intramuscular or subcutaneous dose for the prevention of hypotension is 2–10 mg. The onset of effect after intravenous administration occurs within 1–2 minutes with maximum effect at 10 minutes and lasts 20–60 minutes.

Effects
CVS   Metaraminol causes a sustained increase in the systolic and diastolic blood pressure due to an increase in the systemic vascular resistance; it also increases pulmonary vascular resistance. A reflex bradycardia occurs; the drug has positive inotropic properties and the cardiac output may decrease or remain unchanged in normal subjects. The coronary blood flow is increased by metaraminol by an indirect mechanism.
RS   The drug causes a slight decrease in the respiratory rate and an increase in the tidal volume.
CNS   The cerebral blood flow is decreased by the administration of metaraminol.
GU   The renal blood flow is decreased by metaraminol. The drug causes contraction of the pregnant uterus.
Metabolic/Other   Metaraminol increases glycogenolysis and inhibits insulin release leading to hyperglycaemia. Lipolysis is similarly increased. The drug may also increase oxygen consumption and body temperature.

Toxicity/Side Effects   Headaches, dizziness, tremor and nausea and vomiting may occur with the use of the drug. Rapid and large increases in blood pressure resulting in left ventricular failure and cardiac arrest have been reported after the administration of metaraminol. Extravascular injection of the drug may lead to tissue necrosis and abscess formation at the injection site.

Kinetics   There are no quantitative data available.

Metformin

Uses Metformin is used in the treatment of non-insulin-dependent (type II) diabetes mellitus.

Chemical A biguanide.

Presentation As 500/850 mg tablets of metformin hydrochloride.

Main Action Hypoglycaemia.

Mode of Action Biguanides have no effect in the absence of circulating insulin; they do not alter insulin concentration but do enhance its peripheral action. They appear to act by inhibiting the intestinal absorption of glucose and decreasing the peripheral utilisation of glucose, both by increasing the rate of anaerobic glycolysis and by decreasing the rate of gluconeogenesis.

Route of Administration/Dose The adult oral dose is 1.5–3 g daily, in divided doses. Metformin has a duration of action of 8–12 hours.

Effects
AS Metformin reduces the intestinal absorption of glucose, folate and vitamin B_{12}; it has no effects on gastric motility. The drug may also increase the intestinal utilisation of glucose and cause weight loss.
Metabolic/Other Metformin increases the sensitivity to the peripheral actions of insulin by increasing the number of low-affinity binding sites for insulin in red blood cells, adipocytes, hepatocytes and skeletal muscle cells. The drug does not cause hypoglycaemia in diabetic subjects receiving metformin monotherapy. Metformin inhibits the metabolism of lactate and causes a decrease in the plasma triglyceride, cholesterol and prebeta-lipoprotein concentrations.

Toxicity/Side Effects Metformin is normally well tolerated; gastrointestinal disturbances may occur. Lactic acidosis may complicate the use of the drug rarely.

Kinetics

Absorption The drug is slowly absorbed from the small intestine; the oral bioavailability is 50–60%.

Distribution Metformin is not protein-bound, in the plasma.

Metabolism No metabolites of the drug have been detected in man.

Excretion   The drug is excreted essentially unchanged in the urine. The clearance exceeds the glomerular filtration rate, implying active tubular secretion. The elimination half-life is 1.7–4.5 hours. The drug is not recommended for use in patients with renal impairment.

Methohexitone

Uses Methohexitone is used for the induction and maintenance of anaesthesia.

Chemical A methylated oxybarbiturate.

Presentation As a white crystalline powder in vials containing 0.1/0.5 g of methohexitone sodium mixed with sodium carbonate; this is dissolved in water before administration to yield a clear, colourless solution with a pH of 11 and a pKa of 7.9 which is stable in solution for 6 weeks.

Main Action Hypnotic.

Mode of Action Barbiturates are thought to act primarily at synapses by depressing post-synaptic sensitivity to neurotransmitters and by impairing pre-synaptic neurotransmitter release. Multi-synaptic pathways are depressed preferentially; the reticutar activating system is particularly sensitive to the depressant effects of barbiturates. The action of barbiturates at the molecular level is unknown. They may act in a manner analogous to that of local anaesthetic agents by entering cell membranes in the unionised form, subsequently becoming ionised and exerting a membrane-stabilising effect by decreasing sodium and potassium ion conductance, decreasing the amplitude of the action potential and slowing the rate of conduction in excitable tissue. In high concentrations, barbiturates depress the enzymes involved in glucose oxidation, inhibit the formation of ATP and depress calcium-dependent action potentials. They also inhibit calcium-dependent neurotransmitter release and enhance chloride ion conductance in the absence of GABA.

Routes of Administration/Doses The drug is usually administered intravenously in a dose of 1–1.5 mg/kg; it acts in one arm–brain circulation time and awakening occurs in 2–3 minutes. The drug may also be administered intramuscularly in a dose of 6.6 mg/kg or rectally in a dose of 15–20 mg/kg.

Effects
CVS Methohexitone has negatively inotropic effects and decreases systemic vascular resistance; it may also depress transmission in autonomic ganglia and thus lead to hypotension.
RS Methohexitone is a more powerful respiratory depressant than thiopentone and obtunds the ventilatory response to both hypoxia and hypercarbia. The drug may cause pronounced coughing and hiccuping.
CNS At low doses, methohexitone may cause paradoxical excitement. Induction of anaesthesia with the drug is associated with an increased incidence of excitatory phenomena

when compared to thiopentone. Methohexitone decreases both the cerebral blood flow and intracranial pressure. The drug may cause epileptiform EEG patterns; abnormal muscle movements may also occur due to neurotransmitter release.

AS The drug causes some depression of intestinal activity and constriction of the splanchnic vasculature.

GU Methohexitone decreases renal plasma flow and increases ADH secretion, leading to a decrease in urine output. It has no effect on the tone of the gravid uterus.

Metabolic/Other The drug decreases the production of superoxide anions by polymorphonuclear leucocytes.

Toxicity/Side Effects Methohexitone causes pain on injection in up to 80% of patients. It is less irritant than thiopentone when extravasation occurs, but when administered intra-arterially may lead to arterial constriction and thrombosis. Anaphylactoid reactions occur with a frequency similar to that observed with thiopentone. Nausea and vomiting may complicate the use of methohexitone.

Kinetics

Distribution The drug is 51–65% protein-bound in the plasma, predominantly to albumin; 20% is sequestered in red blood cells; the V_D is 1.13 l/kg. The rapid onset of action of the drug is due to:

1. the high blood flow to the brain
2. the lipophilicity of the drug and
3. its low degree of ionisation – only the non-ionised fraction crosses the blood–brain barrier (methohexitone is 75% non-ionised at pH 7.4: hyperventilation increases the non-bound fraction and increases the anaesthetic effect). The relatively brief duration of anaesthesia following a bolus of methohexitone is due to redistribution to muscle and later to fat. Methohexitone has a shorter duration of action than thiopentone due to its very short distribution half-life and a high clearance, which is four times greater than that of thiopentone.

Metabolism Occurs in the liver, primarily to a 4-hydroxymetabolite.

Excretion The metabolites are excreted in the urine, < 1% of the dose is excreted unchanged. The clearance is 7.9–13.9 ml/min/kg and the elimination half-life is 1.8–6 hours.

Special Points The drug may induce acute clinical and biochemical manifestations in patients with porphyria and is also not recommended for use in epileptics. Methohexitone should be used with caution in patients with fixed cardiac output states, hepatic or renal dysfunction, myxoedema, dystrophia myotonica, myasthenia gravis, familial periodic paralysis, and in the elderly or in patients who are hypovolaemic.

Methoxamine

Uses   Methoxamine is used for:
1. the correction or prevention of hypotension during spinal or general anaesthesia and cardiopulmonary bypass and
2. the treatment of supraventricular tachycardias.

Chemical   A synthetic sympathomimetic amine.

Presentation   As a clear solution containing 20 mg/ml of methoxamine hydrochloride.

Main Actions   Peripheral vasoconstriction and bradycardia.

Mode of Action   Methoxamine is a selective alpha-1 adrenergic agonist.

Routes of Administration/Doses   Methoxamine is administered intravenously at a rate of 1 mg/min to a total dose of 5–10 mg in an adult; it acts within 1–2 minutes and has a duration of action of 1 hour. The corresponding intramuscular dose is 5–20 mg when the onset of action is 15–20 minutes and duration of effect is 90 minutes.

Effects
CVS   Methoxamine commonly produces a reflex and intrinsic bradycardia, accompanied by an increase in the systolic and diastolic blood pressure and central venous pressure. The drug has no effect on the cardiac output, but prolongs the effective refractory period and slows atrio-ventricular conduction.
RS   The drug has no effect on respiratory function.
AS   Contraction of gastrointestinal sphincters follows the administration of methoxamine.
GU   The drug produces renal arterial vasoconstriction leading to a fall in the glomerular filtration rate. Contraction of the pregnant uterus and a decrease in uterine blood flow may occur.
Metabolic/Other   Mydriasis, piloerection and diaphoresis are produced by the drug. Glycogenolysis and gluconeogenesis are stimulated; this is accompanied by a decrease in insulin secretion.

Toxicity/Side Effects   Headaches, projectile vomiting, sensations of coldness and the desire to urinate have been reported in association with the use of methoxamine.

Kinetics   There are no data available.

Special Points   The drug may precipitate severe hypertension in patients with uncontrolled hyperthyroidism or who are receiving monoamine oxidase inhibitors or tricyclic antidepressants.

Methyldopa

Uses   Methyldopa is used in the treatment of:
1. hypertension and
2. pre-eclampsia.

Chemical   A phenylalanine derivative.

Presentation   As 125/250/500 mg tablets and a suspension containing 50 mg/ml of methyldopa. A solution for intravenous administration containing 50 mg/ml of methyldopa hydrochloride is also available.

Main Actions   Antihypertensive.

Mode of Action   Methyldopa is metabolised to alpha-methyl noradrenaline which is stored in adrenergic nerve terminals within the central nervous system; the latter is a potent agonist at alpha-2 (pre-synaptic) nerve terminals and reduces central sympathetic discharge, thereby lowering the blood pressure (cf. clonidine).

Routes of Administration/Dose   The adult oral dose is 0.5–3 g/day in 2–3 divided doses.

Effects
CVS   Methyldopa decreases the systemic vascular resistance with little accompanying change in either cardiac output or heart rate. Postural hypotension occurs uncommonly with the use of the drug.
GU   Methyldopa has little effect on the renal or uteroplacental blood flow, the glomerular filtration rate or filtration fraction.
Metabolic/Other   Plasma renin activity and noradrenaline concentrations decrease after administration of the drug.

Toxicity/Side Effects   The reported side effects after the administration of methyldopa are legion. Cardiovascular disturbances that may result from the use of the drug include orthostatic hypotension, bradycardia and peripheral oedema. Central nervous system disturbances may also occur, including sedation, depression, weakness, paraesthesiae and dizziness. Gastrointestinal, dermatological and haematological disturbances, including thrombocytopenia, a positive Coomb's test (in 10—20%) and haemolytic anaemia have also been reported. Methyldopa may also cause hepatic damage.

Kinetics

Absorption   Methyldopa has a variable absorption when administered orally; the bioavailability is 8–62% by this route, due to a significant first-pass metabolism.

Distribution   The drug is 50% protein-bound in the plasma; the V_D is 0.21–0.37 l/kg.

Metabolism   Methyldopa is conjugated to sulphate as it traverses the intestinal mucosa, and is metabolised in the liver to a variety of poorly characterised metabolites.

Excretion   20–40% of an administered dose is excreted in the urine; two-thirds of this unchanged. The clearance is 2.2–4 ml/min/kg and the elimination half-life is 2.1–2.8 hours.

Special Points   The hypotension effects of the drug are additive with those produced by volatile anaesthetic agents; methyldopa also decreases the apparent MAC of the latter.

   The action of the drug is prolonged in the presence of renal failure; it is removed by haemodialysis.

   Methyldopa commonly produces nasal congestion; care should be exercised during nasal intubation in patients receiving the drug.

Methylphenidate

Uses   Methylphenidate is used for the treatment of:
1. attention-deficit/hyperactivity disorder (ADHD)
2. narcolepsy and has been used for the treatment of
3. post-anaesthetic shivering
4. hiccuping during general anaesthesia
5. depression and
6. brain injury.

Chemical   A piperidine derivative.

Presentation   As 5/10/20 mg tablets of methylphenidate hydrochloride.

Main Actions   Central nervous stimulation.

Mode of Action   Methylphenidate binds to the dopamine transporter in pre-synaptic cell membranes, blocking its re-uptake, thereby increasing extracellular dopamine levels. It also affects norepinephrine re-uptake and binds weakly to 5HT receptors.

Routes of Administration/Doses   The drug is administered orally, to a maximum of 60 mg/day in divided doses.

Effects
CVS   The drug causes dose-dependent hypertension and tachycardia.
CNS   Methylphenidate causes generalised CNS stimulation.
Endocrine/Metabolic   Methylphenidate decreases growth velocity.

Toxicity/Side Effects   Insomnia, nervousness, anorexia, hypertension and tachycardia occur relatively frequently. The drug has significant potential for abuse.

Kinetics

Absorption   Methylphenidate is almost completely absorbed after oral administration.

Distribution   The drug exhibits a low degree of protein binding.

Metabolism   Occurs primarily to deesterification to ritalinic acid.

Excretion   60–80% of the dose is administered in the urine. The elimination half-life is 2.5 hours.

Metoclopramide

Uses Metoclopramide is used in the treatment of:
1. digestive disorders, e.g. hiatus hernia, reflux oesophagitis and gastritis
2. nausea and vomiting due to a variety of causes, e.g. drugs (general anaesthetic agents, opiates and cytotoxic gents), radiotherapy, hepatic and biliary disorders
3. diagnostic radiology of the gastrointestinal tract
4. migraine and
5. post-operative gastric hypotonia.

Chemical A chlorinated procainamide derivative.

Presentation As 10 mg tablets, 15 mg slow-release capsules, a syrup containing 1 mg/ml and as a clear, colourless solution for injection containing 5 mg/ml of metoclopramide hydrochloride.

Main Actions Increased gastrointestinal motility and antiemetic.

Mode of Action The effects of metoclopramide on gastrointestinal motility appear to be mediated by:
1. antagonism of peripheral dopaminergic (D_2-) receptors
2. augmentation of peripheral cholinergic responses and
3. a direct action on smooth muscle to increase tone.

The antiemetic effects of the drug appear to be mediated by:
1. central dopaminergic (D_2-) blockade leading to an increased threshold for vomiting at the chemoreceptor trigger zone and
2. a decrease in the sensitivity of visceral nerves supplying afferent information to the vomiting centre.

Routes of Administration/Doses Metoclopramide may be administered orally, intravenously or intramuscularly; the adult does by all routes is 10 mg 8-hourly. A dose of 1–2 mg/kg is recommended for the treatment of nausea and vomiting associated with cisplatin treatment.

Effects

CVS There have been occasional reports of hypotension during general anaesthesia and cardiac arrest, dysrhythmias and hypertension in patients with phaeochromocytoma following the administration of metoclopramide.

CNS Metoclopramide raises the threshold for vomiting at the chemoreceptor trigger zone and prevents apomorphine-induced vomiting in man. The drug has neuroleptic effects (including an antipsychotic action) as would be expected of a centrally-acting dopamine antagonist.

AS Metoclopramide increases the tone of the lower oesophageal sphincter by about 17 mmHg, accelerates gastric emptying and the amplitude of gastric contractions, and accelerates small intestinal transit time. Its effects on large bowel motility are variable. The drug has no effect on gastric secretion.

GU The drug may increase ureteric peristaltic activity.

Metabolic/Other Metoclopramide stimulates prolactin release and also causes a transient increase in aldosterone secretion.

Toxicity/Side Effects Occur in 11% of patients receiving the drug; drowsiness, dizziness, faintness and bowel disturbances are the most frequently reported side effects. Extrapyramidal side effects occur, the most common manifestations are akathisia and oculogyric crises; extrapyramidal effects occur more frequently with higher doses, in patients with renal impairment and in the elderly. The neuroleptic malignant syndrome has been reported in association with metoclopramide.

Kinetics

Absorption The drug is rapidly absorbed after oral administration and has a bioavailability by this route of 32–97%. This wide variability is due primarily to first-pass conjugation to sulphate.

Distribution Metoclopramide is 13–22% protein bound in the plasma; the V_D is 2.2–3.4 l/kg.

Metabolism Occurs primarily in the liver; the major metabolite is a sulphate derivative. Two other metabolites have been identified in man.

Excretion 80% of an oral dose is excreted in the urine within 24 hours; 20% of this is unchanged and the remainder appears as non-metabolised drug conjugated to a sulphate or glucuronide and as the sulphated metabolite. The clearance is 8.8–11.6 ml/min/kg and the elimination half-life is 2.6–5 hours.

Metoclopramide is not significantly removed by haemodialysis.

Metronidazole

Uses Metronidazole is used for:
1. the treatment and prophylaxis of infections due to anaerobic bacteria, especially *Bacteroides fragilis* and *Clostridia* sp., and the treatment of
2. protozoal infections such as amoebiasis, giardiasis and trichomoniasis
3. acute dental infections and
4. pseudomembranous colitis.

Chemical A synthetic imidazole derivative.

Presentation As 200/400/500 mg tablets; 500 mg or 1 g suppositories and as a clear, colourless, 0.5% solution for intravenous injection of metronidazole.

Main Actions Metronidazole is an antimicrobial agent with a high degree of activity against anaerobes and protozoa.

Mode of Action The drug acts via a reactive intermediate which reacts with bacterial DNA so that the resultant DNA complex can no longer function as an effective primer for DNA and RNA polymerases – all nucleic acid synthesis is thus effectively terminated.

Routes of Administration/Doses The adult oral dose is 200–800 mg, and the corresponding rectal dose is 1 g 8-hourly. The intravenous dose is 500 mg 8-hourly, administered at a rate of 5 ml/min.

Effects
Metabolic/Other Metronidazole decreases the cholesterol content of bile.

Toxicity/Side Effects Unpleasant taste, nausea and vomiting, gastrointestinal disturbances, rashes and darkening of urine have been reported. Peripheral neuropathy and leucopenia may occur with chronic use of the drug.

Kinetics

Absorption The bioavailability of oral metronidazole is 80%, and by the rectal route is 75%.

Distribution Metronidazole is distributed in virtually all tissues and body fluids in concentrations that do not differ markedly from their serum levels. Approximately 10% is protein-bound in the plasma. The V_D is 0.75 l/kg.

Metabolism Occurs by oxidation and glucuronidation in the liver.

Excretion 60% of the dose is excreted unchanged in the urine; the drug does not usually accumulate in renal failure. The clearance is 1.22 ml/kg/min and the elimination half-life is 6–10 hours.

Special Points Metronidazole increases the anticoagulant effect of warfarin and exhibits a disulfiram-like interaction with alcohol producing an acute confusional state.

Prolongation of the action of vecuronium by the co-administration of the drug has been demonstrated in animals.

Metronidazole may cause reddish-brown discoloration of the urine.

Metronidazole is removed by haemodialysis.

Midazolam

Uses Midazolam is used:
1. for induction of anaesthesia
2. for sedation during endoscopy and procedures performed under local anaesthesia and during intensive care
3. as a hypnotic
4. for premedication prior to general anaesthesia and may be of use
5. in the treatment of chronic pain, including deafferentation syndromes.

Chemical A water-soluble imidazobenzodiazepine.

Presentation As a clear, colourless solution of midazolam hydrochloride containing 1/2/5 mg/ml.

Main Actions
1. hypnosis
2. sedation
3. anxiolysis
4. anterograde amnesia
5. anticonvulsant and
6. muscular relaxation.

Mode of Action Benzodiazepines are thought to act via specific benzodiazepine receptors found at synapses through-out the central nervous system, but concentrated especially in the cortex and mid-brain. Benzodiazepine receptors are closely linked with GABA receptors, and appear to facilitate the activity of the latter. Activated GABA receptors.open chloride ion channels which then either hyperpolarise or short-circuit the synaptic membrane. Midazolam has kappa-opioid against activity *in vitro*, which may explain the mechanism of benzo-diazepine-induced spinal analgesia.

Routes of Administration/Doses The intramuscular dose (used for premedication) is 0.07–0.08 mg/kg; the intra-venous dose for sedation is 0.07–0.1 mg/kg, titrated according to response. The end point for sedation is drowsiness and slur-ring of speech – response to commands is, however, maintained. The drug may also be administered intrathecally in an adult dose of 0.3–2 mg or epidurally in a dose of 0.1–0.2 mg/kg.

Effects
CVS Systolic blood pressure decreases by 5% and diastolic pressure by 10% and the systemic vascular resistance falls by 15–33% following the administration of the drug; the heart rate increases by 18%. Midazolam in combination with fen-tanyl obtunds the pressor response to intubation to a greater extent than thiopentone in combination with fentanyl.

RS   Midazolam decreases the tidal volume but this is offset by an increase in the respiratory rare; the minute volume is thus little changed. Apnoea occurs in 10–77% of patients when midazolam is used as an induction agent. The drug impairs the ventilatory response to hypercapnia.

CNS   The drug produces hypnosis, sedation and anterograde amnesia. There have been no studies of the anticonvulsant activity of midazolam in man. The cerebral oxygen consumption and cerebral blood flow are decreased in a dose-related manner, but a normal relationship is maintained between the two. When administered intrathecally or epidurally, the drug has antinociceptive effects.

AS   A midazolam fentanyl induction sequence is associated with a lower incidence of post-operative vomiting than with a thiopentone fentanyl sequence. The drug reduces hepatic blood flow.

GU   Midazolam decreases renal blood flow.

Metabolic/Other   Midazolam decreases the adrenergic but not the cortisol and renin response to stress. The drug causes significant inhibition of phagocytosis and leucocyte bacteriocidal activity.

Toxicity/Side Effects   Side effects are confined to occasional discomfort at the site of injection. Withdrawal phenomena may occur in children after prolonged infusion.

Kinetics

Absorption   The bioavailability when administered by the oral route is 44% and by the intramuscular route is 80–100%.

Distribution   The drug is 96% protein-bound in the plasma; the V_D is 0.8–1.5 l/kg. The V_D may increase to 3.1 l/kg in the critically ill.

Metabolism   Midazolam is virtually completely metabolised in the liver to hydroxylated derivatives which are then conjugated to a glucuronide. Metabolites bind to CNS benzodiazepine receptors and are pharmacologically active.

Excretion   Occurs in the urine, predominantly as the hydroxylated derivatives; renal impairment thus has little effect. The clearance is 5.8–9 ml/min/kg and the elimination half-life is 1.5–3.5 hours. The elimination half-life may increase to 5.4 hours in the critically ill.

Special Points   The short duration of action of midazolam is due to its high lipophilicity, high metabolic clearance and rapid rate of elimination. However, this may not be the case after prolonged dosing on intensive care.

The use of midazolam in premedication decreases the MAC of volatile agents by approximately 15%.

The clinical effects of the drug can be reversed by physostigmine, glycopyrronium and flumazenil.

Mivacurium

Uses Mivacurium is used to facilitate intubation and controlled ventilation.

Chemical A benzylisoquinolinium which is a mixture of three stereoisomers; *trans-trans* (57%), *cis-trans* (36%) and *cis-cis* (4–8%). The *cis-cis* isomer is estimated to have one-tenth of the neuromuscular blocking potency of the other two stereoisomers.

Presentation As a clear, pale-yellow aqueous solution in 5 and 10 ml ampoules containing 2 mg/ml of mivacurium chloride.

Main Action Competitive neuromuscular blockade.

Mode of Action Mivacurium acts by competitive antagonism of acetylcholine at nicotinic (N2) receptors at the postsynaptic membrane of the neuromuscular junction.

Route of Administration/Doses Mivacurium is administered intravenously; the normal intubating dose is 0.07–0.15 mg/kg (0.1–0.2 mg/kg for children aged 2–12 years). Maintenance doses of 0.1 mg/kg are required at approximately 15-minute intervals. The drug may also be infused at a rate of 360–420 µg/hour (600–1000 µg/hour for children aged 2–12). Satisfactory intubating conditions are produced within 2.5 minutes; a single dose will last 10–20 minutes. The mean recovery index is 6.6 minutes. The drug is non-cumulative with repeated administration.

Effects
CVS Mivacurium has minimal cardiovascular effects; a slight (7%) transient decrease in blood pressure and slight (7%) increase in heart rate may occur after rapid intravenous injection. The drug has no significant vagal or ganglion blocking properties in the normal dosage range.
RS Neuromuscular blockade leads to apnoea; bronchospasm may occur secondary to histamine release.

Toxicity/Side Effects Transient cutaneous flushing is the most common side effect. Hypotension, tachycardia, bronchospasm and urticaria may all occur with an incidence of less than 1%.

Kinetics

Distribution The V_D of the *trans-trans* isomer is 0.1 l/kg and that of the *cis-trans* isomer is 0.3 l/kg.

Metabolism The primary mechanism of metabolism of mivacurium is enzymatic hydrolysis by plasma cholinesterases to yield a quaternary alcohol and a quaternary monoester metabolite, which appear to be inactive. Some hydrolysis by liver esterases also occurs.

Excretion   The metabolites are excreted in the bile and urine, together with some unchanged drug. The clearance of the *trans-trans* isomer is 53 ml/kg/minute and the elimination half-life is 2.3 minutes. The clearance of the *cis-trans* isomer is 92 ml/kg/minute and the elimination half-life is 2.1 minutes. Renal failure increases the clinical duration of action of mivacurium by a factor of 1.5 and hepatic failure increases it by a factor of 3.

Special Points   The duration of action of mivacurium is prolonged by isoflurane and enflurane and to a lesser extent by halothane. The following drugs may enhance the neuromuscular effects of mivacurium: aminoglycoside antibiotics, propranolol, calcium channel blockers, diuretics, magnesium and lithium salts. The following drugs may reduce plasma cholinesterase activity and similarly enhance the activity of mivacurium: oral contraceptives, glucocorticoids and monoamine oxidase inhibitors.

Mivacurium does not act as a trigger agent for malignant hyperpyrexia in animal models.

The drug is physically incompatible with alkaline solutions (e.g. barbiturates).

Morphine

Uses Morphine is used:
1. for premedication
2. as an analgesic in the management of moderate to severe pain
3. in the treatment of left ventricular failure
4. to provide analgesia during terminal care and
5. in combination with kaolin in the symptomatic treatment of diarrhoea.

Chemical A phenanthrene derivative.

Presentation As 5/10/30/60/100/200 mg tablets, a syrup containing 2/10/20 mg/ml, as 15/30 mg suppositories and as a clear, colourless solution for injection containing 10/15/30 mg/ml of morphine sulphate, preservative-free morphine must be used for epidural/spinal use.

Main Actions Analgesia and respiratory depression.

Mode of Action Morphine is an agonist at mu- and kappa-opioid receptors. Opioids appear to exert their effects by increasing intracellular calcium concentration, which in turn increases potassium conductance and hyperpolarisation of excitable cell membranes. The decrease in membrane excitability that results may decrease both pre- and post-synaptic responses.

Routes of Administration/Doses The initial adult oral dose is 5–20 mg 4-hourly, increased as required. The dose by the rectal route is 15–30 mg 4-hourly. The corresponding intramuscular or subcutaneous dose is 0.1–0.2 mg/kg and the intravenous dose is 0.05–0.1 mg/kg 3–4 hourly. Morphine may also be administered intrathecally; an adult dose of 0.2–1 mg has been recommended. The drug has a peak analgesic effect 30–60 minutes after intramuscular injection and has a duration of effect of 3–4 hours.

Effects
CVS Morphine has minimal effects on the cardiovascular system; the predominant effect is that of orthostatic hypotension secondary to a decrease in the systemic vascular resistance, at least part of which is mediated by histamine release. The drug may also cause bradycardia when administered in high doses.
RS The principal effect of the drug is respiratory depression, with a decreased ventilatory response to hypoxia and hypercapnia. Morphine also has a potent antitussive action. Bronchoconstriction may occur with the use of high doses of the drug.

CNS   Morphine is a potent analgesic agent, and may also cause drowsiness, relief of anxiety and euphoria. Miosis is produced by the drug as a result of stimulation of the Edinger-Westphal nucleus. Seizures and muscular rigidity may occur with the use of high doses of morphine.

AS   Morphine decreases gastrointestinal motility and decreases gastric acid, biliary and pancreatic secretion; it also increases the common bile duct pressure by causing spasm of the sphincter of Oddi. The drug may also cause nausea, vomiting and constipation.

GU   The drug increases the tone of the ureters, bladder detrusor muscle and sphincter and may precipitate urinary retention.

Metabolic/Other   Mild diaphoresis and pruritus may result from histamine release. Morphine increases the secretion of ADH and may therefore lead to impaired water excretion and hyponatraemia. The drug causes a transient decrease in adrenal steroid secretion.

Toxicity/Side Effects   Respiratory depression, nausea and vomiting, hallucinations and dependence may complicate the use of morphine. Pruritus may occur after epidural or spinal administration of the drug.

Kinetics

Absorption   Morphine is well absorbed when administered orally, the bioavailability by this route is 15–50% due to an extensive first-pass metabolism.

Distribution   The drug is 20–40% protein-bound in the plasma, predominantly to albumin; the V_D is 3.4–4.7 l/kg. Morphine equilibrates slowly between the plasma and CSF; there is no clear correlation between the degree of analgesia and the plasma concentration of the drug.

Metabolism   Occurs in the liver to morphine-3-glucuronide, morphine-6-glucuronide and normorphine. In animal models morphine-6-glucuronide has analgesic effects and morphine-3-glucuronide has effects on arousal. Enterohepatic cycling of the metabolites probably does not occur.

Excretion   Occurs predominantly in the urine as the glucuronide conjugates; 7–10% appears in the faeces as conjugated morphine. The clearance is 12–23 ml/min/kg and the elimination half-life is 1.7–4.5 hours. Cumulation of morphine-6-glucuronide occurs in the presence of renal failure; a reduction in the dose of the drug is necessary under these circumstances.

Special Points   Morphine should be used with caution in the presence of hepatic failure, as the drug may precipitate encephalopathy. Similarly, the use of the drug in patients with hypopituitarism may precipitate coma. In common with

Morphine

other opioids, morphine decreases the apparent MAC of co-administered volatile agents. The actions of the drug are all reversed by naloxone, although the analgesia afforded by the epidural administration of morphine is well preserved after the administration of naloxone.

Morphine is not removed by haemodialysis or by peritoneal dialysis.

Nalbuphine

Uses Nalbuphine is used:
1. for premedication and
2. as an analgesic in the treatment of moderate to severe pain.

Chemical A semi-synthetic phenanthrene derivative.

Presentation As a clear, colourless solution for injection containing 10 mg/ml of nalbuphine hydrochloride.

Main Action Analgesia.

Mode of Action Nalbuphine is an agonist at kappa-opioid receptors and an antagonist at mu-opioid receptors; it thus produces analgesia (a kappa-effect) whilst antagonising both the respiratory depressant effects and the potential for dependency that are associated with the mu-receptor.

Routes of Administration/Doses The drug may be administered intravenously, intramuscularly or subcutaneously in an adult dose of 10–20 mg. Nalbuphine acts within 2–3 minutes when administered intravenously and within 15 minutes when administered intramuscularly. The duration of action is 3–6 hours.

Effects
CVS Nalbuphine has little significant effect on the heart rate, mean arterial pressure, systemic or pulmonary vascular resistance or cardiac output.
RS The drug has a respiratory depressant effect equal to that of morphine, but demonstrates a ceiling effect at a dose of 0.5 mg/kg. It will antagonise the respiratory depressant effects of co-administered pure mu-agonists, whilst adding to the analgesic effect of the latter.
CNS Nalbuphine has an analgesic potency equivalent to that of morphine. It has no euphoriant effects.
AS The drug causes less inhibition of gastrointestinal activity than other opioids.

Toxicity/Side Effects Sedation, dizziness, vertigo, dry mouth and headache may complicate the use of nalbuphine. The drug causes less nausea and vomiting, psychotomimetic effects and dependence than does morphine.

Kinetics

Absorption The bioavailability by the oral route is 12–17% due to a significant first-pass hepatic metabolism. The bioavailability is 80% by the intramuscular and subcutaneous routes.

Distribution   Nalbuphine is 25–40% protein-bound in the plasma; the V_D is 162–498 l.

Metabolism   Occurs predominantly in the liver to two inactive conjugates which are secreted into the bile.

Excretion   The metabolites are predominantly excreted (with some unchanged nalbuphine) via the faeces. A small fraction is excreted unchanged in the urine. The clearance is 0.8–2.3 l/min and the elimination half-life is 110–160 minutes. Care should be exercised during the use of the drug in patients with renal or hepatic impairment.

Special Points   Nalbuphine is ineffective in obtunding the cardiovascular responses to laryngoscopy and intubation. The drug will precipitate withdrawal symptoms in opiate addicts; its effects are reversed by naloxone.

Nalbuphine has been used in the management of postoperative shivering.

Naloxone

Uses Naloxone is used for:
1. the reversal of respiratory depression due to opioids
2. the diagnosis of suspected opioid overdose and has been used in the treatment of
3. clonidine overdose
4. obesity and
5. septic shock.

Chemical A substituted oxymorphone derivative.

Presentation As a clear solution for injection containing 0.02/0.4 mg/ml of naloxone hydrochloride.

Main Actions Reversal of mu-opioid receptor effects, i.e. sedation, hypotension, respiratory depression and the dysphoric effects of partial agonists. The drug will precipitate acute withdrawal symptoms in opiate addicts.

Mode of Action Naloxone is a competitive antagonist at mu-, delta-, kappa- and sigma-opioid receptors.

Routes of Administration/Doses For the reversal of opioid-induced respiratory depression, the drug should be administered intravenously in small incremental doses until the desired end point of reversal of respiratory depression without reversal of analgesia is reached; in adults, 0.1–0.2 mg will normally achieve this effect. In the treatment of known or suspected opioid overdose, 0.4–2.0 mg may be administered intravenously, intramuscularly or subcutaneously. The drug acts within 2 minutes when administered intravenously, and has a duration of effect (approximately 20 minutes) that may be shorter than the opioid whose effects it is desired to counteract. It may therefore be necessary to administer additional doses of naloxone intravenously or intramuscularly.

Effects
CVS The drug has no effect at normal doses; in doses >0.3 mg/kg the blood pressure may increase. Naloxone has been shown to reverse the hypotension associated with endotoxic and hypovolaemic shock in some animal studies.
CNS Naloxone causes slight drowsiness at very high doses. Some forms of stress-induced analgesia are obtunded by naloxone; the drug also decreases the tolerance to pain in subjects with high pain thresholds.
AS Naloxone reverses opioid-induced spasm of the sphincter of Oddi.

Toxicity/Side Effects There are two reports of serious ventricular dysrhythmias occurring in patients with irritable myocardia after the administration of naloxone.

Kinetics

Absorption The drug is 91% absorbed when administered orally, but has a bioavailability by this route of 2%, due to an extensive first-pass metabolism.

Distribution The drug is 46% protein-bound in adult plasma. The V_D is 2 l/kg.

Metabolism The drug is metabolised in the liver, primarily by conjugation to glucuronide.

Excretion The clearance is 25 ml/min/kg and the plasma half-life is 1.2 hours.

Special Points Naloxone is effective in alleviating the pruritus, nausea and respiratory depression associated with the epidural or spinal administration of opioids.

Neostigmine

Uses Neostigmine is used:
1. for the reversal of non-depolarising neuromuscular blockade and in the treatment of
2. myasthenia gravis
3. paralytic ileus and
4. urinary retention.

Chemical A quaternary amine which is an ester of an alkyl carbamic acid.

Presentation As 15 mg tables of neostigmine bromide and as a clear, colourless solution for injection containing 2.5 mg/ml of neostigmine metilsulfate. A fixed dose combination containing 0.5 mg of glycopyrronium and 2.5 mg of neostigmine metilsulfate per ml is also available.

Main Actions Cholinergic.

Mode of Action Neostigmine is a reversible, acid-transferring cholinesterase inhibitor which binds to the esteratic site of acetylcholinesterase and is hydrolysed by the latter, but at a much slower rate than is acetylcholine. The accumulation of acetylcholine at the neuromuscular junction allows the competitive antagonism of any non-depolarising relaxant that may be present.

Routes of Administration/Doses The adult oral dose is 15–50 mg 2–4 hourly. The intravenous dose for the reversal of non-depolarising neuromuscular blockade is 0.05–0.07 mg/kg, administered slowly and in combination with an appropriate dose of an anticholinergic agent. The peak effect of the drug when administered intravenously occurs at 7–11 minutes; a single dose of neostigmine has a duration of action of 40–60 minutes.

Effects
CVS The effects of neostigmine on the cardiovascular system are variable and depend upon the prevailing autonomic tone. The drug may cause bradycardia, leading to a fall in cardiac output; it decreases the effective refractory period of cardiac muscle and increases conduction time in conducting tissue. In high doses, neostigmine may cause hypotension secondary to a central effect.
RS Neostigmine increases bronchial secretion and may cause bronchoconstriction.
CNS In small doses, the drug has a direct action on skeletal muscle leading to muscular contraction. In high doses, neostigmine may block neuromuscular transmission by the combination of a direct effect and by allowing the accumulation of acetylcholine. Miosis and failure of accommodation may be precipitated by the administration of the drug.

AS The drug increases salivation, lower oesophageal and gastric tone, gastric acid output and lower gastrointestinal tract motility. Nausea and vomiting may occur.

GU Neostigmine increases ureteric peristalsis and may lead to involuntary micturition.

Metabolic/Other Sweating and lachrymation are increased.

Toxicity/Side Effects The side effects are manifestations of its pharmacological actions as described above. Cardiac arrest has been reported after the use of neostigmine.

Kinetics Data are incomplete.

Absorption Neostigmine is poorly absorbed when administered orally; the bioavailability by this route is 1–2%.

Distribution The drug is highly ionised and therefore does not cross the blood–brain barrier to any significant extent. Neostigmine is 6–10% protein-bound in the plasma, the V_D is 0.4–1 l/kg.

Metabolism Neostigmine is predominantly metabolised by plasma esterases to a quaternary alcohol; some hepatic metabolism with subsequent biliary excretion may also occur.

Excretion 50–67% of an administered dose is excreted in the urine. The clearance is 5.7–11.1 ml/min/kg and the elimination half-life is 15–80 minutes; the clearance is decreased and the elimination half-life is increased in the presence of renal impairment.

Special Points Neostigmine prolongs the duration of action of suxamethonium. There is some evidence that the use of neostigmine to reverse neuromuscular blockade is associated with an increased incidence of gastrointestinal anastamotic breakdown.

Nifedipine

Uses   Nifedipine is used in the treatment of:
1.   angina
2.   mild to severe hypertension (including pregnancy-induced hypertension)
3.   Raynaud's phenomenon and
4.   coronary artery spasm occurring during coronary angiography or angioplasty.

Chemical   A dihydropyridine derivative.

Presentation   As 5/10 mg capsules and a slow-release preparation containing 10/20/30/60 mg per tablet. A fixed dose combination with atenolol is also available.

Main Actions   Relaxation of arterial smooth muscle in both the coronary and peripheral circulations.

Mode of Action   Nifedipine causes competitive blockade of cell membrane slow calcium channels leading to decreased influx of calcium ions into cells. This produces electromechanical decoupling, inhibition of contraction and relaxation of cardiac and smooth muscle fibres and leads to a negative inotropic effect and vasodilation. It may also act by increasing red cell deformability and preventing platelet clumping and thromboxane release.

Routes of Administration/Doses   The adult oral dose of nifedipine is 10–20 mg 8-hourly (20–40 mg 12-hourly for the slow-release preparation), 100–200 μg may be infused via a coronary catheter over 2 minutes.

Effects
CVS   The mean arterial pressure decreases by 20–33%; this effect is more pronounced in hypertensive patients. This is accompanied by a reflex increase in heart rate by up to 28%. The systemic and pulmonary vascular resistance, left ventricular end-diastolic and pulmonary artery pressure all decrease. Cardiac output is increased; nifedipine also causes a sustained relaxation of epicardial conductance vessels, leading to increased coronary blood flow in patients with ischaemic heart disease. Nifedipine is 3–10 times more effective in inhibiting contraction in coronary artery smooth muscle than in myocardial contractile cells. The drug may also protect the myocardium during reperfusion after cardiac bypass.
RS   Nifedipine demonstrates no intrinsic bronchodilator effect in most studies. The drug appears to inhibit hypoxic pulmonary vasoconstriction.
CNS   The drug causes a marginal increase in the cerebral blood flow due to vasodilation of large cerebral vessels.

AS Contractility throughout the gut and lower oesophageal pressure are decreased by nifedipine. The hepatic blood flow is increased.

GU Nifedipine has no marked effect on the renal blood flow or glomerular filtration rate. Uterine activity is decreased by the drug.

Metabolic/Other Plasma renin activity and catecholamines are increased; short-term use may decrease glucose tolerance. Platelet aggregation is impaired by the drug; thromboxane synthesis is inhibited and nifedipine may thus decrease thromboxane-induced coronary artery spasm.

Toxicity/Side Effects Occur in 20% of patients; head-ache, flushing and dizziness (secondary to vasodilation) are common; oedema of the legs, eye pain and gum hyperplasia have been reported.

Kinetics

Absorption Nifedipine is completely absorbed when administered orally; the bioavailability by this route is 45–68%.

Distribution The drug is 92–98% protein-bound in the plasma, the V_D is 0.62–1.12 l/kg.

Metabolism 95% of the dose is metabolised in the liver to three inactive metabolites.

Excretion 90% of the metabolites are excreted in the urine, the rest in the faeces. The clearance is 27–66 l/hour and the elimination half-life is 1.3–11 hours, dependent upon the route of administration.

Special Points Nifedipine is a safe and effective drug for the treatment of post-surgical hypertension; the reduction in mean arterial pressure is associated with an increase in cardiac index and systemic oxygen transport.

All volatile agents in current use decrease calcium ion release from the sarcoplasmic reticulum and decrease calcium ion flux into cardiac cells; the negatively inotropic effects of nifedipine are thus additive with those of the volatile agents. When used in combination with isoflurane, the negative inotropic effects of the drugs are additive and may result in a profound decrease in cardiac output.

Experiments in animals have demonstrated an increased risk of sinus arrest if volatile agents and calcium antagonists are used concurrently. If withdrawn acutely (especially in the post-operative period) after chronic oral use, severe rebound hypertension may result.

Calcium antagonists may also:
1. reduce the MAC of volatile agents by up to 20% and

Nifedipine

2. increase the efficacy of neuromuscular blocking agents.

Administration of nifedipine immediately prior to induction appears to aggravate redistribution hypothermia.

The drug is not removed by dialysis.

Nimodipine

Uses Nimodipine is used:
1. in the prevention and treatment of cerebral vasospasm secondary to subarachnoid haemorrhage and may be of use in the management of
2. migraine
3. acute cerebrovasular accidents and
4. drug-resistant epilepsy.

Chemical A dihydropyridine.

Presentation As an intravenous infusion containing 200 µg/ml of nimodipine and 30 mg tablets.

Main Action Dilation of cerebral vessels leading to improved cerebral perfusion.

Mode of Action Nimodipine is a calcium antagonist that binds to specific sites in the cell membranes of vascular smooth muscle and prevents calcium ion influx through 'slow' calcium ion channels, leading to vasodilation; the drug has a relatively specific action on cerebral arterioles.

Routes of Administration/Dose The drug should be administered into a running crystalloid infusion via a central vein at the rate of 1 mg/hour for the first two hours and there-after at the rate of 2 mg/hour for 5–14 days.

Effects
CVS In normal subjects, doses of >2 mg/hour decrease the systolic and diastolic blood pressure. In the anaesthetised patient, an infusion of 1 µg/kg/min decreases the systemic vascular resistance by 10–40% and increases cardiac output by 25–45%.
CNS Nimodipine increases the cerebral blood flow by up to 18% with no demonstrable 'steal' effect in patients who have had a subarachnoid haemorrhage. The use of nimodipine in such patients leads to a significant reduction in mortality and morbidity.

Toxicity/Side Effects Side effects occur infrequently, although flushing, headache, nausea, hypotension and reversible abnormalities of liver function tests may complicate the use of the drug.

Kinetics

Absorption Nimodipine is rapidly and well absorbed when administered orally, but has a bioavailability by this route of only 3–28% due to a significant first-pass metabolism.

Distribution The drug is 98% protein-bound in the plasma; the V_D is 0.94–2.3 l/kg.

Metabolism Nimodipine is initially demethylated and dehydrogenated to an inactive pyridine analogue which subsequently undergoes further degradation.

Excretion Half of the dose appears as metabolites in the urine, and a third in the faeces. The clearance is 420–520 l/hour and the elimination half-life is 0.9–7.2 hours (dependent upon the route of administration). The clearance is decreased by hepatic impairment; the effect of renal impairment is unclear.

Special Points Nimodipine has some effect in obtunding the cardiovascular responses to intubation and surgical stimulation; the peak blood pressures post-intubation and post-incision are consistently 10–15% lower in patients receiving the drug than those recorded in untreated patients.

The drug is adsorbed onto polyvinyl chloride tubing and is also light-sensitive; however, it remains stable in diffuse daylight for up to 10 hours.

Nitric oxide

Uses Nitric oxide (NO) is used as a selective pulmonary vasodilator in:
1. acute lung injury and
2. pulmonary hypertension and may be of use in the treatment of
3. bronchospasm and
4. chronic obstructive airways disease.

Chemical An inorganic gas.

Presentation In aluminium or stainless steel cylinders containing 100/1000/2000 p.p.m. nitric oxide in nitrogen; the cylinders are typically of 40 l capacity. Pure nitric oxide is toxic and corrosive. The gas is not licensed for use in the United Kingdom.

Main Action Vasodilation.

Mode of Action Nitric oxide is produced *in vivo* by NO synthase which uses the substrate L-arginine. Nitric oxide diffuses to the vascular smooth muscle layer and stimulates guanylate cyclase; the cGMP produced activates a phosphorylation cascade which leads to smooth muscle relaxation and vasodilation.

Route of Administration/Dose Nitric oxide is administered by inhalation in a dose of 5–80 p.p.m.; the drug is injected into the patient limb of the inspiratory circuit of a ventilator. The delivery system is designed to minimize the oxidation of nitric oxide to nitrogen dioxide. Monitoring of nitric oxide concentrations can be achieved by a chemiluminescent monitor or electrochemical detector.

Effects
CVS Nitric oxide is a potent vasodilator that mediates the hypotension and significant vascular leak characteristic of septic shock. Inhaled nitric oxide is a selective pulmonary vasodilator, since it is avidly bound to haemoglobin and thereby inactivated before reaching the systemic circulation. Nitric oxide released from vascular endothelium inhibits platelet aggregation and attenuates platelet and white cell adhesion. Inhaled nitrous oxide prolongs the bleeding time in volunteers.
RS Nitric oxide inhibits hypoxic pulmonary vasoconstriction and preferentially increases blood flow through well-ventilated areas of the lung, thereby improving ventilation:perfusion relationships.
CNS Nitric oxide increases cerebral blood flow and appears to have a physiological role as a neurotransmitter within the autonomic and central nervous systems.
AS Nitric oxide is a determinant of gastrointestinal motility and appears to modulate morphine-induced constipation.

GU   Nitric oxide may play a role in the regulation of tenin production and sodium homeostasis in the kidney. It is the physiological mediator of penile erection.

Metabolic/Other   Nitric oxide release from macrophages reacts with superoxide ion to form the free radical peroxynitrite, which is toxic to bacteria. Insulin release appears to be modulated by nitric oxide.

Toxicity/Side Effects   Exposure to 500–2000 p.p.m of nitric oxide results in methaemoglobinaemia and pulmonary oedema. Contamination by nitrogen dioxide can similarly lead to pneumonitis and pulmonary oedema.

Kinetics

Absorption   Nitric oxide is highly lipid soluble and diffuses freely across cell membranes.

Metabolism   The gas is rapidly converted to nitrates and nitrites in the presence of oxygen. Inhaled nitric oxide readily reacts with oxidised haemoglobin to yield methaemoglobin; nitric oxide has a half-life <5 seconds.

Special Points   Prolonged inhalation (up to 27 days) of the gas appears safe and is not associated with tachyphylaxis.

Abrupt cessation of nitric oxide can cause a profound decrease in P_aO_2 and increase in pulmonary artery pressure, possibly via down-regulation of endogenous NO production or guanylate cyclase activity.

Mortality does not appear to be affected by the administration of NO in ARDS.

Nitrous oxide

Uses Nitrous oxide is used:
1. as an adjuvant to general anaesthesia
2. as an analgesic during labour and other painful procedures and
3. for cryotherapy.

Chemical An inorganic gas.

Presentation As a liquid in cylinders at a pressure of 44 bar at 15 °C; the cylinders are blue and are available in five sizes (C-G, containing 450–9000 l respectively). Nitrous oxide is a colourless gas with a sweet smell; it is non-flammable but does support combustion. The specific gravity of the gas is 1.53, the boiling point −88°C, the critical temperature 36.5°C and the critical pressure 71.7 atmospheres. The MAC of nitrous oxide is 105, the oil/water solubility coefficient 3.2 and the blood/gas solubility coefficient is 0.47.

Entonox is the trade name given to a 50/50 mixture of oxygen and nitrous oxide. It is available in cylinders which are blue with white shoulders and are of two sizes (G and J, containing 3200 and 6400 l respectively). At normal temperatures, both of the components of Entonox are present in pressurised cylinders in the gaseous phase (due to the Poynting effect); liquefaction of nitrous oxide and separation of the two components may occur at temperatures of −7°C.

Main Actions Analgesia and depression of the central nervous system.

Mode of Action The mode of action of nitrous oxide is unknown; it may act by modulation of enkephalins and endorphins within the central nervous system.

Route of Administration/Dose Nitrous oxide is administered by inhalation; a concentration of 70% in oxygen is conventionally used as a adjunct to general anaesthesia. Entonox is used to provide analgesia for a range of painful procedures.

Effects
CVS Nitrous oxide decreases myocardial contractility *in vitro*; *in vivo*, the mean arterial pressure is usually well maintained by a reflex increase in peripheral vascular resistance. A deterioration in left ventricular function occurs when nitrous oxide is added to a high-dose opioid oxygen anaesthetic sequence, volatile agents or a propofol infusion.
RS The gas causes a slight depression of respiration, with an attendant decrease in tidal volume and increase in respiratory rate. Nitrous oxide is non-irritant and does not cause bronchospasm.

CNS Nitrous oxide is a central nervous system depressant and when administered in a concentration of 80% will cause loss of consciousness in most subjects. The gas is a powerful analgesic in concentrations of >20%. The administration of nitrous oxide increases intracranial pressure.

GU Nitrous oxide has no effect on uterine tone.

Toxicity/Side Effects 15% of patients receiving nitrous oxide will experience nausea and vomiting. The gas is 35 times more soluble than nitrogen in the blood; nitrous oxide will therefore cause an increase in the size of air-filled spaces (e.g. pneumothorax, intestines, air cysts and the middle ear) in the body. A further manifestation of this physical property of the gas is the Fink effect (diffusion hypoxia): when nitrous oxide is discontinued, the ingress of the gas into the alveoli lowers the alveolar oxygen concentration. The prolonged use of high concentrations of nitrous oxide (>6 hours) leads to inactivation of the cobalamin component of methionine synthetase and to a reduction in thymidine and DNA synthesis. The resultant clinical syndrome is akin to pernicious anaemia; megaloblastic anaemia and pancytopenia. Protracted use of the gas may also lead to the development of a peripheral neuropathy. Nitrous oxide is teratogenic in animals when administered during early pregnancy.

Kinetics

Absorption Nitrous oxide diffuses freely across the normal alveolar epithelium. The rate of uptake of the gas is increased by a decreased cardiac output, an increased concentration and by increased alveolar ventilation. Due to its relative insolubility, the alveolar concentration of nitrous oxide approaches the inspired concentration fairly rapidly; 90% equilibration occurring within 15 minutes and 100% equilibration within 5 hours.

Metabolism Little, if any, metabolism occurs in man.

Excretion Nitrous oxide is excreted unchanged through the lungs and skin.

Special Points Nitrous oxide exhibits both the concentration and second gas effects. The concentration effect implies that the greater inspired anaesthetic concentration, the more rapid will be the rise in alveolar concentration. The second gas effect refers to the ability of one gas administered in a high concentration (e.g. nitrous oxide) to accelerate the uptake of another gas (e.g. halothane) that is administered simultaneously, the rapid absorption of the nitrous oxide increasing the alveolar concentration of the halothane.

70% nitrous-oxide in oxygen decreases the MAC of halothane to 0.29, that of enflurane to 0.6 and of isoflurane to 0.5. The use of nitrous oxide appears to be safe in patients susceptible to malignant hyperthermia.

Norepinephrine

Uses Norepinephrine is used in the treatment of refractory hypotension.

Chemical A catecholamine.

Presentation As a clear, colourless solution containing 2 mg/ml of norepinephrine bitartrate for dilution prior to infusion.

Main Action Increased systemic vascular resistance.

Mode of Action Norepinephrine is a directly and indirectly acting sympathomimetic amine that exerts its action predominantly at alpha-adrenergic receptors, with a minor action at beta-receptors.

Route of Administration/Dose Norepinephrine is administered through a central vein as an infusion in dextrose or saline in a concentration of 4 µg/ml at a rate titrated according to the response desired. The drug has a duration of action of 30–40 minutes; tachyphylaxis occurs with prolonged administration.

Effects
CVS Norepinephrine increases the peripheral vascular resistance, leading to an increase in the systolic and diastolic blood pressure; the cardiac output remains unchanged or decreases slightly. Reflex vagal stimulation leads to a compensatory bradycardia. The drug produces coronary vasodilation leading to a marked increase in coronary blood flow. The circulating blood volume is reduced by norepinephrine, due to loss of protein-free fluid to the extracellular fluid. Norepinephrine may also cause nodal rhythm, atrio-ventricular dissociation and ventricular dysrhythmias.
RS The drug causes a slight increase in the minute volume accompanied by a degree of bronchodilatation.
CNS The cerebral blood flow and oxygen consumption are decreased by the administration of norepinephrine; mydriasis also occurs.
AS The hepatic and splanchnic blood flow are decreased by the drug.
GU Norepinephrine decreases the renal blood flow; the glomerular filtration rate is usually well maintained. The tone of the bladder neck is increased. Norepinephrine increases the contactility of the pregnant uterus; this may lead to fetal bradycardia and asphyxia.
Metabolic/Other Norepinephrine may decrease insulin secretion, leading to hyperglycaemia; the concentration of free fatty acids and the plasma renin activity may increase.

Toxicity/Side Effects Anxiety, headache, photophobia, pallor, sweating, gangrene and chest pain may occur with the use of the drug. Extravasation of norepinephrine may lead to sloughing and tissue necrosis.

Kinetics

Absorption Norepinephrine undergoes significant first-pass metabolism and is inactive when administered orally.

Distribution The V_D is 0.09–0.4 l/kg.

Metabolism Exogenous norepinephrine is metabolised by two pathways; by oxidative deamination to the aldehyde by mitochondrial monoamine oxidase (in liver, brain and kidney) and by methylation by cytoplasmic catechol-O-methyl-transferase to normetanephrine. The predominant metabolite appearing in the urine is 3-methoxy, 4-hydroxymandelic acid (VMA).

Excretion 5% of an administered dose of norepinephrine is excreted unchanged; the clearance is 27.9–100 ml/min/kg and the half-life is 0.57–2.4 minutes.

Special Points The use of norepinephrine during halothane anaesthesia may lead to the appearance of serious cardiac dysrhythmias; if co-administered with MAOIs or tricyclic anti-depressants, serious hypertensive episodes may be precipitated.

The drug is pharmaceutically incompatible with barbiturates and sodium bicarbonate.

Omeprazole

Uses Omeprazole is used in the treatment of:
1. peptic ulcer disease
2. peptic oesophagitis and
3. the Zollinger-Ellison syndrome.

Chemical A substituted benzimidazole derivative.

Presentation As capsules containing 10/20/40 mg of omeprazole and in 40 mg vials as a powder of the sodium salt of omeprazole.

Main Actions Inhibition of basal and stimulated gastric acid secretion.

Mode of Action Omeprazole acts via a derivative which binds irreversibly to parietal cell H^+-K^+-ATPase and non-competitively inhibits it. The activity of the parietal cell 'proton pump', which represents the final common pathway of H^+ secretion, is thus inhibited.

Route of Administration/Doses The adult oral dose for the treatment of peptic ulcer disease is 20–40 mg daily for a period of 4–8 weeks; the corresponding dose for the treatment of the Zollinger-Ellison syndrome is 20–120 mg daily. The intravenous dose is administered over 5 minutes.

Effects
AS Omeprazole significantly reduces the volume of gastric juice but has no effect on the rate of gastric emptying. A single 20 mg dose will effectively control acid secretion for 24 hours. In animals, orally administered omeprazole appears to confer protection against stress-induced gastric ulceration.
Metabolic/Other The drug has no demonstrable effect on endocrine function.

Toxicity/Side Effects Omeprazole is usually well tolerated; rashes, nausea, headache, gastrointestinal disturbances, liver dysfunction and arrhythmia may occur.

Kinetics

Absorption Oral omeprazole is rapidly absorbed and has a bioavailability of 40–97%, dependent upon the formulation and dose. The drug may increase its own bioavailability, since degradation occurs under acidic conditions.

Distribution The drug is 95–96% protein-bound in the plasma, predominantly to albumin and alpha-1-acid glycoprotein. The V_D is 0.3–0.4 l/kg.

Metabolism Omperazole is rapidly and completely metabolised by oxidation to a sulphone, reduction to a sulphide and by hydroxylation.

Excretion 80% of an oral dose is excreted in the urine, the remainder in the faeces. The clearance is 533–666 ml/min and the elimination half-life is 0.5–1.5 hours.

Special Points Omeprazole is 2–10 times as potent as cimetidine; furthermore, it heals ulcers significantly more rapidly than conventional H_2-antagonist regimes and may be effective in patients resistant to conventional therapy.

The pharmacokinetics of the drug are unaltered by renal impairment and it is not removed by haemodialysis; no dose reduction is required in patients with renal or hepatic impairment. Omeprazole decreases the clearance of co-administered diazepam, phenytoin and warfarin.

The role of omeprazole in the prevention of stress ulceration in critically ill patients remains to be evaluated. The value of omeprazole in anaesthetic premedication is questionable.

Ondansetron

Uses Ondansetron is used:
1. in the management of nausea and vomiting induced by chemotherapy and radiotherapy and
2. in the prevention and treatment of post-operative nausea and vomiting.

Chemical A synthetic carbazole.

Presentation As a clear, colourless aqueous solution in 2/4 ml ampoules containing 2 mg/ml ondansetron hydrochloride dihydrate and as 4/8 mg tablets.

Main Action Antiemetic.

Mode of Action Ondansetron is a highly selective antagonist at 5-HT_3 receptors and acts both centrally and peripherally. Emetogenic stimuli appear to cause release of 5-HT in the small intestine and initiate a vomiting reflex by activating vagal afferents via 5-HT_3 receptors; ondansetron blocks the initiation of this reflex. Activation of vagal afferents may also result in release of 5-HT in the area postrema, promoting emesis via a central mechanism.

Routes of Administration/Doses For the management of post-operative nausea and vomiting, the adult dose is 8 mg 8-hourly orally or a single intramuscular or intravenous dose of 4 mg.

Effects
CVS Ondansetron has no demonstrable effects on the cardiovascular system.
RS The drug has no effect on the ventilatory response to CO_2.
CNS Ondansetron has no sedative effects and does not impair performance in psychomotor tests.
AS The drug has no effect on gastric motility, but does increase large bowel transit time.
Mecabolic/Other Ondansetron has no effect on serum prolactin concentration or haemostatic function.

Toxicity/Side Effects Constipation, headache and flushing may occur. Anaphylaxis has also been reported.

Kinetics

Absorption Ondansetron is rapidly absorbed after oral administration and has a bioavailability of 60%.

Distribution The drug is 76% protein-bound in the plasma; the V_D is 2 l/kg.

Metabolism Ondansetron is extensively metabolised by hydroxylation or N-demethylation of the indole nucleus, followed by conjugation with glucuronic acid or sulphate.

Excretion   Less than 5% is excreted unchanged in the urine. The clearance is 6.3 ml/min/kg and the elimination half-life is 3 hours.

Special Points   No alteration of dose is needed in patients with renal impairment; hepatic impairment significantly prolongs the serum half-life of ondansetron and the dose should be limited to 8 mg/day.

Ondansetron may reduce the incidence of post-anaesthetic shivering.

Oxygen

Uses   Oxygen is used:
1. in the management of all forms of hypoxia (other than histotoxic)
2. as an adjunct in the management of shock and in the treatment of
3. carbon monoxide poisoning
4. pneumatosis coli
5. decompression sickness and
6. anaerobic infections.

Chemical   A gaseous inorganic element.

Presentation   As a compressed gas in cylinders at a pressure of 137 bar at 15 °C; the cylinders are black with white shoulders and are available in six sizes (C-J, containing 170–88001 respectively). Oxygen is also available commercially in liquid form, one volume of liquid oxygen yielding 840 volumes of gaseous oxygen.

Oxygen is a colourless, odourless, tasteless gas which supports combustion and is explosive in the presence of grease. The specific gravity of the gas is 1.105, the critical temperature −118.4 °C and the critical pressure 50.8 atmospheres.

Main Action   Oxygen's essential role is in the process of oxidative phosphorylation.

Mode of Action   Elemental oxygen is combined with hydrogen ions via mitochondrial cytochrome oxidase; the energy released is used for the synthesis of ATP.

Route of Administration   Oxygen is administered by inhalation; many devices are used for its administration and inspired concentrations of up to 100% may be achieved.

Effects
CVS   The administration of 100% oxygen causes a slight decrease in the heart rate (due to an effect on chemoreceptors), a slight increase in diastolic blood pressure and a decrease of 8–20% in cardiac output, due to myocardial depression. The coronary blood flow decreases secondary to coronary arterial vasoconstriction. In contrast, the pulmonary vascular resistance and the mean pulmonary artery pressure decrease.
RS   Mild respiratory depression (due to a decrease in sensitivity of the respiratory centre to carbon dioxide) results from the administration of 100% oxygen. Nitrogen is eliminated from the lungs within 2 minutes (leading to atelectasis subsequent to the loss of the 'splinting' effect of nitrogen), from the blood within 5 minutes and from the body within 2 hours. The binding of oxygen with haemoglobin tends to displace carbon dioxide from the blood (the Haldane effect).

CNS   The administration of 100% oxygen causes cerebrovascular constriction (due to an increased sensitivity to adrenergic agonists), resulting in a decrease in cerebral blood flow.

Metabolic/Other   The administration of 100% oxygen has no effect on glucose utilisation or the respiratory quotient.

Toxicity/Side Effects   The following toxic effects are associated with the use of high concentrations of oxygen:

1. carbon dioxide retention in patients with respiratory failure who are predominantly dependent upon a hypoxic drive to respiration
2. retrolental fibroplasia
3. acute oxygen toxicity (the Paul-Bert effect) may occur if hyperbaric 100% oxygen is used; the symptoms are altered mood, vertigo, loss of consciousness and convulsions
4. chronic oxygen toxicity may occur when concentrations >60% are used for prolonged periods at atmospheric pressure; the symptoms of this are tracheal irritation, sore throat, substernal pain and the signs are pulmonary congestion, atelectasis and a decreased vital capacity
5. prolonged administration of 100% oxygen may interfere with red cell formation.

Kinetics

Absorption   The gas is freely permeable through normal alveolar tissue.

Distribution   Oxygen is transported in the blood predominantly combined to haemoglobin; in addition each 100 ml of plasma contains 0.3 ml of dissolved oxygen at normal atmospheric pressure and an FiO_2 of 0.21.

Metabolism   Occurs within mitochondria to produce carbon dioxide and water.

Excretion   As exhaled carbon dioxide and metabolic water.

Oxytocin

Uses Oxytocin is used:
1. for the induction and acceleration of labour
2. to promote lactation and in the management of
3. missed and incomplete abortion and
4. post-partum haemorrhage.

Chemical A naturally occurring polypeptide from the posterior lobe of the pituitary gland.

Presentation As a clear solution for injection containing 5/10 Units/ml of synthetic oxytocin (which is free from vasopressin and extraneous animal protein) and in a fixed dose combination for injection containing 5 Units/ml of oxytocin and 500 µg of ergometrine maleate (which has a more sustained effect on the uterus than does oxytocin).

Main Action Stimulation of uterine contraction.

Mode of Action Oxytocin is thought to act by binding to specific receptors on smooch muscle cells and increasing the permeability of the myometrial cell membrane to potassium ions, thereby decreasing the membrane potential and increasing the excitability of uterine smooth muscle.

Routes of Administration/Doses Oxytocin is administered by intravenous infusion at a rate of 1.5–12 mUnits/min, titrated against the frequency and duration of uterine contractions. The intramuscular dose of the oxytocin–ergometrine preparation is 1 ml.

Effects
CVS Bolus intravenous administration of oxytocin causes a decrease in the blood pressure that occurs within 30 seconds and lasts up to 10 minutes – this response is exaggerated in the anaesthetised subject. A reflex tachycardia and an increase in cardiac output by up to 1.5 l/min occur. ECG changes such as prolongation of the Q-T interval and T-wave flattening may reflect poor coronary artery filling.
AS Oxytocin has no effect on lower oesophageal sphincter pressure during pregnancy.
GU Infusions of oxytocin increase the renal blood flow in animal models.
Metabolic/Other Oxytocin has an antidiuretic effect (exerted by a direct action on the renal tubules) which may, when it is administered in high doses with large volumes of electrolyte-free fluid, lead to water intoxication. Oxytocin also causes milk ejection by causing contraction of modified smooth muscle within the mammary gland, forcing milk from alveolar channels into large sinuses.

Toxicity/Side Effects Oxytocin may cause uterine spasm and rupture, leading to fetal asphyxia when infused too rapidly. Anaphylactoid reactions to the drug have also been reported. Water intoxication has been described above.

Kinetics   Data are incomplete.

Absorption   Oxytocin is active when administered by any parenteral route, but is inactivated by chymotrypsin when administered orally.

Metabolism   Oxytocin is rapidly removed from the plasma by hydrolysis in the liver and kidney (by the action of oxytocinase).

Excretion   The elimination half-life is 1–7 minutes.

Special Points   Oxytocin should not be infused through the same intravenous line as blood and plasma as rapid inactivation of the polypeptide by plasma oxytocinase occurs. Infusions of oxytocin may alter the action of co-administered suxamethonium, leading to a decrease in the fasciculations caused by the latter and an increased dose requirement for suxamethonium.

Pancuronium

Uses Pancuronium is used to facilitate intubation and controlled ventilation.

Chemical A bis-quaternary aminosteroid.

Presentation As a clear solution for injection containing 2 mg/ml of pancuronium bromide.

Main Action Competitive neuromuscular blockade.

Mode of Action Pancuronium acts by competitive antagonism of acetylcholine at nicotinic (N2) receptors at the post-synaptic membrane of the neuromuscular junction; it also has some pre-junctional action.

Route of Administration/Dose Pancuronium is administered intravenously; the normal intubating dose is 0.05–0.1 mg/kg with subsequent doses of one-third this amount. Satisfactory intubating conditions are produced within 90–150 seconds according to the dose administered; a single dose lasts 45–60 minutes. The recovery index of the drug is 16–22 minutes.

Effects
CVS Pancuronium causes an increase in the heart rate, blood pressure and cardiac output secondary to a vagolytic action. The systemic vascular resistance remains unchanged after the administration of the drug.
RS Neuromuscular blockade results in apnoea. Pancuronium has a very low potential for histamine release; bronchospasm is extremely uncommon.
Metabolic/Other Pancuronium may decrease the partial thromboplastin time and prothrombin time.

Toxicity/Side Effects There have been rare reports of anaphylactoid reactions associated with the use of the drug.

Kinetics

Distribution Pancuronium is 15–30% protein-bound in the plasma, predominantly to albumin and gamma globulin; the V_D is 0.134–0.162 l/kg. The drug does not cross the placental or blood–brain barrier.

Metabolism 30–45% of an administered dose undergoes hepatic metabolism by deacetylation to 3-hydroxy-, 17-hydroxy- and 3,17-dihydroxy-derivatives with subsequent biliary excretion. The 3-hydroxy-derivative has some neuro-muscular-blocking activity.

Excretion 50% of the dose is excreted in the urine (80% of this as the unchanged drug), with 5–10% appearing in the bile.

The clearance is 1.46–2.22 ml/min/kg and the elimination half-life is 69–129 minutes. The dose should be reduced in the presence of renal or hepatic impairment.

Special Points   The duration of action of pancuronium, in common with other non-depolarising relaxants, is prolonged by hypokalaemia, hypocalcaemia, hypermagnesaemia, hypoproteinaemia, dehydration, acidosis and hypercapnia. Conversely, pancuronium appears to decrease the MAC of halothane; it also tends to counteract the depressant effect of halothane on the blood pressure.

The following drugs, when co-administered with non-depolarising relaxants, increase the effect of the latter: volatile and induction agents, fentanyl, suxamethonium, diuretics, calcium antagonists, alpha- and beta-adenergic antagonists, protamine, metronidazole and the aminoglycoside antibiotics.

The use of pancuronium appears to be safe in patients susceptible to malignant hyperpyrexia.

Papaveretum

Uses   Papaveretum is used:
1. for premedication
2. as an analgesic in the management of moderate to severe pain and
3. to provide analgesia during terminal care.

Chemical   Papaveretum is a standardised mixture of the anhydrous hydrochlorides of the alkaloids of opium. It contains 253 parts of morphine hydrochloride, 23 parts of papaverine and 20 parts of codeine.

Presentation   As a clear, colourless solution for injection containing 7.7/15.4 mg/ml of papaveretum. A fixed-dose combination with scopolamine is also available.

Main Actions   Analgesia and respiratory depression.

Mode of Action   The activity of papaveretum is essentially that of morphine, which is an agonist at mu- and kappa-opioid receptors. Opioids appear to exert their effects by increasing intracellular calcium concentration, which in turn increases potassium conductance and hyperpolarisation of excitable cell membranes. The decrease in membrane excitability that results may decrease both pre- and post-synaptic responses.

Routes of Administration/Doses   The adult intramuscular or intravenous dose is 7.7/15.4 mg/kg 3–4 hourly. Papaveretum is not recommended for intrathecal or epidural administration, due to the presence of hydroxy-benzoate preservatives.

Effects
CVS   Papaveretum has minimal effects on the cardiovascular system; the predominant effect is that of orthostatic hypotension secondary to a decrease in the systemic vascular resistance, at least part of which is mediated by histamine release. The drug may also cause bradycardia when administered in high doses.
RS   The principal effect of the drug is respiratory depression, with a decreased ventilatory response to hypoxia and hypercapnia. Papaveretum also has a potent antitussive action. Bronchoconstriction may occur with the use of high doses of the drug.
CNS   Papaveretum is a potent analgesic agent, and may also cause sedation (to a greater degree than does morphine), relief of anxiety and euphoria. Miosis is produced by the drug as a result of stimulation of the Edinger-Westphal nucleus. Seizures and muscular rigidity may occur with the use of high doses of papaveretum.
AS   Papaveretum decreases gastrointestinal motility and decreases gastric acid, biliary and pancreatic secretion; it also

increases the common bile duct pressure by causing spasm of the sphincter of Oddi. The drug may also cause nausea and vomiting (although to a lesser extent than does morphine) and constipation.

GU   The drug increases the tone of the ureters, bladder detrusor muscle and sphincter and may precipitate urinary retention.

Metabolic/Other   Mild diaphoresis and pruritus may result from histamine release. Papaveretum increases the secretion of ADH and may therefore lead to impaired water excretion and hyponatraemia. The drug causes a transient decrease in adrenal steroid secretion.

Toxicity/Side Effects   Respiratory depression, nausea and vomiting, hallucinations and dependence may complicate the use of papaveretum.

Kinetics   The kinetics of papaveretum are essentially those of morphine (q.v.).

Special Points   Papaveretum should be used with caution in the presence of hepatic failure, as the drug may precipitate encephalopathy. Similarly, the use of the drug in patients with hypopituitarism may precipitate coma. In common with other opioids, papaveretum decreases the apparent MAC of co-administered volatile agents. The actions of the drug are all reversed by naloxone.

Paracetamol

Uses Paracetamol is used:
1. as an analgesic for the relief of pain of mild to moderate severity and
2. as an antipyretic agent.

Chemical An acetanilide derivative.

Presentation As tablets and suppositories containing 120/500 mg of paracetamol and a syrup containing 24/50 mg/ml. A number of fixed dose combinations with dextropropoxyphene, codeine, pentazocine or metaclopramide are also available.

Main Actions Analgesic and antipyretic.

Mode of Action The mode of action of paracetamol is poorly understood. It is apparently a potent inhibitor of prostaglandin synthesis within the central nervous system which accounts for its antipyretic effect – specifically, it inhibits the synthesis of the E series of prostaglandins that are normally produced in the anterior hypothalamus in response to pyrogens. It acts peripherally by blocking impulse generation within the bradykinin-sensitive chemoreceptors responsible for the generation of afferent nociceptive impulses.

Routes of Administration/Doses The adult oral and rectal dose is 500 mg–1 g 4–6 hourly. Analgesic in children may require 90 mg/kg/day in divided doses (30 mg/kg per dose).

Effects
CNS The maximum analgesic effect of paracetamol appears to be greater than that of any other non-opioid analgesic.
AS Paracetamol is occasionally used as a model for drug absorption as its rate of absorption is proportional to the gastric emptying rate. Drugs which alter gastric emptying alter the rate of paracetamol absorption. The drug has no effect on the liver unless taken in overdose and does not cause gastric ulceration.
Metabolic/Other The drug potentiates the effect of antidiuretic hormone. It has no effect on normal haemostatic mechanisms.

Toxicity/Side Effects Gastrointestinal disturbances, skin reactions and idiosyncratic haemopoietic disorders (thrombocytopenia) may occur with therapeutic doses. Approximately 5% of patients who are allergic to aspirin show cross-sensitivity to paracetamol.

Kinetics

Absorption The drug is rapidly absorbed from the upper gastrointestinal tract; the bioavailability when administered by the oral route is 70–90% due to first-pass metabolism. Absorption is variable when administered rectally and the bioavailability by this route is 68–88% of that observed after oral administration.

Distribution At therapeutic levels, paracetamol is 0–5% protein-bound in the plasma; the V_D is 1 l/kg. Being a non-ionised, lipid soluble substance, paracetamol penetrates tissues and the blood–brain barrier well.

Metabolism Occurs predominantly in the liver, 80% being metabolised to glucuronide and sulphate and 10% by cytochrome P-450 to a highly reactive intermediate metabolite which is in turn inactivated by conjugation with glutathione.

Excretion 2–5% is excreted unchanged in the urine; the glucuronide and sulphate metabolites are actively secreted in the renal tubules at low concentrations and actively reabsorbed at high concentrations. The clearance is 5 ml/min/kg and the elimination half-life is 1.9 hours.

Special Points Paracetamol should be used with caution in patients with renal or hepatic impairment.

Hepatic damage occurs readily with doses exceeding 15 g of the drug; with toxic doses the supply of glutathione becomes depleted and the highly reactive intermediate metabolite of paracetamol combines with hepatic cell membranes, leading eventually to centrilobular necrosis. N-acetylcysteine and methionine act as alternative supplies of glutathione and can protect against paracetamol-induced liver damage if administered within 10–12 hours of ingestion of paracetamol. Liver function tests are a poor prognostic indicator under these circumstances; bilirubin levels >4 mg/100 ml and an INR of >2.2 are associated with a poor outcome.

Penicillin

Uses Penicillin is used in the treatment of infections of:
1. the respiratory tract
2. ear, nose and throat
3. skin, bone, soft tissues and wounds and in the treatment of
4. gonorrhoea
5. meningitis and
6. subacute bacterial endocarditis.

Chemical The prototype penicillin.

Presentation The preparation for oral use is phenoxymethylpenicillin (penicillin V), which is presented as 125/250 mg tablets and in an elixir as the potassium salt. The parenteral preparation is benzylpenicillin (penicillin G), which is a white crystalline powder presented in vials containing 0.3/0.6/3/6 g of sodium benzylpenicillin.

Main Actions Penicillin is a bactericidal antibiotic with a narrow spectrum of activity which includes *Streptococcus, Neisseria, Haemophilus, Corynebacterium, Bacillus, Clostridium, Listeria* and *Treponema* sp., some sensitive staphylococcal strains and oral anaerobes. Penicillin is destroyed by beta-lactamases produced by some strains of *Pseudomonas*, Enterobacteriaceae and *Bacteroides*.

Mode of Action Penicillin binds specifically to penicillin-binding proteins (transpeptidases and carboxypeptidases) in the bacterial cell wall and prevents peptidoglycan cross-linking, thereby decreasing the mechanical stability of the bacterial cell wall.

Routes of Administration/Doses The adult oral dose is 125–250 mg 4–6 hourly; the corresponding intravenous and intramuscular dose is 0.6–4.8 g/day in 2–4 divided doses. 1 megaUnit is 600 mg. Penicillin may also be administered intrathecally.

Effects
Metabolic/Other High doses of benzylpenicillin may produce hypernatraemia and hypokalaemia.

Toxicity/Side Effects Gastrointestinal disturbances, allergic phenomena (including anaphylaxis), rashes and haemolytic anaemia may occur with the use of the drug. High parenteral doses of penicillin may cause neuropathy and nephropathy.

Kinetics

Absorption 15–30% of an oral dose of penicillin G (the drug is unstable under acid conditions) and 60% of an oral dose of penicillin V is absorbed. The pharmacokinetics after absorption are similar for both preparations.

Distribution   Penicillin is 59–67% protein-bound in the plasma, predominantly to albumin; the V_D is 0.32–0.81 l/kg.

Metabolism   Penicillin is metabolised to penicilloic acid which is inactive with subsequent transformation to penamaldic and penicillenic acid.

Excretion   60–90% of a dose is excreted in the urine by active tubular secretion; up to 25% is excreted unchanged. The elimination half-life is 0.7 hours.

Special Points   Penicillin is removed by haemodialysis.

Pentazocine

Uses Pentazocine is used for the relief of moderate to severe pain.

Chemical A benzmorphan derivative.

Presentation As tablets containing 25/50 mg of pentazocine hydrochloride, as 50 mg suppositories, and a clear solution for injection containing 30 mg/ml of pentazocine lactate.

Main Action Analgesia.

Mode of Action Pentazocine appears to exert its analgesic effects by an agonistic effect at kappa-opioid receptors; it has weak antagonistic activity at mu-opioid receptors.

Routes of Administration/Doses The adult oral dose is 50–100 mg 3–4 hourly; the corresponding parenteral dose is 30–60 mg 3–4 hourly. The drug is irritant when injected intramuscularly or subcutaneously. Pentazocine acts within 2–3 minutes when administered intravenously and within 20 minutes when administered intramuscularly; the duration of action is 3–4 hours.

Effects
CVS High doses of the drug may lead to a slight increase in the heart rate and blood pressure; this may lead to an increase in cardiac work.
RS Pentazocine causes an equal degree of respiratory depression as an equipotent dose of morphine; however, a 'ceiling effect' limits the degree of respiratory depression produced with doses in excess of 60 mg.
CNS The drug is approximately one-third as potent an analgesic as morphine; it cause sedation and does not exhibit any euphoriant properties.
AS Pentazocine appears to cause less nausea and vomiting and a less marked rise in biliary tract pressure than an equipotent dose of morphine. The drug decreases both gastric and small intestinal motility.
GU Pentazocine decreases the renal plasma flow but has no effect on glomerular filtration rate. The drug increases uterine activity.
Metabolic/Other The drug causes an increase in the plasma catecholamine concentration.

Toxicity/Side Effects Respiratory depression, dizziness, nausea, sweating, dysphoria and hallucinations may complicate the use of the drug. Tolerance and dependence may occur with prolonged use.

Kinetics

Absorption   The drug is well absorbed when administered orally; the bioavailability is 20% due to a significant hepatic first-pass metabolism.

Distribution   Pentazocine is 60–70% protein-bound in the plasma; the V_D is 4.9 l/kg.

Metabolism   Occurs in the liver by oxidation and glucuronidation.

Excretion   60% of the dose is excreted in the urine within 24 hours, 2–12% unchanged. The clearance is 1320 ml/min and the elimination half-life is 2 hours.

Special Points   Pentazocine, being a weak antagonist at mu-opioid receptors, can precipitate withdrawal symptoms in opiate addicts. The respiratory depressant effects of the drug are reversed by naloxone.

   Pentazocine is pharmaceutically incompatible with thiopentone, methohexitone and diazepam.

   The drug is removed by haemodialysis.

Pethidine

Uses Pethidine is used:
1. for premedication
2. as an analgesic in the management of moderate to severe pain and
3. as an antispasmodic agent in the treatment of renal and biliary colic.

Chemical A synthetic phenylpiperidine derivative.

Presentation As 50 mg tablets and a clear, colourless solution for injection containing 10/50 mg/ml of pethidine hydrochloride.

Main Actions Analgesia and respiratory depression.

Mode of Action Pethidine is an agonist at mu- and kappa-opioid receptors. Opioids appear to exert their effects by increasing intracellular calcium concentration, which in turn increases potassium conductance and hyperpolarisation of excitable cell membranes. The decrease in membrane excitability that results may decrease both pre- and post-synaptic responses.

Routes of Administration/Doses The adult oral dose is 50–150 mg 4-hourly; the corresponding dose by the intramuscular route is 25–150 mg and by the intravenous route 25–100 mg. Pethidine may also be administered via the epidural route; a dose of 25 mg is usually employed. The drug acts within 15 minutes when administered orally and within 10 minutes when administered intramuscularly; the duration of action is 2–3 hours.

Effects
CVS Pethidine causes orthostatic hypotension due to the combination of histamine release and alpha-adrenergic blockade that it produces. The drug also has a mild quinidine-like effect and anticholinergic properties, which may lead to the development of a tachycardia.
RS The drug is a potent respiratory depressant, having a greater effect on tidal volume than on the respiratory rate. Pethidine obtunds the ventilatory response to both hypoxia and hypercapnia. Chest wall rigidity may occur with the use of the drug. It has little antitussive activity.
CNS Pethidine is one-tenth as potent an analgesic as morphine. It appears to cause more euphoria and less nausea and vomiting than an equipotent dose of morphine. Miosis and corneal anaesthesia follow the use of the drug.
AS In common with other opioids, pethidine decreases the rate of gastric emptying. The drug appears to cause a less marked increase in bile duct pressure and less depression of

intestinal activity (and therefore constipation) than equipotent doses of morphine.

GU The drug decreases ureteric tone; it may increase the amplitude of contractions of the pregnant uterus.

Metabolic/Other Pethidine increases ADH secretion and decreases adrenal steroid secretion.

Toxicity/Side Effects Respiratory depression, nausea and vomiting, hallucinations and dependence may complicate the use of pethidine. The drug evokes less histamine release than morphine.

Kinetics

Absorption The bioavailability when administered orally is 45–75%, due to a significant first-pass effect. The drug has a bioavailability of 100% when administered intramuscularly (into the deltoid muscle).

Distribution Pethidine is 49–67% protein-bound in the plasma; the V_D is 3.5–5.3 l/kg. The drug crosses the placenta; the mean cord blood concentration at delivery is 75–90% of the maternal venous concentration.

Metabolism Occurs in the liver by N-demethylation to norpethidine and by hydrolysis to pethidinic acid; norpethidine is further hydrolysed to norpethidinic acid. The acid metabolites are further conjugated prior to excretion. Norpethidine may accumulate in the presence of renal failure and has 50% the analgesic potency of the parent compound and marked convulsant properties.

Excretion 1–25% of the administered dose is excreted unchanged in the urine, dependent upon the urinary pH. Norpethidine is excreted in the urine; cumulation may occur in the presence of renal or hepatic impairment. The clearance is 12–22 ml/min/kg and the elimination half-life is 2.4–7 hours. The clearance is reduced by the co-administration of halothane.

Special Points Pethidine may precipitate a severe hypertensive episode in patients receiving MAOIs. The drug reduces the apparent MAC of co-administered volatile agents. By convention, pethidine is used in asthmatic patients although there is no published evidence that the drug causes bronchospasm less frequently than morphine in this group of patients.

Pethidine effectively inhibits post-anaesthetic shivering.

Phenelzine

Uses Phenelzine is used in the treatment of:
1. non-endogenous depression and
2. phobic disorders.

Chemical A substituted hydrazine.

Presentation As tablets containing 15 mg of phenelzine sulphate.

Main Action Antidepressant.

Mode of Action Phenelzine is an irreversible inhibitor of mitochondrial monoamine oxidase, an enzyme involved in the metabolism of catecholamines and 5-hydroxytryptamine. It is assumed that the antidepressant activity of the drug is related to the increased concentration of monoamines in the central nervous system that results from the use of the drug.

Route of Administration/Dose The adult oral dose is 15 mg 6–8 hourly; this is reduced once a satisfactory response has been obtained. The maximum inhibition of enzyme activity is achieved within a few days, but the antidepressant effect of the drug may take 3–4 weeks to become established.

Effects
CVS The predominant effect of the drug is orthostatic hypotension; MAOIs were formerly used as antihypertensive agents.
CNS Phenelzine is an effective antidepressant which may also produce stimulation of the central nervous system resulting in tremor and insomnia. The MAOIs suppress REM sleep very effectively.
AS Constipation occurs commonly with the use of the drug – the mechanism of this effect is unknown.
Metabolic/Other Inappropriate secretion of ADH has been reported in association with the use of phenelzine.

Toxicity/Side Effects Disturbances of the central nervous system (including convulsions and peripheral neuropathy), anticholinergic side effects and hepatotoxicity may complicate the use of the drug. More importantly, a host of serious and potentially fatal interactions may occur between MAOIs and tyramine-containing substances, sympathomimetic agents and central nervous system depressants (*v.i.*).

Kinetics Data are incomplete.

Absorption Phenelzine is readily absorbed when administered orally.

Metabolism   80% of the dose is metabolised by oxidation and hydroxylation to phenylacetic acid and parahydroxy-phenylacetic acid. The drug may inhibit its own metabolism.

Excretion   Occurs predominantly in the urine as free and unconjugated aromatic forms of the drug.

Special Points   MAOIs demonstrate several important drug interactions:
1. drugs such as pethidine, fentanyl, morphine and barbiturates whose action is terminated by oxidation have a more profound and prolonged effect in the presence of MAOIs; this is particularly marked in the case of pethidine. Marked hyperpyrexia, possibly due to 5-HT release, may also occur when pethidine is administered to a patient who is already receiving MAOIs
2. indirectly – acting sympathomimetic agents (e.g. ephedrine) produce an exaggerated pressor response in the presence of co-administered MAOIs – severe hypertensive episodes (which are best treated with phentolamine) may result from this interaction.
3. MAOIs markedly exaggerate the depressant effects of volatile anaesthetic agents on the blood pressure and central nervous system
4. MAOIs inhibit plasma cholinesterase and may therefore prolong the duration of action of co-administered suxamethonium
5. MAOIs may also potentiate the effects of antihypertensive and hypoglycaemic agents, anti-Parkinsonian drugs and local anaesthetics.

A period of two weeks is required to restore amine metabolism to normal after the cessation of administration of phenelzine. This is the recommended period that should elapse between discontinuation of MAOI therapy and elective surgery. Post-operative analgesia for patients who are still receiving MAOI therapy has been safely provided using chlorpromazine and codeine.

Phenoxybenzamine

Uses   Phenoxybenzamine is used in the treatment of:
1. hypertensive crises
2. Raynaud's phenomenon and
3. in the pre-operative preparation of patients due for the removal of a phaeochromocytoma.

Chemical   A tertiary amine which is a halo-alkylamine.

Presentation   As 10 mg tablets and a clear, colourless solution for injection containing 50 mg/ml of phenoxybenzamine hydrochloride.

Main Actions   Vasodilation (predominantly arterial).

Mode of Action   Phenoxybenzamine acts via a highly reactive carbonium ion derivative which binds covalently to alpha-adrenergic receptors to produce irreversible competitive alpha-blockade. The drug increases the rate of peripheral turnover of noradrenaline and the amount of noradrenaline released per impulse by blockade of pre-synaptic alpha-2 receptors. Haloalkylamines also inhibit the response to serotoninergic, histaminergic and cholinergic stimulation.

Routes of Administration/Doses   The adult dose by the oral route is 10–60 mg/day in divided doses. The corresponding dose by intravenous infusion (diluted in dextrose or saline) over 1 hour is 10–40 mg. After intravenous administration, the drug acts in 1 hour and has a duration of action of 3–4 days.

Effects
CVS   Phenoxybenzamine produces a decrease in the peripheral vascular resistance which leads to a decrease in the diastolic blood pressure and pronounced orthostatic hypotension. A reflex tachycardia and an increase in cardiac output follow the administration of the drug. Phenoxybenzamine inhibits catecholamine-induced cardiac dysrhythmias. The drug causes a shift of fluid from the interstitial to the vascular compartment due to vasodilation of pre- and post-capillary resistance vessels.
CNS   The drug decreases cerebral blood flow only if marked hypotension occurs. Motor excitability may follow the administration of phenoxybenzamine; however, sedation is the usual effect observed. Miosis occurs commonly.
AS   Phenoxybenzamine produces little change in gastrointestinal tone or splanchnic blood flow.
GU   The drug causes little alteration of renal blood flow; it decreases the motility of the non-pregnant uterus.

Toxicity/Side Effects   Dizziness, sedation, a dry mouth, paralytic ileus and impotence may result from the use of phenoxybenzamine. The drug is irritant if extravasation occurs.

Kinetics   Data are incomplete.

Absorption   Phenoxybenzamine is incompletely absorbed after oral administration; the bioavailability by this route is 20–30%.

Distribution   The drug is highly lipophilic.

Metabolism   Phenoxybenzamine is predominantly metabolised in the liver by deacetylation.

Excretion   Occurs via the urine and bile; the half-life is 24 hours.

Special Points   Systemic administration of the drug may lead to an increase in the systemic absorption of co-administered local anaesthetic agents. Phenoxybenzamine causes marked congestion of the nasal mucosa and this may make nasal instrumentation more traumatic if topical vasoconstrictors are not used.

Phentolamine

Uses   Phentolamine is used for:
1. the diagnosis and peri-operative management of patients with phaeochromocytoma
2. the acute treatment of hypertension occurring during anaesthesia and
3. the treatment of left ventricular failure complicating myocardial infarction.

Chemical   An imidazoline.

Presentation   As a clear solution for injection containing 10 mg/ml of phentolamine mesilate.

Main Actions   Hypotension, positive inotropism and chronotropism.

Mode of Action   Phentolamine acts by transient competitive alpha-adrenergic blockade (it is 3–5 times as active at alpha-1 as at alpha-2 receptors); it also has some beta-adrenergic agonist and anti-serotoninergic activity.

Routes of Administration/Doses   The adult intramuscular dose for the control of paroxysmal hypertension is 5–10 mg; the drug may also be administered by intravenous infusion (diluted in dextrose or saline) at the rate of 0.1–0.2 mg/min.

Effects
CVS   Phentolamine causes a marked reduction in the systemic vascular resistance, producing a decrease in blood pressure and a reflex tachycardia. The drug has a positive inotropic action, which is probably an indirect effect due to alpha-2 blockade leading to noradrenaline release. The coronary blood flow increases; the drug also has class I antiarrhythmic effects. In patients with heart failure, phentolamine causes an increase in the heart rate and cardiac output, with a concomitant decrease in the pulmonary arterial pressure, systemic vascular resistance and left ventricular end-diastolic pressure.
RS   The drug increases the vital capacity, FEV_1 and maximum breathing capacity in normal subjects, and prevents histamine-induced bronchoconstriction. Respiratory tract secretions are increased by the drug. Phentolamine is a pulmonary arterial vasodilator.
AS   The drug increases salivation, gastric acid and pepsin secretion and gastrointestinal motility.
Metabolic/Other   The drug increases insulin secretion.

Toxicity/Side Effects   Phentolamine is generally well tolerated, but may cause orthostatic hypotension, dizziness, abdominal discomfort and diarrhoea. Cardiovascular collapse and death have followed the administration of phentolamine when it is used as a diagnostic test for phaeochromocytoma.

Kinetics   Data are incomplete.

Absorption   The bioavailability is 20% when administered orally.

Excretion   10% of the dose is excreted in the urine unchanged. The plasma half-life is 10–15 minutes.

Special Points   Phentolamine causes marked congestion of the nasal mucosa and this may make nasal instrumentation more traumatic if topical vasoconstrictors are not used.

Phenytoin

Uses   Phenytoin is used:
1. in the prophylaxis and treatment of generalised tonic-clonic and partial epilepsies and in the treatment of
2. fast atrial and ventricular dysrhythmias resulting from digoxin toxicity and
3. trigeminal neuralgia.

Chemical   A hydantoin derivative.

Presentation   As 25/50/100/300 mg capsules, a syrup containing 6 mg/ml and as a clear, colourless solution for injection containing 50 mg/ml of phenytoin sodium.

Main Actions   Anticonvulsant and antiarrhythmic.

Mode of Action   Phenytoin has membrane stabilising activity and slows inwards sodium and calcium ion flux during depolarisation in excitable tissue; it also delays outwards potassium ion flux. There appears to be a high-affinity binding site within the central nervous system for phenytoin which suggests the existence of an endogenous ligand.

Routes of Administration/Doses   The adult oral dose is 200–600 mg/day; a small dose should be used initially and gradually increased thereafter. The corresponding intramuscular dose is 100–200 mg 4-hourly for 48–72 hours, decreasing to 300 mg daily. The intravenous loading dose for the management of epilepsy is 10–15 mg/kg (administered slowly), followed by a maintenance dose of 100 mg 6–8-hourly. When used in the treatment of cardiac dysrhythmias, the corresponding intravenous dose is 3.5 mg/kg. The therapeutic range is 10–20 mg/l.

Effects

CVS   Phenytoin exhibits class I antiarrhythmic properties and enhances atrio-ventricular nodal conduction. Hypotension may complicate rapid intravenous administration of the drug; complete heart block, ventricular fibrillation and asystole have also been reported under these circumstances.

CNS   80% of newly diagnosed epileptics can be controlled with phenytoin monotherapy. The drug acts as an articovulsant by stabilising rather than raising the seizure threshold and by preventing the spread of seizure activity rather than by abolishing a primary discharging focus.

Metabolic/Other   Hyperglycaemia, hypocalcaemia and alterations in liver function tests have been described consequent to phenytoin therapy. The drug suppresses ADH secretion.

Toxicity/Side Effects   Phenytoin has both idiosyncratic and concentration-dependent side effects. The idiosyncratic side effects include acne, gum hyperplasia, hirsutism, coarsened facies, folate-dependent megaloblastic anaemia and other blood dyscrasias, osteomalacia, erythroderma, lymphadenopathy, systemic lupus erythematosus, hepatotoxicity and allergic phenomena. The concentration-dependent side effects include nausea and vomiting, drowsiness, behavioural disturbances, tremor, ataxia, nystagmus, paradoxical seizures, peripheral neuropathy and cerebellar damage. The drug is irritant if extravasation occurs when given intravenously and may cause muscular damage when administered intramuscularly.

Kinetics

Absorption   Absorption is very slow by both the intramuscular and oral routes. The oral bioavailability is 85–95%.

Distribution   Phenytoin is 90–93% protein-bound in the plasma; the V_D is 0.5–0.7 l/kg.

Metabolism   There is a large genetic variation in the rate of metabolism of phenytoin, which occurs in the liver predominantly to a hydroxylated derivative which is subsequently conjugated to glucuronide. Phenytoin exhibits zero-order elimination kinetics just above the therapeutic range; the implication of this is that the dose required to produce a plasma concentration within the therapeutic range is close to that which will produce toxicity.

Excretion   70–80% of the dose is excreted in the urine by active tubular secretion as the major metabolite; <5% is excreted unchanged. The clearance is 5.5–9.5 ml/kg/day and the elimination half-life is 9–22 hours in the first-order kinetics range; the latter increases at higher dose ranges when the capacity of the hepatic mono-oxygenase system becomes saturated. The dose of phenytoin should be reduced in the presence of hepatic impairment, but renal impairment requires little alteration of dosage (despite the fact that the free fraction of the drug increases in the presence of uraemia, an increase in the clearance and V_D tend to offset this).

Special Points   Phenytoin is a potent enzyme inducer and demonstrates a plethora of drug interactions, amongst which the most important are the precipitation of phenytoin toxicity by metronidazole and isoniazid and a reduced effectiveness of benzodiazepines, pethidine and warfarin caused by the co-administration of phenytoin. The drug may also decrease the MAC of volatile agents and enhance the central nervous system toxicity of local anaesthetics; it appears to increase the dose requirements of all the non-depolarising relaxants (with the exception of atracurium) by 60–80%.

The parenteral preparation of phenytoin precipitates in the presence of most crystalloid solutions.

The drug is not removed by dialysis.

Piperacillin

Uses   Piperacillin is used in the treatment of:
1. urinary and respiratory tract infections
2. intra-abdominal and biliary tract sepsis
3. gynaecological and obstetric infections
4. infections of skin, soft tissue, bone and joints
5. septicaemia
6. meningitis and for
7. peri-operative prophylaxis.

Chemical   A semi-synthetic penicillin.

Presentation   In vials containing 1/2 g and infusion bottles containing 4 g of piperacillin sodium. A fixed dose combination with tazobactam is also available.

Main Actions   Piperacillin is a bactericidal broad spectrum antibiotic that is effective against many beta-lactamase-producing organisms. *In vitro*, it shows activity against the Gram-negative organisms *Escherichia coli, Haemophilus influenzae* and *Klebsiella, Neisseria, Proteus, Shigella* and *Serratia* sp.; anaerobes including *Bacteroides* and *Clostridium* sp. and the Gram-positive enterococci, *Staphylococcus* and *Streptococcus* sp. It is particularly effective against *Pseudomonas*, indole-positive *Proteus, Streptococcus faecalis* and *Serratia marcescens*.

Mode of Action   Piperacillin binds to cell wall penicillin-binding proteins (PBPs) and inhibits their activity; specifically, it affects PBP 1A/B which are involved in the cross-linking of cell wall peptidoglycans, PBP 2 which is involved in the maintenance of the rod shape and PBP 3 which is involved in septal synthesis.

Routes of Administration/Doses   The adult intravenous dose is 4 g 6–8 hourly (each gram should be infused over 3–5 minutes) and the intramuscular dose 2 g 6–8 hourly.

Effects
Metabolic/Other   Piperacillin has a lower sodium content than other disodium penicillins and causes less fluid and electrolyte derangements; serum potassium levels may decrease after the administration of the drug.

Toxicity/Side Effects   Gastrointestinal upsets, abnormalities of liver function tests, allergic reactions and transient leucopenia and neutropenia may complicate the use of the drug. Deterioration in renal function has been reported in patients with pre-existent severe renal impairment treated with piperacillin.

Kinetics

Absorption Piperacillin is poorly absorbed when administered orally and is hydrolysed by gastric acids.

Distribution The drug is 16% protein-bound in the plasma; the V_D is 0.32 l/kg. High concentrations are found in most tissues and body fluids.

Metabolism Piperacillin is not metabolised in man.

Excretion 20% is excreted in the bile; the remainder is excreted in the urine by glomerular filtration and tubular secretion. The elimination half-life is 36–72 minutes.

Special Points The dose of piperacillin should be reduced in the presence of renal impairment; the drug is 30–50% removed by haemodialysis.

Polygeline

Uses Polygeline is used:
1. for plasma volume replacement in haemorrhage, burns or excessive fluid and electrolyte loss
2. for extracorporeal circulation, isolated organ perfusion and plasma exchange and
3. as a carrier solution for insulin.

Chemical Polygeline is a polypeptide produced by the thermal degradation of bovine gelatin – the hydrolysate thus formed consists of small polypeptides of molecular weight 12 000–15 000 daltons. These are then cross-linked via urea bridges to yield molecules with an average molecular weight of 35 000 and subsequently dissolved in water. The ionic composition is then adjusted to yield the formulation described below.

Presentation Polygeline is presented in 500 ml plastic bottles containing a sterile, pyrogen-free, straw-coloured solution of pH 7.2. Each litre contains 35 g of polygeline, 145 mmol of sodium and chloride ions, 5.1 mmol of potassium ions and 6.25 mmol of calcium ions.

Main Action Plasma volume expansion.

Mode of Action Polygeline equilibrates throughout the body (28% in circulating blood, 27–31% in the interstitial space and 40–46% in urine) to restore the haemodynamic status after a period of hypovolaemia.

Route of Administration/Dose Polygeline is administered intravenously as required to restore the circulating volume: it should not be used to restore greater than 25% of the total circulating blood volume.

Effects
CVS The haemodynamic effects of polygeline are proportional to the prevailing volaemic status.
GU Renal perfusion is restored towards normal in hypovolaemic subjects transfused with the colloid; in addition, polygeline has an osmotic diuretic effect.
Metabolic/Other Polygeline has no effect on the blood sugar concentration, and no specific effect on coagulation or fibrinolysis.

Toxicity/Side Effects A degree of histamine release occurs in 1 in 1000 patients who receive the colloid; since the preparation is non-immunogenic, it is assumed that this is an anaphylactoid response. Severe, life-threatening reactions are very rare.

Kinetics

Distribution The distribution of polygeline has been described earlier; the V_D is 9–13 l.

Metabolism *In vitro* studies suggest that polygeline is degraded by proteolytic enzymes to smaller peptides and amino acids.

Excretion 74% is excreted in the urine within 4 days; about 10% is excreted in the faeces. Excretion is complete after 12 days. Two fractions are recognised – 30% consists of a small molecular weight fraction which is rapidly excreted (with an elimination half-life of 0.2–0.4 hours in animals) and the remaining 70% consists of a larger molecular weight fraction which is excreted with an elimination half-life of 8.4 hours in man.

Special Points Polygeline contains ionic calcium and may thus enhance the toxicity of digoxin administered concurrently and may also cause coagulation of citraced blood (with which it should not be mixed). It has no effect on blood cross-matching.

The use of polygeline is not recommended as a prophylactic measure against the occurrence of hypotension in patients undergoing spinal or epidural anaesthesia.

Prazosin

Uses Prazosin is used in the treatment of:
1. hypertension
2. Raynaud's phenomenon and may be of use in the treatment of
3. congestive cardiac failure
4. aortic and mitral regurgitation
5. phaeochromocytoma and
6. bladder neck obstruction.

Chemical A quinazoline derivative.

Presentation As tablets containing 0.5/1/2/5 mg of prazosin hydrochloride.

Main Actions Arterial and venous vasodilation.

Mode of Action Prazosin is a highly selective competitive antagonist of alpha-1 (post-synaptic) adrenoceptors, thereby causing relaxation of vascular smooth muscle.

Routes of Administration/Doses The adult dose is 1 mg 8–12 hourly (introduced cautiously) increased to a total of 20 mg daily.

Effects
CVS Prazosin dilates coronary arteries, peripheral arterioles and veins, leading to a decrease in the pulmonary and systemic vascular resistance and blood pressure. Relatively little reflex tachycardia occurs; the drug may have a direct negative chronotropic effect on the sinus node. The cardiac output may increase in patients with heart failure who receive the drug.
RS Prazosin produces clinically insignificant bronchodilatation in some asthmatic subjects.
GU Prazosin has little effect on the renal blood flow or glomerular filtration rate. The drug causes relaxation of the bladder trigone and sphincter muscle.
Metabolic/Other Prazosin may cause a significant increase in the plasma noradrenaline concentration; it has little effect on plasma renin activity.

Toxicity/Side Effects Prazosin is generally well tolerated. Postural hypotension, drowsiness, fatigue, nausea and urinary urgency may occur. The 'first-dose phenomenon' consists of dizziness and faintness, possibly accompanied by palpitations, occurring as a result of profound hypotension, bradycardia and decreased venous return.

Kinetics

Absorption The oral absorption is variable; the bioavailability by this route is 43–62%.

Distribution   Prazosin is 92% protein-bound in the plasma, predominantly to an acid glycoprotein. The V_D is 0.5–0.89 l/kg.

Metabolism   Occurs via dealkylation in the liver – the metabolites are active.

Excretion   Excretion occurs predominantly in the bile and faeces; less than 10% is excreted unchanged. The clearance is 3.5–4 ml/kg/min and the elimination half-life is 2.5–2.9 hours.

Special Points   False positive results may occur in patients undergoing screening tests for phaeochromocytoma. An additive hypocensive effect should be expected with co-administered volatile anaesthetic agents.

The drug is not removed by dialysis.

Prednisolone

Uses Prednisolone is used:
1. as replacement therapy in adrenocortical deficiency states and in the treatment of
2. allergy and anaphylaxis
3. hypercalcaemia
4. asthma
5. a panoply of autoimmune disorders
6. some forms of red eye and
7. in leukaemia chemotherapy regimes and
8. for immunosupression after organ transplantation.

Chemical A synthetic glucocorticosteroid.

Presentation As 1/2.5/5/20 mg tablets of prednisolone, a solution for injection containing 25 mg/ml of prednisolone acetate and as eye/ear drops and retention enemas.

Main Action Anti-inflammatory.

Mode of Action Corticosteroids act by controlling the rate of protein synthesis; they react with cytoplasmic receptors to form a complex which directly influences the rate of RNA transcription. This directs the synthesis of lipocortins.

Routes of Administration/Doses The adult oral dose is 5–60 mg/day in divided doses, using the lowest dose that is effective and on alternate days if possible to limit the development of side effects. The intramuscular or intra-articular dose is 25–100 mg once or twice weekly.

Effects
CVS In the absence of corticosteroids vascular permeability increases, small blood vessels demonstrate an inadequate motor response and cardiac output decreases. Steroids have a positive effect on myocardial contractility and cause vasoconstriction by increasing the number of alpha-1 adrenoreceptors and beta-adrenoreceptors and stimulating their function.
CNS Corticosteroids increase the excitability of the central nervous system; the absence of glucocorticoid leads to apathy, depression and irritability.
AS Prednisolone increases the likelihood of peptic ulcer disease. It decreases the gastrointestinal absorption of calcium.
GU Prednisolone has weak mineralocorticoid effects and produces sodium retention and increased potassium excretion; the urinary excretion of calcium is also increased by the drug. The drug increases the glomerular filtration rate and stimulates tubular secretory activity.

Metabolic/Other   Prednisolone exerts profound effects on carbohydrate, protein and lipid metabolism. Glucocorticoids stimulate gluconeogenesis and inhibit the peripheral utilisation of glucose; they cause a redistribution of body fat, enhance lipolysis and also reduce the conversion of amino acids to protein. Prednisolone is a potent anti-inflammatory agent which inhibits all stages of the inflammatory process by inhibiting neutrophil and macrophage recruitment, blocking the effect of lymphokines and inhibiting the formation of plasminogen activator. Corticosteroids increase red blood cell, neutrophil and haemoglobin concentrations, whilst depressing other white cell lines and the activity of lymphoid tissue.

Toxicity/Side Effects   Consist of an acute withdrawal syndrome and a syndrome (Cushing's) produced by prolonged use of excessive quantities of the drug. Cushing's syndrome is characterised by growth arrest, a characteristic appearance consisting of central obesity, a moon face and buffalo hump, striae, acne, hirsutism, skin and capillary fragility together with the following metabolic derangements: altered glucose tolerance, fluid retention, a hypokalaemic alkalosis and osteoporosis. A proximal myopathy, cataracts, mania and an increased susceptibility to peptic ulcer disease may also complicate the use of the drug.

Kinetics

Absorption   Prednisolone is rapidly and completely absorbed when administered orally or rectally; the bioavailability by either route is 80–100%.

Distribution   The drug is reversibly bound in the plasma to albumin and a specific corticosteroid binding globulin; the drug is 80–90% protein-bound at low concentrations but only 60–70% protein-bound at higher concentrations. The V_D is 0.35–0.7 l/kg according to the dose.

Metabolism   Occurs in the liver by hydroxylation with subsequent conjugation.

Excretion   11–14% of the dose is excreted unchanged in the urine. The clearance is dose-dependent and ranges from 170–200 ml/min; the elimination half-life is 2.6–5 hours.

Special Points   Prednisone and prednisolone are metabolically interconvertible; only the latter is active. The conversion of prednisone to prednisolone is rapid and extensive and occurs as a first-pass effect in the liver. Prednisolone is 4 times as potent as hydrocortisone and 6 times less potent than dexamethasone. It has been recommended that peri-operative

Prednisolone

steroid cover be given:
1. to patients who have received steroid replacement therapy for >2 weeks prior to surgery or for >1 month in the year prior to surgery and
2. to patients undergoing pituitary or adrenal surgery. Glucocorticoids antagonise the effects of anticholine-sterase drugs.

Prilocaine

Uses Prilocaine is used as a local anaesthetic.

Chemical A secondary amine which is an amide derivative of toluidine.

Presentation As a clear, colourless 0.5/1/2/4% solution for injection of prilocaine hydrochloride and a 3% solution with 0.03 IU of felypressin per ml.

Main Action Local anaesthetic.

Mode of Action Local anaesthetics diffuse in their uncharged base form through neural sheaths and the axonal membrane to the internal surface of cell membrane sodium ion channels; here they combine with hydrogen ions to form a cationic species which enters the internal opening of the sodium ion channel and combines with a receptor. This produces blockade of the sodium ion channel, thereby decreasing sodium ion conductance and preventing depolarisation of the cell membrane.

Routes of Administration/Doses Prilocaine may be administered topically, by infiltration, or epidurally; the toxic dose of prilocaine is 6 mg/kg (8 mg/kg with felypressin). Prilocaine has a duration of action 1.5 times that of lignocaine.

Effects

CVS Prilocaine has few haemodynamic effects when used in low doses, except to cause a slight increase in the systemic vascular resistance leading to a mild increase in the blood pressure. In toxic concentrations, the drug decreases peripheral vascular resistance and myocardial contractility, producing hypotension and possibly cardiovascular collapse.

RS The drug causes bronchodilatation at subtoxic concentrations. Respiratory depression occurs in the toxic dose range.

CNS The principal effect of prilocaine is reversible neural blockade; this leads to a characteristically biphasic effect in the central nervous system. Initially, excitation (lightheadedness, dizziness, visual and auditory disturbances and fitting) occurs, due to the blockade of inhibitory pathways in the cortex; with increasing doses, depression of both facilitatory and inhibitory pathways occur, leading to central nervous system depression (drowsiness, disorientation and coma). Local anaesthetic agents block neuromuscular transmission when administered intra-arterially; it is thought that a complex of neurotransmitter, receptor and local anaesthetic is formed which has negligible conductance.

AS Local anaesthetics depress contraction of the intact bowel.

Toxicity/Side Effects Prilocaine is intrinsically less toxic than lignocaine. Allergic reactions to the amide-type local anaesthetic agents are extremely rare. The side effects are predominantly correlated with excessive plasma concentrations of the drug. Methaemoglobinaemia may occur if doses in excess of 600 mg are administered to an adult (*v.i.*).

Kinetics Data are incomplete.

Absorption The absorption of local anaesthetic agents is related to:
1. the site of injection (intercostal > epidural > brachial plexus > subcutaneous)
2. the dose – a linear relationship exists between the total dose and the peak blood concentrations achieved and
3. the presence of vasoconstrictors, which delay absorption.

Distribution Prilocaine is 55% protein-bound in the plasma, predominantly to alpha-1 acid glycoprotein.

Metabolism Prilocaine is rapidly metabolised in the liver, initially to O-toluidine which is in turn metabolised to 4- and 6-hydroxytoluidine. Some metabolism occurs also in the lung and kidney. Excessive plasma concentrations of O-toluidine may lead to the development of methaemoglobinaemia, which responds to the intravenous administration of 1–2 mg/kg of methylene blue.

Excretion Occurs as inactive metabolites in the urine, <1% unchanged.

Special Points The onset and duration of conduction blockade is related to the pKa, lipid solubility and extent of protein binding of the drug. A low pKa and a high lipid solubility are associated with a rapid onset time; a high degree of protein binding is associated with a long duration of action. The pKa of prilocaine is 7.9 and the heptane:buffer partition coefficient is 0.9.

Local anaesthetic agents significantly increase the duration of action of both depolarising and non-depolarising relaxants.

EMLA (Eutectic Mixture of Local Anaesthetics) is a white cream used to provide topical anaesthesia prior to venepuncture, and has also been used to provide anaesthesia for split-skin grafting. It contains 2.5% lignocaine and 2.5% prilocaine in an oil–water emulsion. When applied topically under an occlusive dressing, local anaesthesia is achieved after 1–2 hours and lasts for up to 5 hours. The preparation causes temporary blanching and oedema of the skin; detectable methaemoglobinaemia may also occur.

Prochlorperazine

Uses Prochlorperazine is used in the treatment of:
1. nausea and vomiting
2. vertigo
3. psychotic states, including mania and schizophrenia and
4. in premedication.

Chemical A phenothiazine of the piperazine subclass.

Presentation As tablets containing 3/5/25 mg, suppositories containing 5/25 mg, as a clear, colourless solution for injection containing 12.5 mg/ml of prochlorperazine maleate, and as a syrup containing 1 mg/ml of prochlorperazine mesylate.

Main Actions Antiemetic.

Mode of Action The antiemetic and neuroleptic effects of the drug appear to be mediated by central dopaminergic (D_2-) blockade leading to an increased threshold for vomiting at the chemoreceptor trigger zone; in higher doses, prochlorperazine appears to have an inhibitory effect at the vomiting centre.

Routes of Administration/Doses The adult dose is 5–20 mg 8–12 hourly and the corresponding intramuscular dose is 12.5 mg 6-hourly.

Effects
CVS Prochlorperazine may cause orthostatic hypotension secondary to alpha-adrenergic blockade. ECG changes, including an increased Q-T interval, ST depression and T- and U-wave changes, may also occur.
RS The drug may cause mild respiratory depression.
CNS Prochlorperazine has neuroleptic properties but appears to be less soporific than perphenazine.
AS Lower oesophageal tone is increased by the drug.
Metabolic/Other In common with other phenothiazines, prochlorperazine has antiadrenergic, anti-inflammatory, antipruritic, anticholinergic and antihistaminergic effects. The drug may also cause hyperprolactinaemia.

Toxicity/Side Effects Prochlorperazine may cause extrapyramidal reactions, jaundice, leucopenia and rashes. The neuroleptic malignant syndrome (a complex of symptoms that include catatonia, cardiovascular lability, hyperthermia and myoglobinaemia) which has a mortality in excess of 10% has been reported in association with the use of the drug.

Kinetics Data are incomplete.

Absorption The drug is slowly absorbed when administered orally; the bioavailability is 0–16% by this route.

Distribution   The degree of protein-binding of prochlorperazine is unknown; the V_D is 20–22 l/kg.

Metabolism   Prochlorperazine undergoes significant first-pass metabolism in the liver; its metabolic pathways remain poorly elucidated. Metabolism may occur by S-oxidation to a sulphoxide.

Special Points   Prochlorperazine is not removed by haemodialysis.

Promethazine

Uses   Promethazine is used in the treatment of:
1. nausea and vomiting (including motion sickness)
2. allergic reactions
3. pruritus and for
4. sedation in children.

Chemical   A phenothiazine.

Presentation   As 10/25 mg tablets, an elixir containing 1 mg/ml and a clear, colourless solution for injection containing 25 mg/ml of promethazine hydrochloride.

Main Actions   Antihistaminergic, sedative and antiemetic.

Mode of Action   Promethazine acts primarily as a reversible competitive antagonist at H1 histaminergic receptors; it also has some anticholinergic, antiserotoninergic and antidopaminergic activity.

Routes of Administration/Doses   The adult oral dose is 20–75 mg daily in divided doses; the corresponding intramuscular and intravenous dose is 25–50 mg. The drug acts within 15 minutes and has a duration of action of 8–20 hours.

Effects
CVS   When normal therapeutic doses are used, promethazine has no significant cardiovascular effects. Rapid intravenous administration may cause transient hypotension.
RS   The drug causes bronchodilatation, a reduction in respiratory tract secretions and has antitussive properties.
CNS   Promethazine is a potent sedative and anxiolytic; it also has a slight antanalgesic effect. It reduces motion sickness by suppression of vestibular end-organ receptors and by an inhibitory action at the chemoreceptor trigger zone. The drug has local anaesthetic properties.
AS   Promethazine decreases the tone of the lower oesophageal sphincter.

Toxicity/Side Effects   The drug exhibits predictable anticholinergic side effects and may produce extra-pyramidal reactions when used in high doses. Jaundice, photosensitivity, excitatory phenomena, gastrointestinal and haemopoietic disturbances may complicate the use of promethazine.

Kinetics

Absorption   Promethazine is well absorbed when administered orally, but undergoes an extensive first-pass metabolism.

Distribution   The drug is 93% protein-bound in the plasma; the V_D is 2.5 l/kg.

Metabolism   Promethazine is metabolised in the liver by sulphoxidation and N-dealkylation.

Excretion   Occurs predominantly in the urine, 2% unchanged. The clearance is 1.41 l/min and the elimination half-life is 7.5–10 hours.

Special Points   The depressant effects of the drug on the central nervous system are additive with those produced by anaesthetic agents.

Promethazine is not removed by haemodialysis.

Propofol

Uses Propofol is used:
1. for the induction and maintenance of general anaesthesia
2. for sedation during intensive care and regional anaesthesia and has been used
3. in the treatment of refractory nausea and vomiting in patients receiving chemotherapy and
4. in the treatment of status epilepticus.

Chemical Propofol is 2,6-diisopropylphenol; a phenol derivative.

Presentation As a white oil-in-water emulsion containing 1% or 2% w/v of propofol in soybean oil, purified egg phosphatide, and sodium hydroxide.

Main Action Hypnotic.

Mode of Action The mode of action of propofol is unclear. It potentiates the inhibitory transmitters glycine and GABA which enhance spinal inhibition during anaesthesia.

Routes of Administration/Doses Propofol is administered intravenously in a bolus dose of 1.5–2.5 mg/kg for induction and as an infusion of 4–12 mg/kg/hour for maintenance of anaesthesia. For children, the induction dose should be increased by 50% and the maintenance infusion by 25–50%. Consciousness is lost in about 30 seconds and waking occurs about 10 minutes after a single dose. Plasma concentrations of 2–6 µg/ml and 0.5–1.5 µg/ml are associated with hypnosis and sedation respectively.

Effects
CVS Propofol produces a 15–25% decrease in the blood pressure and systemic vascular resistance without a compensatory increase in heart rate; the cardiac output decreases by 20%. In fit patients, the drug attenuates the haemodynamic response to laryngoscopy. Vasodilation occurs secondary to propofol-stimulated production and release of nitric oxide. Profound bradycardia and asystole may complicate the use of the drug.
RS Bolus administration of propofol produces apnoea of variable duration and suppression of laryngeal reflexes. Infusion of the drug produces a decrease in tidal volume, tachypnoea and a depressed ventilatory response to hypercarbia and hypoxia. Propofol causes bronchodilation possibly via a direct effect on bronchial smooth muscle. The drug does not increase intrapulmonary shunting and may preserve the mechanism of hypoxic pulmonary vasoconstriction.
CNS Propofol produces a smooth, rapid induction with rapid and clear-headed recovery. Intracranial pressure, cerebral

perfusion pressure and cerebral oxygen consumption all decrease following administration of the drug. In animal models, propofol exhibits anticonvulsant properties. There is no evidence that the drug produces epileptiform activity in non-epileptic patients. Involuntary movements after propofol are not accompanied by seizure activity on EEG recordings.

AS Propofol appears to possess intrinsic antiemetic properties which may be mediated by antagonism of dopamine D_2 receptors.

GU In animals, propofol causes a reduction in the excretion of sodium ions.

Metabolic/Other Long-term use of propofol infusions may result in hypertriglyceridaemia. The 1% preparation has a calorific value of 1 Cal/ml. Clinically significant impairment of adrenal steroidogenesis does not occur. Propofol is a free-radical scavenger.

Toxicity/Side Effects Pain on injection occurs in up to 28% of subjects. The incidence may be reduced by addition of lignocaine, cooling the drug and the use of large veins. There are case reports of epileptiform movements, facial parasthesiae and bradycardia following the administration of propofol, although the incidence of allergic phenomena is low. The use of propofol appears to be safe in patients susceptible to porphyria (although urinary porphyrin concentrations may increase) and malignant hyperpyrexia. There are reports of neurological sequelae and increased mortality complicating long-term use of propofol for sedation of children receiving intensive therapy. The quinol metabolites may occasionally cause green discoloration of the urine and green hair.

Kinetics

Distribution Propofol is 97% protein-bound in the plasma; the V_D is 700–1500 l. The distribution half-life is 1.3–4.1 minutes, resulting in a brief duration of anaesthesia following bolus administration of the drug.

Metabolism Propofol is rapidly metabolised in the liver, primarily to inactive glucuronide (49–73%), and sulphate and glucuronide conjugates of the hydroxylated metabolite via cytochrome P-450. Interpatient variability determines the ratio between glucuronide and hydroxylated pathway. Extrahepatic mechanisms may contribute to the metabolism of the drug. Renal and hepatic disease have no clinically significant effect on the metabolism of propofol.

Excretion The metabolites are excreted in the urine; 0.3% is excreted unchanged. The clearance is 18.8–40.3 ml/kg/min and the elimination half-life is 9.3–69.3 minutes. The clearance is decreased in the presence of renal failure. Under normal conditions, propofol is non-cumulative.

Propofol

Special Points   Propofol may increase the energy required for successful cardioversion. The. drug causes shortened duration of seizure activity during electroconvulsive therapy, although it does not decrease the efficacy of the treatment. Propofol is physically incompatible with atracurium. Aqueous emulsions of the drug support both bacterial and fungal growth.

Propranolol

Uses Propranolol is used in the treatment of:
1. hypertension
2. angina
3. a variety of cardiac tachydysrhythmias
4. essential tremor and in the adjunctive management of
5. anxiety
6. thyrotoxicosis
7. hypertrophic obstructive cardiomyopathy
8. phaeochromocytoma and in the prophylaxis of
9. recurrence of myocardial infarction and
10. migraine.

Chemical An aromatic amine.

Presentation As tablets containing 10/40/80/160 mg, and as a clear solution for injection containing 1 mg/ml of propranolol hydrochloride.

Main Actions Negative inotropism and chronotropism.

Mode of Action Propranolol acts by competitive antagonism of beta-1 and beta-2 adrenoceptors; it has no intrinsic sympathomimetic activity. It also exerts a membrane stabilising effect when used in very high doses by the inhibition of sodium ion currents.

Routes of Administration/Doses The adult oral dose is 30–320 mg/day in 2–3 divided doses, according to the condition requiring treatment. The corresponding dose by the intravenous route is 1–10 mg, titrated according to response.

Effects
CVS Propranolol is negatively inotropic and chronotropic and leads to a decrease in myocardial oxygen consumption; the mechanism of the drug's antihypertensive action remains poorly defined. Blockade of beta-2 adrenoceptors produces an increase in the peripheral vascular resistance.
RS Propranolol causes a decrease in FEV_1 by increasing airways resistance; it also attenuates the ventilatory response to hypercapnia.
CNS The drug crosses the blood–brain barrier; its central effects may be involved in the mechanism of the drug's antihypertensive action. Propranolol diminishes physiological tremor and decreases intraocular pressure.
GU Propranolol decreases uterine tone, especially during pregnancy.
Metabolic/Other The drug decreases plasma renin activity and suppresses aldosterone release. Propranolol causes a decrease in the plasma free fatty acid concentration and may

also cause hypoglycaemia due to blockade of gluconeogenesis. The drug increases total body sodium concentration and thus the extracellular fluid volume.

Toxicity/Side Effects The side effects of propranolol are predictable manifestations of non-specific beta-adrenergic blockade. The drug may thus precipitate heart failure or heart block, exacerbate peripheral vascular disease, lead to bronchospasm, sleep disturbances and nightmares, mask the symptoms of hypoglycaemia and cause impaired exercise tolerance.

Kinetics

Absorption 90% of an oral dose of propranolol is absorbed; the bioavailability is 30–35% due to an extensive first-pass metabolism.

Distribution The drug is 90–96% protein-bound in the plasma, predominantly to alpha-1 acid glycoprotein; the V_D is 3.6 l/kg.

Metabolism Propranolol undergoes extensive hepatic metabolism by oxidative deamination and dealkylation with subsequent glucuronidarion; the 4-hydroxy metabolite is active.

Excretion Occurs via the urine; less than 1% of the dose is excreted unchanged. The clearance is 0.5–1.2 l/min and the elimination half-life is 2–4 hours. The dose should be reduced in the presence of hepatic failure; no alteration in dose is necessary in the presence of renal impairment.

Special Points Beta-adrenergic blockade should be continued throughout the peri-operative period; abrupt withdrawal of propranolol may precipitate angina, ventricular dysrhythmias, myocardial infarction and sudden death. The co-administration of propranolol and non-depolarising relaxants may lead to a slight potentiation of the latter.

The drug is not removed by dialysis.

Protamine

Uses   Protamine is used:
1.   to neutralise the anticoagulant effects of heparin and
2.   to prolong the effects of insulin.

Chemical   A purified mixture of low-molecular-weight cationic proteins prepared from fish sperm.

Presentation   As a clear, colourless solution for injection containing 10 mg/ml of protamine sulphate.

Main Actions   Neutralisation of the anticoagulant effect of heparin; in high doses, protamine has a weak intrinsic anticoagulant effect.

Mode of Action   Both *in vitro* and *in vivo*, the strongly basic compound protamine complexes with the strongly acidic compound heparin to form a stable salt – this complex is inactive. The intrinsic anticoagulant effect of the drug appears to be due to the inhibition of the formation and activity of thromboplastin.

Route of Administration/Dose   Protamine is administered by slow intravenous injection; the dose should be adjusted according to the amount of heparin that is to be neutralised, the time that has elapsed since the administration of heparin and the Activated Coagulation Time (ACT). 1 mg of protamine will neutralise 100 units of heparin. A maximum adult dose of 50 mg of the drug should be administered in any 10-minute period.

Effects
CVS   Protamine is a myocardial depressant and may cause bradycardia and hypotension secondary to complement activation and leukotriene release. The pulmonary artery pressure may increase, leading to an impairment of right ventricular output.

Toxicity/Side Effects   Rapid intravenous administration of protamine may be complicated by acute hypotension, bradycardia, dyspnoea and flushing. Anaphylactoid reactions may also occur; antibodies to human protamine often develop in vasecromised males and may predispose to hypersensitivity phenomena.

Kinetics   Data are incomplete.

Metabolism   The metabolic fate of the protamine heparin complex has not been well elucidated; it may undergo partial degradation, thereby freeing heparin.

Ranitidine

Uses   Ranitidine is used in the treatment of:
1. peptic ulcer disease
2. reflux oesophagitis
3. the Zollinger-Ellison syndrome and
4. for the prevention of stress ulceration in critically ill patients and
5. prior to general anaesthesia in patients at risk of acid aspiration, especially during pregnancy and labour.

Chemical   A furan derivative.

Presentation   As a clear solution for intravenous or intramuscular injection containing 25 mg/ml, as 150/300 mg tablets and as a syrup containing 15 mg/ml of ranitidine hydrochloride.

Main Actions   Inhibition of gastric acid secretion.

Mode of Action   Ranitidine acts via competitive blockade of histaminergic H2 receptors. Histamine appears to be necessary to potentiate the action of gastrin and acetylcholine on the gastric parietal cell, as well as acting directly as a secretogogue.

Routes of Administration/Doses   Ranitidine may be administered by slow intravenous or intramuscular injection, the dose being 50 mg 6–8-hourly. The oral dose is 150 mg twice daily.

Effects
CVS   No effect is seen with normal clinical dosages.
RS   The drug has no effect on respiratory parameters.
AS   Ranitidine profoundly inhibits gastric acid secretion, reducing the volume, hydrogen ion and pepsin content. The drug has a longer duration of antisecretory activity than cimetidine. Ranitidine has been reported to cause a dose-related increase in lower oesophageal sphincter tone.
Metabolic/Other   Ranitidine does not show the antiandrogenic, antidopaminergic or effects on cytochrome P-450 mediated metabolism that are associated with cimetidine. The drug crosses the placenta, but no adverse effects on the fetal well-being have been demonstrated.

Toxicity/Side Effects   Reversible abnormalities of liver function tests, rashes and anaphylactoid reactions have been reported following the use of ranitidine. Reversible confusion, thrombocytopenia and leucopenia occur rarely after administration of the drug.

Kinetics

Absorption   Ranitidine has an oral bioavailability of 50–60%.

Distribution The drug is approximately 15% protein-bound in the plasma; the V_D is 1.2–1.8 l/kg.

Metabolism A small fraction of the drug is metabolised by oxidation and methylation.

Excretion Ranitidine is predominantly excreted unchanged by the kidney. The clearance is 10 ml/min/kg and the elimination half-life is 1.6–2.5 hours.

Special Points A reduced dosage of the drug should be used in patients with renal failure; the drug is removed by haemodialysis.

Ranitidine may be associated with an increase in nosocomial pneumonia is ventilated critically ill patients.

Remifentanil

Uses Remifentanil is used to provide the analgesic component of general anaesthesia, and in intensive care.

Chemical A synthetic anilidopiperidine derivative.

Presentation As a clear, colourless solution for injection, containing remifentanil hydrochloride in a glycine buffer in 1/2/5 mg vials for dilution prior to infusion.

Main Actions Analgesia and respiratory depression.

Mode of Action Remifentanil is a pure mu-agonist; the mu-opioid receptor appears to be specifically involved in the mediation of analgesia. Opioids appear to exert their effects by increasing intracellular calcium concentration which, in turn, increases potassium conductance and hyperpolarisation of excitable cell membranes. The decrease in membrane excitability that results may decrease both pre- and post-synaptic responses.

Route of Administration/Doses Remifentanil is administered intravenously in boluses of 1 µg/kg and may be infused at a rate of 0.0125–1 µg/kg/min. The peak effect of the drug occurs within 1–3 minutes. The offset is rapid and predictable, even after prolonged infusion.

Effects
CVS Remifentanil decreases mean arterial pressure and heart rate by 20%. Myocardial contractility and cardiac output may also decrease.
RS Remifentanil is a potent respiratory depressant, causing a decrease in both the respiratory rate and tidal volume; it also diminishes the ventilatory response to hypoxia and hypercarbia. Chest wall rigidity (the 'wooden chest' phenomenon) may occur after the administration of remifentanil – this may be an effect of the drug on mu-receptors located on GABA-ergic interneurones. The drug does not cause histamine release and thus does not precipitate bronchospasm.
CNS Remifentanil has a centrally mediated vagal activity. It has an analgesic potency similar to fentanyl and possesses minimal hypnotic or sedative activity. It produces EEG effects similar to those of other opioids – high-amplitude, low-frequency activity. Miosis is produced as a result of stimulation of the Edinger-Westphal nucleus.
AS The drug decreases gastrointestinal motility; there is a relatively low incidence of nausea and vomiting associated with its use.

Toxicity/Side Effects Respiratory depression, bradycardia, nausea and vomiting may all complicate the use of remifentanil. Because of its short duration of action, post-operative discomfort may be pronounced if remifentanil is used as a sole analgesic agent peri-operatively.

Kinetics   Data are incomplete.

Distribution   The V_D is 25–40 l/kg.

Metabolism   Remifentanil rapidly undergoes ester hydrolysis by non-specific plasma esterases to a carboxylic acid derivative which is 300–1000 fold less potent than remifentanil and is excreted in the urine. N-dealkylation is a minor metabolic pathway.

Excretion   The clearance is 4.2–5 l/min and the elimination half-life is 10–21 minutes. The clearance appears to be independent of renal and hepatic function.

Special Points   Remifentanil causes an age-related decrease in the MAC of isoflurane. Remifentanil has glycine in the preparation and therefore it should not be used by the epidural or spinal route.

Rocuronium

Uses Rocuronium is used to facilitate intubation and controlled ventilation.

Chemical An aminosteroid which is structurally related to vecuronium.

Presentation As a clear, colourless solution containing 10 mg/ml of rocuronium bromide. The drug is available in 5 and 10 ml ampoules.

Main Action Competitive neuromuscular blockade.

Mode of Action Rocuronium acts by competitive antagonism of acetylcholine at nicotinic (N2) receptors at the postsynaptic membrane of the neuromuscular junction; it also has some pre-junctional action.

Route of Administration/Doses Rocuronium is administered intravenously; the normal intubating dose is 0.6 mg/kg with subsequent doses of one-quarter this amount. The drug may also be infused at a rate of 300–600 µg/kg/hour. Satisfactory intubating conditions are produced within 1 minute – 'priming' does not decrease the onset time of rocuronium. The recovery index is 8–17 minutes. The drug is non-cumulative with repeated administration.

Effects
CVS Rocuronium has minimal cardiovascular effects; with large doses a mild vagolytic effect leads to a slight (9%) increase in heart rate and an increase in mean arterial pressure of up to 16%.
RS Neuromuscular blockade leads to apnoea. Rocuronium does not cause significant histamine release; bronchospasm is extremely uncommon.

Toxicity/Side Effects Fatal anaphylactoid reactions to rocuronium have been reported. Rocuronium causes pain on injection.

Kinetics

Distribution The drug is 30% protein-bound in the plasma; the V_D is 0.27 l/kg.

Metabolism No metabolites of rocuronium have been detected in plasma or urine.

Excretion Rocuronium is excreted primarily by hepatic uptake and hepatobiliary excretion. 30–40% of the dose is excreted unchanged in the bile; 13–31% in the urine. The clearance is 3.9 ml/kg/min and the elimination half-life is 97 minutes. The pharmacokinetics of rocuronium are not significantly altered in the presence of renal failure. The elimination half-life and duration of action of rocuronium are increased in the presence of hepatic dysfunction.

Special Points   The duration of action of rocuronium, in common with other non-depolarising relaxants, may be prolonged by hypokalaemia, hypocalcaemia, hypermagnesaemia, hypoproteinaemia, dehydration, acidosis and hypercapnia. The following drugs, when co-administered with non-depolarising relaxants, increase the effect of the latter: volatile and induction agents, fentanyl, suxamethonium, diuretics, calcium antagonists, alpha- and beta-adrenergic antagonists, protamine, metronidazole and the aminoglycoside antibiotics.

Rocuronium is physically incompatible with thiopentone, methohexitone and diazepam. In animal studies, rocuronium does not appear to be a triggering factor for malignant hyperpyrexia.

Rocuronium causes significantly less rise in intraocular pressure compared to suxamethonium.

Rofecoxib

Uses Rofecoxib is used in the treatment of:
1. osteoarthritis
2. post-operative and dental pain
3. primary dysmenorrhoea and
4. rheumatoid arthritis.

Chemical Furanone.

Presentation As 12.5/25 mg tablets and a suspension containing 2.5/5 mg/ml of rofecoxib.

Main Actions Analgesic, anti-inflammatory and antipyretic.

Mode of Action Rofecoxib is a selective and potent inhibitor of COX-2 enzyme which converts arichidonic acid to cyclic endoperoxides, and thus prevents the formation of prostaglandins and endoperoxides.

Routes of Administration/Doses Rofecoxib is administered orally, in doses of 12.5 mg/day for the treatment of osteoarthritis and up to 50 mg once daily for the management of acute pain.

Toxicity/Side-Effects The drug is generally well tolerated. Insomnia, dizziness, diarrhoea, nausea, headaches and pruritus have been reported. COX-2 inhibitors have a lower incidence of upper gastrointestinal side effects than non-selective NSAIDS.

Effects
GU The drug causes sodium retention and a decrease in the glomerular filtration rate.
Metabolic/Other Naturally occurring pyrexia is reduced by rofecoxib. The drug has no effect on platelet aggregation.

Kinetics

Absorption The drug is well absorbed after oral administration with an oral bioavailability of 93%.

Distribution Rofecoxib is 87% protein-bound in the plasma. The V_D is 1.3 l/kg.

Metabolism The drug is extensively metabolised in the liver, primarily to dihydro derivatives.

Excretion 14% is excreted unchanged in the faeces, 1% unchanged in the urine and the remainder as urinary metabolites. The clearance is 8 l/hr and the elimination half-life is 17 hours.

Special Points Rofecoxib appears to be safe to use in patients with NSAID-induced asthma.

Ropivacaine

Uses Ropivacaine is used as a local anaesthetic.

Chemical An aminoamide which is a member of the pipecoloxylidide group of local anaesthetics.

Presentation As a clear, colourless solution containing 0.2/0.75/1.0% ropivacaine hydrochloride.

Main Action Local anaesthetic.

Mode of Action Local anaesthetics diffuse in their uncharged base form through neural sheaths and the axonal membrane to the internal surface of cell membrane sodium ion channels; here they combine with hydrogen ions to form a cationic species which enters the internal opening of the sodium ion channel and combines with a receptor. This produces blockade of the sodium ion channel, thereby decreasing sodium ion conductance and preventing depolarisation of the cell membrane.

Routes of Administration/Doses Ropivacaine may be administered topically, by infiltration or epidurally; the drug is not currently intended for use in spinal anaesthesia. Sensory blockade is similar in time course to that produced by bupivacaine; motor blockade is slower in onset and shorter in duration than after an equivalent dose of bupivacaine. Alkalinisation of 0.75% ropivacaine significantly increases the duration of epidural blockade.

Effects
CVS Ropivacaine is less cardiotoxic than bupivacaine; in toxic concentrations the drug decreases myocardial contractility, resulting in cardiovascular collapse. Ropivacaine has a biphasic vascular effect causing vasoconstriction at low, but not at high, concentrations.
CNS The principal effect of ropivacaine is reversible neural blockade; this leads to a characteristically biphasic effect in the central nervous system. Initially, excitation (lightheadedness, dizziness, visual and auditory disturbances and fitting) occurs, due to the blockade of inhibitory pathways in the cortex. With increasing doses, depression of both facilitatory and inhibitory pathways occur, leading to central nervous system depression (drowsiness, disorientation and coma). Local anaesthetic agents block neuromuscular transmission when administered intra-arterially; it is thought that a complex of neuro-transmitter, receptor and local anaesthetic is formed which has negligible conductance.
GU Ropivacaine does not compromise uteroplacental circulation.

Toxicity/Side Effects Allergic reactions to the amide-type local anaesthetic agents are extremely rare. The side effects are predominantly correlated with excessive plasma concentrations of the drug, as described above.

Kinetics

Absorption The absorption of local anaesthetic agents is related to:
1. the site of injection (intercostal > epidural > brachial plexus > subcutaneous)
2. the dose – a linear relationship exists between the total dose and the peak blood concentrations and
3. the presence of vasoconstrictors, which delay absorption.

Distribution Ropivacaine is 94% protein-bound to alpha-1 acid glycoprotein in the plasma; the V_D is 52–66 l/kg.

Metabolism Occurs in the liver via cytochrome P-450 to 2,6-pipecoloxylidide.

Excretion The clearance is 0.82 l/min and the terminal elimination half-life is 59–173 minutes. 86% is excreted in the urine, 1% unchanged.

Special Points The onset and duration of conduction blockade is related to the pKa, lipid solubility and extent of protein binding of the drug. A low pKa and a high lipid solubility are associated with a rapid onset time; a high degree of protein binding is associated with a long duration of action. The pKa of ropivacaine is 8.1 and the heptane: buffer partition coefficient is 2.9.

Salbutamol

Uses   Salbutamol is used in the treatment of:
1. asthma
2. chronic obstructive airways disease and
3. uncomplicated preterm labour.

Chemical   A synthetic sympathomimetic amine.

Presentation   As 2/4/8 mg tablets, a syrup containing 0.4/2.5 mg/ml, an aerosol delivering 100 µg/puff, a dry powder for inhalation in capsules containing 200/400 µg, a solution for nebulisation containing 2.5/5 mg/ml and as a clear, colourless solution for injection containing 1 mg/ml of salbutamol sulphate.

Main Actions   Bronchodilatation and uterine relaxation.

Mode of Action   Salbutamol is a beta-adrenergic agonist (with a more pronounced effect at beta-2 than beta-1 receptors) that acts by stimulation of membrane-bound adenyl cyclase in the presence of magnesium ions to increase intracellular cAMP concentrations. It also directly inhibits antigen-induced release of histamine and Slow Releasing Substance of Anaphylaxis from mast cells.

Routes of Administration/Doses   The adult oral dose is, 2–4 mg 6–8 hourly. One or two metered puffs of 200–400 µg of the powder may be inhaled 6–8 hourly. 2.5–5 mg of the nebulised solution may similarly be inhaled 6-hourly. The drug may also be administered subcutaneously or intramuscularly in a dose of 0.5 mg 4-hourly. Salbutamol should be administered intravenously as an infusion diluted in dextrose or saline at a rate not exceeding 0.5 µg/kg/min. Bronchodilatation is observed 5–15 minutes after inhalation and 30 minutes after ingestion of the drug and lasts for up to 4 hours.

Effects
CVS   In high doses, the beta-1 actions of the drug lead to positive inotropic and chronotropic effect. At lower doses, the beta-2 effects predominate and cause a decrease in the peripheral vascular resistance leading to a decrease in the diastolic blood pressure of 10–20 mmHg.
RS   Bronchodilatation, leading to an increased PEFR and FEV_1, occurs after the administration of salbutamol. This is additive to the bronchodilatation produced by phosphodiesterase inhibitors. The drug interferes with the mechanism of hypoxic pulmonary vasoconstriction; an adequate inspired oxygen concentration should be ensured when the drug is used.
GU   Salbutamol decreases the tone of the gravid uterus; 10% of an administered dose crosses the placenta and may lead to tachycardia in the fetus.

Metabolic/Other   Salbutamol may decrease the plasma potassium concentration by causing a shift of the ion into cells. It may also cause an increase in the plasma concentrations of free fatty acids and glucose; insulin release is therefore stimulated.

Toxicity/Side Effects   Anxiety, insomnia, tremor (with no attendant change in motor strength), sweating, palpitations, ketosis, hypokalaemia, postural hypotension and nausea and vomiting may occur following the use of the drug.

Kinetics   Data are incomplete.

Absorption   10% of the dose administered by inhalation reaches the bronchial tree, the remainder being swallowed.

Distribution   Salbutamol is 8–64% protein-bound in the plasma; the V_D is 156 l.

Metabolism   Salbutamol undergoes a significant first-pass metabolism in the liver; the major metabolite is salbutamol 4-O-sulphate.

Excretion   30% of the dose is excreted unchanged in the urine, the remainder in faeces and as the sulphate derivative in the urine. The clearance is 28 l/hour and the elimination half-life is 2.7–5 hours.

Special Points   Salbutamol appears to potentiate non-depolarising muscle relaxants.

Sevoflurane

Uses   Sevoflurane is used for the induction and maintenance of general anaesthesia.

Chemical   A halogenated ether.

Presentation   As a clear, colourless liquid which is non-flammable; the commercial preparation contains no additives or stabilisers. The molecular weight of sevoflurane is 200, the boiling point 58.5 °C and the saturated vapour pressure is 21.3 kPa at 20 °C. The MAC of sevoflurane ranges from 1.71 to 2.05 (0.7–2.0 in the presence of 65% nitrous oxide), the oil/gas solubility coefficient is 53 and the blood/gas solubility coefficient 0.6. Sevoflurane is unstable in the presence of moist soda lime, producing small amounts of a sevo-olefin called 'Compound A'. Sevoflurane has a low solubility in rubber and plastics.

Main Action   General anaesthesia (reversible loss of both awareness and recall of noxious stimuli).

Mode of Action   The mechanism of general anaesthesia remains to be fully elucidated. General anaesthetics appear to disrupt synaptic transmission (especially in the area of the ventrobasal thalamus). The mechanism may include potentiation of gamma-amino-butylic acid and glycine receptors and antagonism at NMDA receptors. Their mode of action at the molecular level appears to involve expansion of hydrophobic regions in the neuronal membrane, either within the lipid phase or within hydrophobic sites in cell membrane proteins.

Route of Administration/Dose   Sevoflurane is administered by inhalation; the agent has a pleasant, non-irritant odour. The concentration used for the inhalational induction of anaesthesia is 5–7% and for maintenance 0.5–3%.

Effects
CVS   Sevoflurane causes a dose-related decrease in myocardial contractility and mean arterial pressure; systolic pressure decreases to a greater degree than diastolic pressure. The drug has little effect on the heart rate and does not sensitize the myocardium to the effects of catecholamines. Sevoflurane does not appear to cause 'coronary steal'.
RS   Sevoflurane causes an increase in respiratory rate; minute volume remains unchanged. The drug depresses the ventilatory response to CO_2 and inhibits hypoxic pulmonary vasoconstriction. Sevoflurane appears to relax bronchial smooth muscle constricted by histamine or acetylcholine.
CNS   The principal effect of sevoflurane is general anaesthesia. The drug decreases cerebral vascular resistance and cerebral metabolic rate and increases intracranial pressure in a

dose-related manner. Sevoflurane does not cause epileptiform
EEG activity.
GU   Sevoflurane reduces renal blood flow and leads to a
modest increase (comparable to that caused by enflurane) in
fluoride ion concentrations. There is no evidence that sevoflurane causes gross changes in human renal function.
Metabolic/Other   In animal models the drug decreases liver
synthesis of fibrinogen, transferrin and albumin.

Toxicity/Side Effects   Sevoflurane acts as a trigger agent
for the development of malignant hyperthermia. There are no
reports of renal toxicity occurring in patients who have
received the drug.

Kinetics

Absorption   The major factors affecting the uptake of
volatile anaesthetic agents are solubility, cardiac output and
the concentration gradient between the alveoli and venous
blood. Sevoflurane is exceptionally insoluble in blood; alveolar
concentration therefore reaches inspired concentration very
rapidly, resulting in a rapid induction of (and emergence from)
anaesthesia. An increase in the cardiac output increases the
rate of alveolar uptake and slows the induction of anaesthesia.
The concentration gradient between alveoli and venous blood
approaches zero at equilibrium; a large concentration gradient
favours the onset of anaesthesia.

Distribution   The drug is initially distributed to organs
with a high blood flow (the brain, heart, liver and kidney) and
later to less well-perfused organs (muscle, fat and bone).

Metabolism   Sevoflurane is metabolised by hepatic
cytochrome P-450IIEI to yield hexafluoroisopropanol, which
is further conjugated to its glucuronide. Approximately 3% of
the absorbed dose of sevoflurane is metabolised.

Excretion   Excretion is via the lungs, predominantly
unchanged. Elimination of sevoflurane is rapid due to its low
solubility. Peak excretion of hexafluoroisopropanol glucuronide
occurs within 12 hours; the elimination half-life is 55 hours.

Special Points   Sevoflurane potentiates the action of
co-administered depolarising and non-depolarising relaxants
to a greater extent than either halothane or enflurane.

Sodium bicarbonate

Uses Sodium bicarbonate is used:
1. for the correction of profound metabolic acidosis, especially that complicating cardiac arrest
2. for the alkalinisation of urine and
3. as an antacid.

Chemical An inorganic salt.

Presentation As 300 mg tablets and as a clear, colourless sterile solution containing 1.26/4.2/8.4% w/v sodium bicarbonate in an aqueous solution. The 8.4% solution contains 1 mmol/ml of sodium and bicarbonate ions and has a calculated osmolarity of 2000 mOsm/l.

Mode of Action The compound freely dissociates to yield bicarbonate ions, which represent the predominant extracellular buffer system. Each gram of sodium bicarbonate will neutralise 12 mEq of hydrogen ions.

Routes of Administration/Doses The adult oral dose for the relief of dyspepsia is 600–1800 mg as required. For the alkalinisation of urine, an oral dose of 3 g is administered every 2 hours until the pH of the urine is >7.

When administered intravenously for the treatment of profound metabolic acidosis, the dose required to restore the pH to normal is usually calculated from the formula:

$$\text{dose (mmol)} = \frac{\text{base deficit (mEq/l)} \times \text{body weight (kg)}}{3}$$

and half this amount administered, before the acid-base status is reassessed.

Effects
CVS Overenthusiastic correction of an acidosis will result in a metabolic alkalosis, which may result in myocardial dysfunction and peripheral tissue hypoxia due to a shift in the oxygen dissociation curve to the left.
RS Metabolic alkalosis diminishes pulmonary ventilation by an effect on the respiratory centre.
CNS The major clinical effect of metabolic alkalosis is excitability of the central nervous system, manifested as nervousness, convulsions, muscle weakness and tetany.
AS Oral administration of the drug results in the release of carbon dioxide with subsequent belching.
Metabolic/Other Hypernatraemia, hyperkalaemia and hypocalcaemia may all result from the intravenous administration of sodium bicarbonate.

Toxicity/Side Effects Hypernatraemia and hyperosmolar syndromes may complicate the use of sodium bicarbonate. The compound is highly irritant to tissues when extravasated and may cause skin necrosis and sloughing.

Kinetics Data are incomplete.

Metabolism Bicarbonate ions react with hydrogen ions to yield carbon dioxide and water.

Excretion Occurs via renal excretion of bicarbonate and exhalation of carbon dioxide.

Special Points Sodium bicarbonate is physically incompatible with calcium salts (which it precipitates) and may cause inactivation of co-administered adrenaline, isoprenaline and suxamethonium.

The use of sodium bicarbonate should be avoided in patients with renal, hepatic or heart failure due to its high sodium content.

Sodium chloride

Uses Sodium chloride is used:
1. to provide maintenance fluid and extracellular fluid replacement
2. to replace sodium and chloride ions under circumstances of reduced intake or excessive loss
3. in the management of hyperosmolar diabetic coma
4. as a priming fluid for haemodialysis and cardiopulmonary bypass machines
5. for rehydration of neonates and infants (0.45% solutions)
6. in the management of severe salt depletion (1.8% solutions)
7. for the dilution of drugs and
8. for interspinous ligament injection in the treatment of chronic neck and back pain (10% solutions).

Chemical An inorganic salt.

Presentation As clear, colourless, sterile 0.45/0.9/1.8/5% solutions in bags of various capacities. The 0.9% solution contains 154 mmol of both sodium and chloride ions per litre. The pH ranges from 4.5–7; they contain no preservative or antimicrobial agents.

Main Action Volume expansion.

Route of Administration/Dose Sodium chloride solutions are administered intravenously at a rate titrated against the patient's clinical status.

Effects
CVS The haemodynamic effects of sodium chloride are proportional to the prevailing circulating volume and are short-lived.
GU Renal perfusion is temporarily restored towards normal in hypovolaemic patients transfused with the crystalloid.

Toxicity/Side Effects The predominant hazard is that of overtransfusion, leading to hypernatraemia or pulmonary oedema.

Kinetics Data are incomplete.

Absorption Sodium chloride is rapidly and completely absorbed when administered orally.

Distribution 0.9% solution is isotonic with extracellular fluid; it is initially distributed into the intravascular compartment where it remains for approximately 30 minutes before being distributed uniformly throughout the extracellular space.

Excretion In the urine.

Sodium nitroprusside

Uses Sodium nitroprusside is used in the management of:
1. hypertensive crises
2. aortic dissection prior to surgery
3. left ventricular failure and
4. to produce hypotension during surgery.

Chemical An inorganic complex.

Presentation As an intravenous solution 10 mg/ml of sodium nitroprusside for dilution prior to infusion it must be protected from light.

Main Actions Vasodilation and hypotension.

Mode of Action Sodium nitroprusside dilates both resistance and capacitance vessels by a direct action on vascular smooth muscle. It appears to act by interacting with sulphydryl groups in the smooth muscle cell membrane, thereby stabilising the membrane and preventing the calcium ion influx necessary for the initiation of contraction.

Route of Administration/Dose Sodium nitroprusside should be administered through a dedicated vein using a controlled infusion device at the rate of 0.5–6 µg/kg/min, titrated according to response. Invasive arterial pressure measurement during the use of the drug is considered mandatory. Onset of action is almost immediate; the desired response is usually achieved in 1–2 minutes.

Effects
CVS In hypertensive and normotensive patients, infusion of the drug causes a decrease in the systemic blood pressure and a compensatory tachycardia; the cardiac output is usually well maintained. In patients with heart failure, cardiac output increases due to a decrease in both venous return and systemic vascular resistance. The myocardial wall tension is decreased and myocardial oxygen consumption falls; the heart rate tends to decrease due to improved haemodynamics with the use of the drug. The blood pressure is usually well maintained under these circumstances. Myocardial contractility is unaltered by the drug.
RS Sodium nitroprusside causes a reversible decrease in P_aO_2 due to attenuation of hypoxic pulmonary vasoconstriction; an increased inspired oxygen concentration may be necessary.
CNS The drug causes cerebral vasodilation, leading to an increase in intracranial pressure in normocapnic patients; a 'steal' phenomenon may occur. The autoregulatory curve is shifted to the left.
AS Sodium nitroprusside decreases to lower oesophageal sphincter pressure and may cause a paralytic ileus.

GU   The renal blood flow and glomerular filtration rate are well maintained during infusions of the drug.

Metabolic/Other   A compensatory increase in plasma catecholamine concentration and plasma renin activity occur during the use of the drug. A metabolic acidosis may also occur.

Toxicity/Side Effects   The major disadvantage of the drug is its liability to produce cyanide toxicity, the likelihood of which is increased by hypothermia, malnutrition, vitamin B_{12} deficiency and severe renal or hepatic impairment. Cyanide ion toxicity is related to the rate of infusion of sodium nitroprusside rather than to the total dose used; however, it is recommended that no more than 1.5 mg/kg of the drug is infused acutely, and no more than 4 μg/kg/min is used chronically. The cyanide ion combines with cytochrome C and leads to impairment of aerobic metabolism; metabolic acidosis due to an increased serum lactic acid concentration may result. The signs of cyanide ion toxicity are tachycardia, dysrhythmias, hyperventilation, sweating and the development of a metabolic acidosis; these occur at plasma cyanide ion concentrations in excess of 8 μg/ml. Treatment of cyanide ion toxicity involves curtailing the infusion of sodium nitroprusside, general supportive measures and the administration of sodium thiosulphate or dicobalt edetate.

Additionally, profound hypotension produced by the drug may manifest itself as nausea and vomiting, abdominal pain, restlessness, headache, dizziness, palpitations and retrosternal pain.

Kinetics   Pharmacokinetic data are difficult to obtain, due to the very short duration of action of the drug.

Absorption   The drug is not absorbed orally.

Distribution   Sodium nitroprusside in the blood is confined essentially to the plasma; scarcely any is present within red blood cells. The V_D is approximately the same as the extracellular space (15 l).

Metabolism   Occurs by two separate pathways: in the presence of low plasma concentrations of sodium nitroprusside, the predominant route appears to be by reaction with the sulphydryl groups of amino acids present in the plasma. In the presence of higher plasma concentrations of the drug, rapid non-enzymatic hydrolysis occurs within red blood cells. Five cyanide ions are produced by the degradation of each molecule of sodium nitroprusside; one reacts with methaemoglobin to form cyanomethaemoglobin. The remaining four cyanide ions enter the plasma; 80% of these react with thiosulphate in a reaction catalysed by hepatic rhodanese to form thiocyanate. The remainder of the cyanide ions react with hydroxy-cobalamin to form cyanocobalamin (vitamin B_{12}).

Sodium nitroprusside

Excretion Both thiocyanate and cyanocobalamin are excreted unchanged in the urine. The elimination half-life of the former is 2.7 days.

Special Points Sodium nitroprusside is removed by haemodialysis.

Sodium valproate

Uses Sodium valproate is used in the treatment of:
1. primary generalised epilepsies, especially petit mal epilepsy, myoclonic seizures, infantile spasms and tonic-clonic epilepsy
2. chronic pain of non-malignant origin.

Chemical Sodium valproate is the sodium salt of valproic acid, a fatty (carboxylic) acid.

Presentation As 100/200/500 mg tablets, a syrup containing 40 mg/ml and in ampoules containing 400 mg of lyophilised soium valproate for dilution in 4 ml of water.

Main Action Anticonvulsant.

Mode of Action The most likely mode of action is via GABA-ergic inhibition; sodium valproate increases brain GABA levels by inhibition of succinic semialdehyde dehydrogenase in the GABA shunt. Alternatively it may:
1. mimic the action of GABA at post-synaptic receptors and
2. reduce excitatory inhibition (especially that due to aspartate).

Routes of Administration/Doses The adult oral dose is 600–2500 mg daily in two divided doses. The intravenous dose is 400–2500 mg daily in divided doses. The effective plasma range is 40–100 mg/l.

Effects
CNS The drug has anticonvulsant properties as described. Sodium valproate produces minimal sedation; an essential tremor may occasionally develop with the use of the drug.
Metabolic/Other Hyperammonaemia occurs infrequently.

Toxicity/Side Effects Sodium valproate is generally well tolerated. Hepatic dysfunction, acute pancreatitis, gastrointestinal upsets, hair loss, oedema and weight gain may occur following administration of the drug. There are also reports of platelet disturbances (decreased platelet aggregation and thrombocytopenia) and coagulation disturbances (increased bleeding time, prothrombin time and partial activated thromboplastin time) complicating the administration of sodium valproate.

Kinetics

Absorption Sodium valproate is rapidly and completely absorbed; the oral bioavailability is virtually 100%.

Distribution The drug is 90% protein-bound in the plasma, predominantly to albumin; the V_D is 0.1–0.41 l/kg. Brain concentrations are 7–28% of plasma levels.

Metabolism Sodium valproate is almost completely metabolised in the liver by oxidation and glucuronidation; some of the metabolites are active.

Excretion 1–3% is excreted unchanged in the urine. The clearance is 7–11 ml/kg/hour and the elimination half-life is 8–20 hours.

Special Points High concentrations of sodium valproate displace thiopentone from its binding sites *in vitro* and similarly displace diazepam *in vivo*. Platelet function may need to be monitored prior to surgery or epidural or spinal anaesthesia.

The drug is contraindicated in patients with acute liver disease, and liver function should be monitored during chronic therapy. The sedative effects of the drug are additive with those of other central nervous system depressants.

Sodium valproate is not removed by dialysis.

Spironolactone

Uses   Spironolactone is used in the treatment of:
1. congestive cardiac failure
2. hepatic cirrhosis with ascites and oedema
3. refractory oedema
4. hypertension
5. the nephrotic syndrome
6. in combination with loop or thiazide diuretics to conserve potassium and
7. in the diagnosis and treatment of Conn's syndrome.

Chemical   A synthetic steroid.

Presentation   As 25/50/100 mg tablets of spironolactone. Fixed-dose combinations with hydroflumethiazide or frusemide are also available.

Main Action   Diuretic.

Mode of Action   Spironolactone acts as a competitive antagonist of aldosterone at the latter's receptor site in the distal convoluted tubule; consequently, sodium ion reabsorption is inhibited and potassium ion reabsorption is increased. The drug thus promotes saliuresis and also potentiates that produced by other diuretic agents.

Routes of Administration/Doses   The adult oral dose of spironolactone is 100–400 mg daily; the corresponding dose of potassium canrenoate is 200–800 mg administered by slow intravenous infusion. The drug has a slow onset of action; the diuretic effect takes 3 to 4 days to become established.

Effects
CVS   The drug has an antihypertensive effect that may be mediated by alteration of the extracellular:intracellular sodium ion gradient or by antagonism of the effect of aldosterone on arteriolar smooth muscle.
CNS   Spironolactone may produce both sedation and muscular weakness, presumably secondarily to electrolyte derangements.
GU   The principal effect of the drug is diuresis, with retention of potassium ions. The renal blood flow and glomerular filtration rate are unaffected although the free water clearance may increase.
Metabolic/Other   Spironolactone has an antiandrogenic effect, due to inhibition of ovarian androgen secretion and interference with the peripheral action of endogenous androgens. The drug increases renal calcium ion excretion, and may also lead to a reversible hyperchloraemic metabolic acidosis and an increased plasma urea concentration.

Toxicity/Side Effects The predominant side effect of spironolactone is hyperkalaemia, especially in the presence of renal impairment. The use of the drug is also associated with an appreciable incidence of nausea and vomiting and other gastrointestinal disturbances. Menstrual irregularities in the female and gynaecomastia in the male may result from the antiandrogenic effects of spironolactone.

Kinetics

Absorption Spironolactone is incompletely absorbed when administered orally and has a bioavailability by this route of 70%; the drug undergoes extensive first-pass hepatic metabolism.

Distribution The drug is >90% protein-bound in the plasma.

Metabolism Spironolactone is rapidly and extensively metabolised by deacetylation and dethiolation; some of the metabolites, including canrenone, are active.

Excretion The metabolites are principally excreted in the urine, with a small proportion undergoing biliary excretion. The elimination half-life of spironolactone is 1–2 hours.

Special Points Spironolactone decreases the responsiveness to co-administered pressor agents and increases the effects of co-administered cardiovascular depressants, including anaesthetic agents. The drug increases the serum concentrations of co-administered digoxin and may interfere with digoxin assay techniques.

Streptokinase

Uses Streptokinase is used:
1. in the treatment of acute myocardial infarction
2. for the intravascular dissolution of thrombi and emboli, e.g. deep vein thrombosis and pulmonary embolus and
3. in the treatment of acute or subacute occlusion of peripheral arteries.

Chemical A protein obtained from Group C beta-haemolytic streptococci.

Presentation As a freeze-dried powder in vials containing 250 000/750 000/1.5 million units of streptokinase.

Main Actions Fibrinolysis.

Mode of Action Streptokinase acts indirectly on plasmin; the first phase is the formation of a streptokinase–plasminogen activator complex which then converts further plasminogen molecules to active plasmin. Plasmin then digests fibrin to produce lysis of thrombi.

Routes of Administration/Doses Streptokinase is infused intravenously (either peripherally or centrally at the site of occlusion) in 50–200 ml of saline, dextrose or gelatin. For the treatment of acute myocardial infarction, 1.5 million units are infused over a period of 1 hour. For the dissolution of thrombi or emboli, 250 000 units are infused over 30 minutes; subsequently, 100 000 units are infused per hour for 24–72 hours. Therapy should be monitored by either the thrombin time (which should be 2–5 times the control value) or prothrombin time.

Effects
CVS Transient hypotension and dysrhythmias may occur following the administration of streptokinase.
Metabolic/Other Fibrinolysis is produced by the action of the drug on plasmin.

Toxicity/Side Effects Excessive haemorrhage may complicate the use of the drug; if serious, this should be treated by cessation of Streptokinase therapy, resuscitation and intravenous tranexamic acid (10 mg/kg). Pyrexia occurs commonly. Allergic reactions may occur, particularly on repeated exposure, as streptokinase is markedly antigenic. This can be minimised by steroid and antihistamine pretreatment. Poly-neuropathy has occasionally been reported following the use of the drug.

Kinetics Data are incomplete.

Excretion The elimination half-life is 83 minutes.

Special Points Clotting factors return to normal values 24 hours after cessation of therapy; this is the time interval advisable before invasive procedures are undertaken.

Treatment with anticoagulants (including dextrans) or any drug which affects platelet function or formation increases the danger of haemorrhage.

Heparinisation may be indicated to prevent further thrombosis after initial treatment with streptokinase.

Sucralfate

Uses   Sucralfate is used:
1. in the treatment of peptic ulcer disease and
2. for the prevention of stress ulceration in the critically ill.

Chemical   An aluminium salt of sulphated sucrose.

Presentation   As tablets containing 1 g sucralfate and a white, viscous suspension containing 200 mg/ml of sucralfate.

Main Actions   Cytoprotection of the upper gastrointestinal tract.

Mode of Action   At acid pH sucralfate forms a viscous paste which adheres preferentially to peptic ulcers via ionic binding. It acts by providing a physical barrier to the diffusion of acid, pepsin and bile salts and also by forming complexes with proteins at the ulcer surface which resist peptic hydrolysis.

Routes of Administration/Doses   The adult dose for the prophylaxis of stress ulceration is 1 g 6-hourly.

Effects
AS   Sucralfate has weak intrinsic antacid activity. It has no effect on gastric emptying time. The drug increases gastric blood flow and enhances gastric epithelial proliferation via stimulation of gastric mucosal epidermal growth factor and fibroblast growth factor.
Metabolic/Other   In uraemic patients sucralfate increases aluminium absorption and therefore should be used with care. It acts as a phosphate binder which may induce hypophosphataemia.

Toxicity/Side Effects   Sucralfate is essentially non-toxic. Constipation occurs in 2%.

Kinetics

Absorption   Sucralfate is minimally (3–5%) absorbed after oral administration.

Distribution   85–95% of an oral dose remains in the gastrointestinal tract. The V_D and percentage protein binding are unknown.

Metabolism   No metabolism of the drug occurs in man.

Excretion   Predominantly unchanged in the faeces. The fraction that is absorbed is excreted primarily in the urine.

Sufentanil

Uses Sufentanil is used for:
1. the induction and maintenance of general anaesthesia and has been used for
2. post-operative analgesia.

Chemical A phenylpiperidine which is the thienyl derivative of fentanyl.

Presentation As a clear solution containing 50 µg/ml of sufentanil citrate. The drug is not commercially available in the United Kingdom.

Main Action Analgesia and respiratory depression.

Mode of Action Sufentanil is a highly selective mu-agonist; the mu-opioid receptor appears to be specifically involved in the mediation of analgesia. Part of the analgesic effect of the drug may be attributable to stimulation of 5-HT release. Opioids appear to exert their effects by increasing intracellular calcium concentration which, in turn, increases potassium conductance and hyperpolarisation of excitable cell membranes. The decrease in membrane excitability that results may decrease both pre- and post-synaptic responses.

Routes of Administration/Doses The intravenous dose is 0.5–50 µg/kg and the adult dose via the epidural route is 10–100 µg (the optimal post-operative dose being 30–50 µg. When administered intravenously, the drug acts in 1–6 minutes and the duration of effect is 0.5–8 hours, dependent on the other components of the anaesthetic.

Effects
CVS Sufentanil causes little haemodynamic disturbance. Heart rate and blood pressure tend to decrease immediately post-induction. Venous pooling may lead to orthostatic hypotension.
RS The drug produces dose-dependent respiratory depression, which may be delayed in onset. Chest wall rigidity (the 'wooden chest' phenomenon) may occur after the administration of sufentanil – this may be an effect of the drug on mu-receptors located on GABA-ergic interneurones.
CNS Sufentanil is 2000–4000 times as potent an analgesic as morphine. The EEG changes produced by the drug are similar to those produced by fentanyl: initial beta activity is decreased and alpha activity is increased; subsequently alpha activity disappears and delta activity predominates. The drug has no intrinsic effect on intracranial pressure. Miosis is produced as a result of stimulation of the Edinger-Westphal nucleus.
AS Sufentanil appears to cause less nausea than fentanyl. The drug may cause spasm of the sphincter of Oddi.

Metabolic/Other The drug tends to obtund the stress response to surgery, although it does not completely abolish it. Sufentanil may cause histamine release and may have less effect on immune function than fentanyl.

Toxicity/Side Effects Hypotension, tachycardia, brady-cardia, nausea and the 'wooden chest' phenomenon are the side effects most commonly reported with the use of sufentanil. Tonic/clonic movements of the limbs have also been reported.

Kinetics

Absorption The drug is normally administered intra-venously; the drug is, however, 20% absorbed when adminis-tered transdermally.

Distribution Sufentanil is 92% protein-bound in the plasma, predominantly to alpha-1 acid glycoprotein. The drug is highly lipophilic; the V_D is 1.74–5.17 l/kg.

Metabolism The metabolic pathways are unknown in man, although two metabolites (norsufentanil and desmethyl-sufentanil) have been identified in the urine.

Excretion 60% of an administered dose appear in the urine and 10% in bile. The clearance is 11–21 ml/min/kg; the elimina-tion half-life is 119–175 minutes.

Special Points Sufentanil decreases the MAC of co-administered volatile agents by 60–70%. The drug should be used with caution in the presence of renal or hepatic failure although the kinetics appear to be unaltered.

The drug increases the effect of non-depolarising muscle relaxants to a similar extent to halothane.

Suxamethonium

Uses Suxamethonium is used:
1. wherever rapid and profound neuromuscular blockade is required, e.g. to facilitate tracheal intubation and
2. for the modification of fits after electroconvulsive therapy.

Chemical The dicholine ester of succinic acid (equivalent to two acetylcholine molecules joined back-to-back).

Presentation As a clear aqueous solution containing 50 mg/ml of suxamethonium chloride – the preparation should be stored at 4 °C.

Main Actions Neuromuscular blockade of brief duration in skeletal muscle.

Mode of Action Suxamethonium causes prolonged depolarisation of skeletal muscle fibres to a membrane potential above which an action potential can be triggered.

Routes of Administration/Doses The intravenous dose is 0.5–2.0 mg/kg; the onset of action occurs within 30 seconds and the duration of action is 3–5 minutes. Infusion of a 0.1% solution at 2–15 mg/kg/hr will yield 90% twitch depression. The intramusular dose is up to 2.5 mg/kg. Equal doses on a mg/kg basis have a shorter duration of action in infants.

Effects
CVS With repeated doses of suxamethonium, bradycardia and a slight increase in mean arterial pressure may occur.
RS Apnoea occurs subsequent to skeletal muscle paralysis.
CNS The administration of suxamethonium may initially cause fasciculations which are then followed by a phase I depolarising block. The characteristics of this during partial paralysis are:
1. a well-sustained tetanus during stimulation at 50–100 Hz
2. the absence of post-tetanic facilitation
3. a train-of-four ratio of greater than 0.7 and
4. potentiation by anticholinesterases.
    With repeated administration or a large total dose a phase II block may develop. The characteristics of this during partial paralysis are:
1. a poorly sustained tetanus
2. post-tetanic facilitation
3. a train-of-four ratio of less than 0.3
4. reversal by anticholinesterases and
5. tachyphylaxis.
    Intracranial and intraocular pressure are both raised following the administration of suxamethonium.
AS The intragastric pressure increases by 7–12 cmH$_2$O; the lower oesophageal sphincter tone simultaneously decreases

with the use of suxamethonium. Salivation and gastric secretion are increased.

Metabolic/Other Serum potassium concentration is briefly increased in normal individuals by 0.2–0.4 mmol/l.

Toxicity/Side Effects Bradycardia and other dysrhythmias may occur with single or repeated dosing. The hyperkalaemic response is markedly exaggerated in patients with burns or major denervation of muscle and acute or chronic renal failure; this may lead to cardiac arrest. Postoperative muscular pains are common, especially in women, the middle-aged and those ambulant early in the post-operative period. Intraocular pressure is transiently raised following the use of suxamethonium – the drug should be used with caution in patients with penetrating eye injuries. Suxamethonium is a potent trigger agent for the development of malignant hyperthermia, and may cause generalised contractures in those patients exhibiting myotonia. Prolonged apnoea may occur in susceptible individuals (*v.i.*).

Kinetics

Distribution An initial rapid redistribution phase may contribute to the brief duration of action of the drug. Suxamethonium appears to be protein-bound to an unknown extent.

Metabolism The drug is hydrolysed by plasma cholinesterase (EC 3.1.1.8) to succinylomonocholine (which is weakly active) and choline; the former is further hydrolysed by plasma cholinesterase to succinic acid and choline. 80% of an administered dose is hydrolysed before it reaches the neuromuscular junction.

Excretion 2–10% of an administered dose is excreted unchanged in the urine. The *in vivo* hydrolysis rate is 3–7 mg/l/min and the half-life 2.7–4.6 minutes.

Special Points The incidence of muscle pains after the administration of suxamethonium may be decreased by pretreatment with:
1. a low (0.2 mg/kg) dose of suxamethonium
2. a small dose of a non-depolarising relaxant
3. diazepam
4. dantrolene
5. aspirin or
6. vitamin C.

Plasma cholinesterase activity may be influenced by both genetic and acquired factors, leading to an altered pattern of response to suxamethonium. The normal gene encoding for plasma cholinesterase is E_I^u (usual); three abnormal genes also exist: E_I^a (atypical), E_I^s (silent) and E_I^f (fluoride-resistant).

Suxamethonium

Simple Mendelian genetics are involved; 94% of the population are heterozygous for the usual gene and are clinically normal in their response to suxamethonium. E_I^a homozygotes comprise 0.03%, E_I^s homozygotes 0.001% and E_I^f homozygotes 0.0003% of the population and all remain apnoeic for 1–2 hours after receiving the drug and develop a phase II block during this period (fresh frozen plasma may be used to provide a source of plasma cholinesterase under these circumstances). All possible combinations of heterozygote exist – they constitute 3.8% of the population and remain apnoeic for approximately 10 minutes after receiving suxamethonium.

In addition, plasma cholinesterase concentrations may be reduced in pregnancy, liver disease, cardiac or renal failure, hypoproteinaemic states, carcinomatosis, thyrotoxicosis, tetanus, muscular dystrophy and in patients with burns, and suxamethonium may have a prolonged action in these states. Drugs which decrease the activity of plasma cholinesterase include ecothiopate, tacrine, procaine, lignocaine, lithium and magnesium salts, ketamine, pancuronium, the oral contraceptive pill, and cytotoxic agents. Suxamethonium does not appear to be potentiated by volatile agents, although phase II block may appear more readily in their presence.

Suxamethonium is pharmaceutically incompatible with thiopentone. The effects of digoxin may be enhanced by suxamethonium, leading to enhanced ventricular excitability.

Temazepam

Uses   Temazepam is used:
1.   as a hypnotic and
2.   for anaesthetic premedication.

Chemical   A 3-hydroxy benzodiazepine which is a minor metabolite of diazepam.

Presentation   As capsules containing 10/15/20/30 mg, and an elixir containing 2 mg/ml of temazepam.

Main Actions   Temazepam has anxiolytic, hypnotic, anti-convulsant and muscle-relaxant properties.

Mode of Action   Benzodiazepines are thought to act via specific benzodiazepine receptors found at synapses throughout the central nervous system, but concentrated especially in the cortex and mid-brain. Benzodiazepine receptors are closely linked with GABA receptors, and appear to facilitate the activity of the latter. Activated GABA receptors open chloride ion channels which then either hyperpolarise or short-circuit the synaptic membrane.

Route of Administration/Dose   Temazepam is administered orally; the adult dose is 10–60 mg.

Effects
CVS   Benzodiazepines have minimal effects on cardiovascular parameters; an insignificant decrease in blood pressure may occur. Benzodiazepines can dilate coronary blood vessels whilst simultaneously reducing myocardial oxygen consumption.
RS   High doses (>40 mg) decrease the ventilatory response to hypercapnia.
CNS   The drug causes muscular relaxation, sedation, hypnosis and axiolysis; it also has anticonvulsant properties.
Metabolic/Other   High (>40 mg) doses cause a slight fall in temperature.

Toxicity/Side Effects   Temazepam is normally well tolerated; gastrointestinal upsets, headaches, dreams, paraesthesiae and a 'hangover effect' (in 10–15%) may occur. Tolerance and dependence may occur with prolonged use of benzodiazepines; acute withdrawal of benzodiazepines in these circumstances may produce insomnia, anxiety, confusion, psychosis and perceptual disturbances.

Kinetics

Absorption   Absorption of oral temazepam is virtually complete; antacids delay the absorption of benzodiazepines.

Distribution   Temazepam is 76% protein-bound *in vitro*. The V_D is 0.8 l/kg.

Metabolism   The drug is predominantly metabolised in the liver by direct conjugation to glucuronide; active metabolites are not formed to any great extent.

Excretion   80% of an administered dose appears in the urine as inactive conjugates; 12% is excreted in the faeces. The clearance is 6.6 l/hour and the elimination half-life is 5–11 hours.

Special Points   The drug is not removed by haemodialysis. Temazepam is a drug of abuse and has controlled drug status.

Terbutaline

Uses   Terbutaline is used in the treatment of:
1. asthma
2. chronic obstructive airways disease and
3. uncomplicated preterm labour.

Chemical   An alcohol.

Presentation   As 5/7.5 mg tablets, a syrup containing 0.3 mg/ml, a clear solution for injection containing 0.5 mg/ml, a respirator solution containing 2.5/10 mg/ml and as an inhaler delivering 0.25/0.5 μg per actuation of terbutaline sulphate. It can be administered intravenously 250–500 μg 6-hourly, and by infusion at a rate up to 5 μg/min per adults.

Main Actions   Bronchodilatation and uterine relaxation.

Mode of Action   Terbutaline is a beta-adrenergic agonist (with a more pronounced effect at beta-2 than beta-1 receptors) that acts by stimulation of membrane-bound adenyl cyclase in the presence of magnesium ions to increase intracellular cAMP concentrations.

Routes of Administration/Doses   The adult oral dose is 2.5–5 mg 8-hourly; the subcutaneous, intramuscular and intravenous dose is 0.25–0.5 mg once or twice a day. Terbutaline may be administered by intravenous infusion diluted in dextrose or saline at the rate of 1.5–5 μg/min for 8–10 hours. The dose by inhalation is 0.25–0.5 μg 4-hourly or 2–5 mg 8–12-hourly if nebulised.

Effects
CVS   When used in large doses, terbutaline has positive inotropic and chronotropic effects.
RS   Bronchodilatation, leading to an increased PEFR and FEV_1, occurs after administration of the drug. This is additive to the bronchodilatation produced by phosphodiesterase inhibitors. The drug interferes with the mechanism of hypoxic pulmonary vasoconstriction; an adequate inspired oxygen concentration should be ensured when terbutaline is used.
GU   Terbutaline relaxes uterine musculature. An increased tendency to bleeding has been reported in association with Caesarean section.
Metabolic/Other   Hyperinsulinaemia, leading to hypoglycaemia and hypokalaemia, may follow administration of the drug. Antepartum administration of terbutaline stimulates release of surface-active material into the alveolar space of the fetus, improving the function of the neonatal lung.

Toxicity/Side Effects   Tremor, palpitations, cramps, anxiety and headache occur uncommonly after the administration of terbutaline.

Kinetics

Absorption   The drug is incompletely absorbed after oral administration; the bioavailability is 7–26%. Less than 10% is absorbed after inhalation, the remainder being swallowed.

Distribution   Terbutaline is 25% protein-bound in the plasma; the V_D is 1.6 l/kg.

Metabolism   Terbutaline has an extensive first-pass metabolism; the drug is predominantly metabolised to a sulphate conjugate.

Excretion   60–70% is excreted unchanged in the urine; the remainder as the sulphated conjugate. The clearance is 1.75–2.75 ml/min/kg and the elimination half-life is 11.5–23 hours.

Tetracycline

Uses   Tetracycline is used in the treatment of infections of:
1. the respiratory, gastrointestinal and urinary tracts
2. ear, nose and throat
3. soft tissues and in the treatment of
4. venereal diseases, including non-specific urethritis
5. typhus fever
6. psittacosis
7. cholera
8. acne rosacea and for
9. the treatment of recurrent pleural effusions and
10. the prophylaxis of subacute bacterial endocarditis.

Chemical   A napthacenecarboxamide derivative.

Presentation   As 250 mg tablets, a syrup containing 25 mg/ml, in vials containing 100 mg (with procaine) for intramuscular injection and 250/500 mg (with ascorbic acid) for intravenous injection of tetracycline hydrochloride. An ointment for topical use is also available.

Main Actions   Tetracycline is a broad spectrum bacteriostatic antibiotic which is active against Gram-positive and Gram-negative bacteria, including *Clostridium, Streptococcus, Neisseria, Brucella* and *Vibrio* sp., *Haemophilus influenzae, Yersinia pestis* and rickettsiae, *Mycoplasma, Chlamydia, Leptospira* and *Treponema* sp.

Mode of Action   Tetracycline inhibits bacterial protein synthesis by binding to bacterial 30S ribosomes (in the same manner as do aminoglycosides) and preventing the access of aminoacyl tRNA to the mRNA-ribosome complex, thereby preventing further elongation of the polypeptide chain.

Routes of Administration/Doses   The adult oral dose is 250–500 mg 6-hourly. The corresponding intramuscular dose is 100 mg 4–8-hourly and the intravenous dose is 0.5–1 g 12-hourly. The intrapleural dose is 500 mg (of the intravenous preparation). Intramuscular injection of the drug is painful.

Effects
CVS   Tetracycline may increase intracranial pressure.
Metabolic/Other   The drug may cause an increase in the plasma urea concentration and decrease the plasma prothrombin activity.

Toxicity/Side Effects   Occur in 1–5% of patients. The drug may cause renal and hepatic impairment, gastrointestinal and haematological disturbances, moniliasis, rashes, photosensitivity and thrombophlebitis. Tetracycline may also cause tooth staining in infancy.

Kinetics

Absorption Tetracycline is incompletely absorbed when administered orally (it chelates with iron, calcium and aluminium in the gut). The bioavailability is 77% by the oral route.

Distribution The drug is widely distributed and exhibits good tissue penetration. The drug is 62–68% protein-bound in the plasma; the V_D is 0.75–1.37 l/kg.

Metabolism 5% of the dose is metabolised to epitetracycline, the remainder is excreted unchanged.

Excretion 95% of the dose is excreted unchanged; 60% is excreted in the urine by glomerular filtration, the remainder in the faeces. The clearance is 1.43–1.91 ml/min/kg and the half-life is 10–16 hours. A decreased dose should be used in the presence of renal failure.

Special Points Tetracycline has been demonstrated to increase the action of non-depolarising relaxants. It is pharmaceutically incompatible with a host of other drugs, including thiopentone, sodium bicarbonate and autologous blood.

Thiopentone

Uses Thiopentone is used:
1. for the induction of anaesthesia
2. in the management of status epilepticus and has been used
3. for brain protection.

Chemical A thiobarbiturate.

Presentation As a hygroscopic yellow powder, containing thiopentone sodium and 6% sodium carbonate stored under an atmosphere of nitrogen. The drug is reconstituted in water prior to use to yield a 2.5% solution with a pH of 10.8 and pKa of 7.6 which is stable in solution for 24–48 hours.

Main Actions Hypnotic and anticonvulsant.

Mode of Action Barbiturates are thought to act primarily at synapses by depressing post-synaptic sensitivity to neurotransmitters and by impairing pre-synaptic neurotransmitter release. Multi-synaptic pathways are depressed preferentially; the reticular activating system is particularly sensitive to the depressant effects of barbiturates. The action of barbiturates at the molecular level is unknown. They may act in a manner analogous to that of local anaesthetic agents by entering cell membranes in the unionised form, subsequently becoming ionised and exerting a membrane-stabilising effect by decreasing sodium and potassium ion conductance, decreasing the amplitude of the action potential and slowing the rate of conduction in excitable tissue. In high concentrations, barbiturates depress the enzymes involved in glucose oxidation, inhibit the formation of ATP and depress calcium-dependent action potentials. They also inhibit calcium-dependent neurotransmitter release and enhance chloride ion conductance in the absence of GABA.

Routes of Administration/Doses The dose by the intravenous route is 2–7 mg/kg; following bolus administration, thiopentone acts in one arm–brain circulation time and lasts for 5–15 minutes; it is cumulative with repeated administration. The drug may also be administered rectally in a dose of 1 g/22 kg body weight, when it acts within 15 minutes.

Effects
CVS Thiopentone is a negative inotrope and decreases cardiac output by approximately 20%; the blood pressure usually decreases as a result of both this effect and a decrease in systemic vascular resistance.
RS Thiopentone is a potent respiratory depressant; following intravenous administration a period of apnoea may occur, followed by a more prolonged period of respiratory depression with a decrease in ths ventilatory response to hypercapnia.

Laryngeal spasm is occasionally seen in association with the administration of thiopentone; the drug may also produce a degree of bronchoconstriction.

CNS Thiopentone produces a smooth, rapid induction of anaesthesia. Cerebral blood flow, intracranial pressure and intraocular pressure are all decreased after the administration of the drug. As with all barbiturates, thiopentone has anticonvulsant properties. The drug is antanalgesic when used in small doses. The characteristic EEG changes observed after thiopentone administration are initially a fast activity which is subsequently replaced by synchronised low-frequency waves.

AS The drug causes some depression of intestinal activity and constriction of the splanchnic vasculature.

GU Thiopentone decreases renal plasma flow and increases ADH secretion, leading to a decrease in urine output. It has no effect on the tone of the gravid uterus.

Metabolic/Other A slight transient decrease in the serum potassium concentration may occur following the administration of thiopentone.

Toxicity/Side Effects Severe anaphylactoid reactions may occur with the use of the drug, with a reported incidence of 1 in 20 000. Extravasation of the drug may lead to tissue necrosis; inadvertent intra-arterial injection may lead to arterial constriction and thrombosis. The treatment of the latter includes the administration of analgesia and alpha-adrenergic antagonists, sympathetic blockade of the limb and anticoagulation.

Kinetics

Absorption Thiopentone is absorbed when administered orally or rectally.

Distribution The drug is 65–86% protein-bound in the plasma, predominantly to albumin; 40% is sequestered in red blood cells; the V_D is 1.96 l/kg. The rapid onset of action of the drug is due to:
1. the high blood flow to the brain
2. the lipophilicity of the drug and
3. its low degree of ionisation – only the non-ionised fraction crosses the blood–brain barrier (thiopentone is 61% non-ionised at pH 7.4: hyperventilation increases the non-bound fraction and increases the anaesthetic effect).

The relatively brief duration of anaesthesia following a bolus of thiopentone is due to redistribution to muscle and later to fat.

Metabolism Occurs in the liver by side-arm oxidation, oxidation to pentobarbitone and ring cleavage to form urea and 3-carbon fragments. 15% of the dose of the drug is metabolised per hour; 30% may remain in the body 24 hours after administration.

Thiopentone

Excretion Occurs predominantly in the urine as inactive metabolites; 0.5% is excreted unchanged. The clearance is 2.7–4.1 ml/kg/min and the elimination half life is 3.4–22 hours.

Special Points Volatile agents and surgery have no effect on the V_D or clearance of thiopentone; morphine increases the hypnotic effect of the drug and increases its brain half-life. The drug may induce acute clinical and biochemical manifestations in patients with porphyria. Thiopentone should be used with caution in patients with fixed cardiac output states, hepatic or renal dysfunction, myxoedema, dystrophia myotonica, myasthenia gravis, familial periodic paralysis, and in the elderly or in patients who are hypovolaemic.

Thiopentone is not removed by dialysis.

Thyroxine/ Triiodothyronine

Uses Thyroid hormones are used in the treatment of:
1. hypothyroidism
2. myxoedema coma and
3. goitre.

Chemical Both hormones are iodine-containing amino acid derivatives of thyronine.

Presentation Thyroxine is presented as tablets containing 50/100 µg of thyroxine sodium. Triiodothyronine is presented as 20 µg tablets and a white lyophilised powder for reconstitution in water containing 20 µg of triiodothyronine.

Main Actions Modulation of growth and metabolism.

Mode of Action The thyroid hormones, probably predominantly triiodothyronine, combine with a 'receptor protein' within the cell nucleus and thereby activate the DNA transcription process leading to an increase in the rate of RNA synthesis and a generalised increase in protein synthesis.

Routes of Administration/Doses The adult oral dose of thyroxine is 25–300 µg daily in divided doses, titrated according to the clinical response and results of thyroid function tests. The corresponding dose of triiodothyronine is 10–60 µg daily; the dose by the intravenous route is 5–20 µg 4–12 hourly; close monitoring is essential during intravenous administration. There is a 24 hour latency period before the effects of thyroxine are manifested; the peak effect occurs in 6–7 days. Triiodothyronine acts in 6 hours and the peak effect is observed within 24 hours.

Effects
CVS The thyroid hormones are positively inotropic and chronotropic; these effects may be mediated by an increase in the number of myocardial beta-adrenergic receptors. The systolic blood pressure is increased by 10–20 mmHg; the diastolic blood pressure decreases and mean arterial pressure remains unchanged. Vasodilation results from the increase in peripheral oxygen consumption; the circulating blood volume also increases slightly.
RS The thyroid hormones increase the rate and depth of respiration secondary to the increase in the basal metabolic rate.
CNS The hormones have a stimulatory effect on central nervous system function; tremor and hyperreflexia may result. Their physiological function also includes mediation of negative feedback on the release of Thyroid Stimulating Hormone from the pituitary.

AS   Appetite is increased following the administration of thyroxine or triiodothyronine; the secretory activity and motility of the gastrointestinal tract are also increased.

GU   The thyroid hormones are involved in the control of sexual function and menstruation.

Metabolic/Other   Thyroid hormones promote gluconeogenesis and increase the mobilisation of glycogen stores. Lipolysis is stimulated leading to an increase in the concentration of free fatty acids; hypercholesterolaemia may result from increased cholesterol turnover. The rate of protein synthesis is enhanced.

Toxicity/Side Effects   Excessive administration of the thyroid hormones results in the clinical state of thyrotoxicosis.

Kinetics

Absorption   Both thyroxine and triiodothyronine are completely absorbed when administered orally.

Distribution   Both hormones are bound to thyroid-binding globulin and thyroid-binding pre-albumin in the plasma; thyroxine is 99.97% bound and triiodothyronine is 99.5% bound. The V_D of thyroxine is 0.2 l/kg and that of triiodothyronine is 0.5 l/kg.

Metabolism   35% of thyroxine is converted to triiodothyronine in the periphery (predominantly in the liver and kidney) and some to inactive reverse T3. Both thyroxine and triiodothyronine undergo conjugation to glucuronide and sulphate and are excreted in the bile; some enterohepatic circulation occurs.

Excretion   20–40% of an administered dose is excreted in the faeces unchanged. The clearance of thyroxine is 1.7 ml/min and the elimination half-life is 6–7 days; the clearance of triiodothyronine is 17 ml/min and the elimination half-life is 2 days.

Special Points   The thyroid hormones increase the anticoagulant activity of co-administered warfarin. Beta-adrenergic antagonists interfere with the conversion of thyroxine to triiodothyronine and lead to a relative increase in the inactive reverse T3 fraction.

Tolbutamide

Uses Tolbutamide is used in the treatment of non-insulin-dependent (type II) diabetes mellitus.

Chemical A sulphonylurea.

Presentation As 500 mg tablets of tolbutamide.

Main Action Hypoglycaemia.

Mode of Action Tolbutamide acts by liberating insulin from pancreatic beta-cells; it appears to act by binding to the plasma membrane of the beta-cell and producing prolonged depolarisation, reducing the permeability of the membrane to potassium. This in turn leads to opening of calcium channels; the resulting influx of calcium causes triggering of insulin release. Sulphonylureas may also act by altering peripheral insulin-receptor number and sensitivity.

Route of Administration/Dose The adult oral dose is 0.5–2 g daily.

Effects

Metabolic/Other Tolbutamide causes a prompt and prolonged (6–12 hour) decrease in the blood sugar concentration; healthy subjects show a smaller decrease than do diabetic subjects. Sulphonylureas are ineffective in pancreatectomised patients and insulin-dependent diabetics. The drug also causes a decrease in the plasma free fatty acid concentration.

Toxicity/Side Effects Occur in about 3% of patients who receive the drug. Gastrointestinal disturbances, cholestatic jaundice and alterations in liver function tests may occur. Tolbutamide has a disulfiram-like interaction when taken with alcohol. Rashes, reversible leucopenia, haemolytic anaemia and paraesthesiae have also been reported.

Kinetics

Absorption The drug is 90% absorbed when administered orally; marked variations occur.

Distribution Tolbutamide is 93% protein-bound in the plasma, predominantly to albumin; the V_D is 0.15 l/kg.

Metabolism The drug is extensively metabolised in the liver by hydroxylation and carboxylation to active metabolites. There are genetically determined differences between individuals in the rate of metabolism.

Excretion 33% is excreted in the urine as the hydroxylated derivative; 66% as the carboxylated derivative. The clearance is 0.3 ml/min/kg and the elimination half-life is 7–10 hours.

Special Points It is generally recommended that oral hypoglycaemic agents are omitted on the morning of proposed surgery.

The drug should not be used in patients with hepatic or renal impairment. Tolbutamide is not removed by haemodialysis. An increase in cardiovascular mortality has been demonstrated in adults taking a fixed-dose regime of tolbutamide over a period of years.

The following drugs may potentiate the effect of sulphony-lureas either by displacement from plasma proteins or by inhibition of their hepatic metabolism and result in hypoglycaemia: NSAIDs, salicylates, sulphonamides, oral anticoagulants, MAOIs, and beta-adrenergic antagonists. Conversely, the following drugs tend to counteract the effect of sulphonylureas and result in loss of diabetic control: thiazide and other diuretics, steroids, phenothiazines, phenytoin, sympathomimetic agents and calcium antagonists.

Tramadol

Uses Tramadol is used in the management of moderate to severe pain.

Chemical A synthetic opioid of the aminocyclohexanol group. The drug is a racemic mixture of two enantiomers, $(+)$ and $(-)$ tramadol.

Presentation As a clear aqueous solution for injection containing 50 mg/ml and tablets containing 50/100/150/200/300/400 mg of tramadol hydrochloride.

Main Actions Centrally mediated analgesia.

Mode of Action Tramadol is a non-selective agonist at mu-, kappa- and delta-opioid receptors (with a higher relative affinity for mu-receptors). It also inhibits neuronal reuptake of noradrenaline and enhances serotonin (5-HT) release; inhibition of pain perception partly involves activation of descending serotonergic and noradrenergic pathways.

Routes of Administration/Doses Tramadol may be administered orally, intramuscularly or by slow intravenous injection or infusion. The adult dose is 50–100 mg 4–6-hourly for all routes of administration. The paediatric dose is 1–2 mg/kg 4–6 hourly.

Effects
CVS Tramadol has no clinically significant cardiovascular effects after intravenous administration.
RS Respiratory rate, minute volume and P_aCO_2 remain essentially unchanged following intravenous administration of therapeutic doses of the drug.
CNS Tramadol has an analgesic potency equivalent to pethidine. The analgesic effect is only partially (30%) reversed by naloxone.
AS Tramadol has no demonstrable effect on bile duct sphincter activity. Constipation occurs uncommonly.

Toxicity/Side Effects The principal side effects of tramadol are nausea, dizziness, sedation and diaphoresis. The potential for tolerance and dependence appear to be low.

Kinetics

Absorption The bioavailability following oral administration of the drug is 68–100%.

Distribution The drug is 20% protein-bound in the plasma; the V_D is 2.9–4.37 l/kg. 80% of an administered dose crosses the placenta.

Metabolism   85% of an administered dose is metabolised by demethylation in the liver. One metabolite (O-demethyl tramadol) is active.

Excretion   90% of the dose is excreted in the urine and 10% in the faeces. The clearance is 6.7–10.1 ml/kg/min and the elimination half-life is 270–450 minutes. The elimination half-life is doubled in patients with impaired renal or hepatic function.

Special Points   The use of tramadol is not recommended in patients with end-stage renal failure; the dosage interval should be increased to 12 hours in patients with renal or hepatic impairment.

The drug is not licensed for intraoperative use as it may enhance intraoperative recall during enflurane/nitrous oxide anaesthesia.

Tramadol appears to be effective in the treatment of post-operative shivering.

The drug precipitates when mixed with diazepam or midazolam.

The drug is only slowly removed by haemodialysis or haemofiltration.

Tranexamic acid

Uses Tranexamic acid is used:
1. as a short-term adjunct to the management of haemor-rhage due to increased fibrinolysis or fibrinogenolysis, e.g. post-prostatectomy bleeding, epistaxis or bleeding from cerebral aneurysms
2. prior to dental extraction in haemophiliacs
3. prior to repeat cardiac surgery
4. for the reversal of thrombolytic therapy and
5. in the chronic treatment of menorrhagia and
6. hereditary angioneurotic oedema.

Chemical Derivative of lysine.

Presentation A clear, colourless solution for intravenous use containing 100 mg/ml of tranexamic acid, in 500 mg tablet form and as a syrup containing 100 mg/ml.

Main Action Inhibition of fibrinolysis.

Mode of Action Tranexamic acid competitively inhibits the activation of plasminogen to plasmin.

Routes of Administration/Doses The intravenous dose is 15–25 mg/kg administered over 5 minutes. The correspond-ing oral dose is 1 g 6–8-hourly.

Effects
Metabolic/Other The thrombin time is increased; tranexamic acid has no effect on other coagulation parameters. Inhibition of complement pathways occurs following administration of the drug.

Toxicity/Side Effects Gastrointestinal disturbances may complicate the use of tranexamic acid.

Kinetics Data are incomplete.

Absorption Tranexamic acid is rapidly absorbed when administered orally; its bioavailability by this route is 34%.

Metabolism Little metabolism of tranexamic acid occurs.

Excretion 95% of an intravenously administered dose is excreted unchanged in the urine. The clearance is 1.6 ml/min/kg and elimination half-life is 1–2 hours.

Trichloroethylene

Uses   Trichloroethylene is used:
1. for the induction and maintenance of general anaesthesia and has been used
2. for pain relief during labour.

Chemical   A halogenated hydrocarbon.

Presentation   As a blue liquid (that should be protected from light) that is coloured with waxoline blue to enable differentiation from chloroform. The commercial preparation contains 0.01% thymol which prevents decomposition on exposure to light; it is non-flammable in normal anaesthetic concentrations. The molecular weight of trichloroethylene is 131.4, the boiling point 67 °C and the saturated vapour pressure is 8 kPa at 20 °C. The MAC of trichloroethylene is 0.17, the oil/water solubility coefficient 400 and the blood/gas solubility coefficient 9.

Main Actions   General anaesthesia (reversible loss of both awareness and recall of noxious stimuli) and analgesia.

Mode of Action   The mechanism of general anaesthesia remains to be fully elucidated. General anaesthetics appear to disrupt synaptic transmission (especially in the area of the ventrobasal thalamus), predominantly by inhibiting neurotransmitter release and by interfering with the interaction of neurotransmitters with post-synaptic receptors. Their mode of action at the molecular level appears to involve expansion of hydrophobic regions in the neuronal membrane, either within the lipid phase or within hydrophobic sites in cell membrane proteins.

Route of Administration/Dose   Trichloroethylene is administered by inhalation, conventionally via a calibrated vaporiser. The concentration used for the induction and maintenance of anaesthesia is 0.2–2%.

Effects
CVS   Trichloroethylene is noted for its cardiovascular stability; the heart rate, blood pressure and cardiac output are little altered by the administration of the drug. Trichloroethylene has a marked propensity to cause dysrhythmias and sensitises the myocardium to the effects of circulating catecholamines.
RS   The drug is moderately irritant to the respiratory tract and characteristically causes tachypnoea associated with a decreased tidal volume which may lead to both hypoxia and hypercapnia.
CNS   The principal effect of trichloroethylene is general anaesthesia; the drug also has a marked analgesic effect. The drug increases cerebral blood flow, leading to an increase in

intracranial pressure. A slight decrease in skeletal muscle tone results from the use of trichloroethylene.

AS   Nausea and vomiting occur commonly with the use of the drug.

GU   Trichloroethylene reduces the tone of the pregnant uterus when used in concentrations >0.5%.

Toxicity/Side Effects   Trichloroethylene may provoke the appearance of myocardial dysrhythmias, particularly in the presence of hypoxia, hypercapnia or excessive catecholamine concentrations.

Kinetics

Absorption   The major factors affecting the uptake of volatile anaesthetic agents are solubility, cardiac output and the concentration gradient between the alveoli and venous blood. Trichloroethylene is relatively soluble in blood; alveolar concentration therefore reaches inspired concentration relatively slowly, resulting in a slow induction of anaesthesia. An increase in the cardiac output increases the rate of alveolar uptake and slows the induction of anaesthesia. The concentration gradient between alveoli and venous blood approaches zero at equilibrium; a large concentration gradient favours the onset of anaesthesia.

Distribution   The drug is initially distributed to organs with a high blood flow (the brain, heart, liver and kidney) and later to less well-perfused organs (muscles, fat and bone).

Metabolism   20% of an administered dose is metabolised in the liver to yield trichloroacetic acid, monochloroacetic acid and trichloroethanol (which is subsequently conjugated with glucuronide) and inorganic chloride.

Excretion   80% is exhaled unchanged; the metabolites are excreted in the urine over several days.

Special Points   Trichloroethylene should not be used in a closed circuit with soda lime, since it decomposes in the presence of heat and alkali to form hydrochloric acid, carbon monoxide, dichloroacetylene and phosgene, all of which are toxic.

D-Tubocurarine

Uses Tubocurarine is used to facilitate intubation and controlled ventilation.

Chemical A monoquaternary alkaloid which is a derivative of isoquinoline.

Presentation As a clear, colourless solution for injection containing 10 mg/ml of tubocurarine chloride.

Main Action Competitive neuromuscular blockade.

Mode of Action Tubocurarine acts by competitive antagonism of acetylcholine at nicotinic (N2) receptors at the post-synaptic membrane of the neuromuscular junction; it also has some pre-junctional action.

Route of Administration/Dose Tubocurarine is administered intravenously; the normal intubating dose is 0.3–0.5 mg/kg with subsequent doses of one-third this amount. Satisfactory incubating conditions are produced within 3–5 minutes; a single dose lasts 20–30 minutes. The recovery index of the drug is 19–26 minutes.

Effects
CVS Hypotension and tachycardia may follow the administration of tubocurarine, resulting from the combined effects of histamine release, ganglion blockade and a decreased venous return caused by the loss of skeletal muscle tone. The drug appears to be concentrated in myocardial tissue and to protect against the development of cardiac dysrhythmias.
RS Neuromuscular blockade leads to apnoea. Tubocurarine has a marked potential for histamine release; bronchospasm is not uncommon. The drug also tends to increase bronchial secretions.
AS Tubocurarine increases salivation and decreases the tone and motility of the gastrointestinal tract.
Metabolic/Other The drug may cause decreased blood co-agulability as a result of the release of histamine from mast cells.

Toxicity/Side Effects Anaphylactoid reactions and profound hypotension may occur with the use of the drug. There are two reports of the development of malignant hyperpyrexia in patients who had received tubocurarine.

Kinetics

Absorption The drug is poorly and erratically absorbed after oral administration.

Distribution Tubocurarine is 42–58% protein-bound in the plasma, predominantly to albumin. The V_D is 0.19–0.41 l/kg. The drug does not cross the placental or blood–brain barrier.

Metabolism   Little metabolism of the drug occurs in man; 1% of the dose is demethylated in the liver.

Excretion   60–70% of an administered dose appears in the urine; the remainder is excreted in the bile. The clearance is 1.6–3 ml/min/kg and the elimination half-life is 0.9–3.1 hours. The drug is cumulative in the presence of renal impairment.

Special Points   The duration of action of tubocurarine, in common with other non-depolarising relaxants, is prolonged by hypokalaemia, hypocalcaemia, hypermagnesaemia, hypo-proteinaemia, dehydration, acidosis and hypercapnia. The following drugs, when co-administered with non-depolarising relaxants, increase the effect of the latter: volatile and induction agents, fentanyl, suxamethonium, diuretics, calcium antagonists, alpha- and beta-adrenergic antagonists, prota-mine, metronidazole and the aminoglycoside antibiotics.

Neonates and infants have an increased sensitivity to tubocurarine, as determined by the plasma tubocurarine concentration at which 50% depression of EMG twitch height occurs. A decreased dose should not, however, be used in the very young, as the drug has a larger volume of distribution in this group. Additionally, the longer elimination half-life of the drug in neonates and infants carries the implication that the dose interval should be increased as the age of the patient decreases.

Vecuronium

Uses Vecuroniurn is used to facilitate intubation and controlled ventilation.

Chemical A bis-quaternary aminosteroid which is the mono-quaternary analogue of pancuronium.

Presentation As a lyophilised powder (containing a citrate phosphate buffer and mannitol) which is diluted in water prior to use to yield a clear, colourless solution containing 2 mg/ml of vecuronium bromide; the solution is stable for 24 hours.

Main Action Competitive neuromuscular blockade.

Mode of Action Vercuronium acts by competitive antagonism of aceylcholine at nicotinic (N2) receptors at the postsynaptic membrane of the neuromuscular junction; it also has some pre-junctional action.

Route of Administration/Dose Vecuronium is administered intravenously; the normal intubating dose is 0.08–0.1 mg/kg with subsequent doses of one-third this amount. The drug may also be infused at a rate of 50–80 µg/kg/hour. Satisfactory intubating conditions are produced within 2 minutes; there is a linear relationship between the dose and the duration of action. The recovery rate following administration by infusion is a similar to that observed after bolus administration; the recovery index is 14–30 minutes, according to dose. The drug is non-cumulative with repeated administration.

Effects
CVS Vecuronium has minimal cardiovascular effects; with large doses, a slight (9%) increase in cardiac output and (12%) decrease in systemic vascular resistance may occur. Unlike pancuronium, the drug does not antagonise fentanyl-induced bradycardia.
RS Neuromuscular blockade leads to apnoea. Vecuronium has a very low potential for histamine release; bronchospasm is extremely uncommon.
CNS The drug has no effect on intracranial or intraocular pressure.
AS Lower oesophageal sphincter pressure remains unaltered after the administration of vecuronium.
Metabolic/Other Vecuronium may decrease the partial thromboplastin time and prothrombin time.

Toxicity/Side Effects There have been rare reports of anaphylactoid reactions in association with vecuronium.

Kinetics

Distribution The drug is 60–90% protein-bound in the plasma; the V_D is 0.18–0.27 l/kg. The drug does not cross the placental or blood–brain barrier.

Metabolism Vecuronium is metabolised by deacetylation in the liver to the active metabolites 3- and 17-hydroxy and 3,17-dihydroxyvecuronium; they are present in very low concentrations and may be of clinical significance after prolonged dosing.

Excretion 25% of the dose is excreted unchanged in the urine and 20% unchanged in the bile; the clearance is 3–6.4 ml/kg/min and the elimination half-life is 31–80 minutes. Renal failure leads to a prolongation of the elimination half-life but to no clinically significant increase in the duration of action of vecuronium; hepatic failure causes a significant decrease in the clearance and consequent increase in the duration of action of the drug.

Special Points The duration of action of vecuronium, in common with other non-depolarising relaxants, is prolonged by hypokalaemia, hypocalcaemia, hypermagnesaemia, hypoproteinaemia, dehydration, acidosis and hypercapnia. The following drugs, when co-administered with non-depolarising relaxants, increase the effect of the latter: volatile and induction agents, fentanyl, suxamethonium, diuretics, calcium antagonists, alpha- and beta-adrenergic antagonists, protamine, metronidazole and the aminoglycoside antibiotics.

The use of vecuronium appears to be safe in patients susceptible to malignant hyperpyrexia.

Verapamil

Uses Verapamil is used in the treatment of:
1. hypertension of mild to moderate severity
2. angina and
3. paroxysmal supraventricular tachycardia, atrial fibrillation and flutter.

Chemical A synthetic papaverine derivative.

Presentation As 40/80/120/160/180/240 mg tablets and as a clear solution for injection of a racemic mixture of verapamil hydrochloride containing 2.5 mg/ml.

Main Actions Antihypertensive and antianginal.

Mode of Action Verapamil causes competitive blockade of cell membrane slow calcium ion channels leading to a decreased influx of calcium ions into vascular smooth muscle and myocardial cells. This results in electromechanical decoupling, inhibition of contraction and relaxation of cardiac and smooth muscle fibres leading to coronary and systemic arterial vasodilation.

Routes of Administration/Doses The adult oral dose is 240–480 mg daily in 2–3 divided doses. The corresponding intravenous dose in 5–10 mg administered over 30 seconds; the injection should cease as soon as the desired effect is achieved. The peak effect after intravenous administration occurs at 3–5 minutes and the duration of action is 10–20 minutes.

Effects
CVS Verapamil is a class IV antiarrhythmic agent; it decreases automaticity and conduction velocity and increases the refractory period. Atrio-ventricular conduction is slowed; the drug appears to be taken, up and bound specifically by atrio-ventricular nodal tissue. The drug causes a decrease in the systemic vascular resistance and is a potent coronary artery vasodilator. Verapamil has negative dromotropic and inotropic effects which are enhanced by acidosis.
CNS Cerebral vasodilation occurs after the administration of verapamil. The drug has local anaesthetic properties.
GU Verapamil decreases renovascular resistance.

Toxicity/Side Effects Oral administration of the drug may lead to dizziness, flushing, nausea and first- or second-degree heart block. Intravenous administration may precipitate heart failure in patients with impaired left ventricular function and precipitate ventricular tachycardia or fibrillation in patients with the Wolff-Parkinson-White syndrome.

Kinetics

Absorption Verapamil is, completely absorbed when administered orally; the bioavailability is 10–22% due to a significant first-pass metabolism.

Distribution The drug is 90% protein-bound in the plasma; the V_D is 3.1–4.9 l/kg.

Metabolism Occurs by demethylation and dealkylation in the liver – the metabolites possess some activity.

Excretion 70% of the dose is excreted in the urine and 16% in the faeces. The clearance is 6.8–16.8 ml/min/kg and the elimination half-life is 3–7 hours. The dose should be reduced in patients with significant hepatic impairment.

Special Points The effects of volatile agents and beta-adrenergic antagonists on myocardial contractility and conduction are synergistic with those of verapamil; caution Should be exercised when these combinations are used. The drug increases the serum concentrations of co-administered digoxin.

Verapamil and dantrolene administered concurrently in animals cause hyperkalaemia leading to ventricular fibrillation; these drugs are not recommended for use together in man. The drug decreases the MAC of halothane in animal models; chronic exposure to the drug may potentiate the actions of both depolarising and non-depolarising relaxants. Verapamil attenuates the pressor response to laryngoscopy and intubation.

Verapamil is not removed by haemodialysis.

Warfarin

Uses   Warfarin is used:
1. in the prophylaxis of systemic embolisation in patients with rheumatic heart disease and atrial fibrillation and in patients with prosthetic heart valves and
2. in the prophylaxis and treatment of deep vein thrombosis and pulmonary embolism.

Chemical   A synthetic coumarin derivative.

Presentation   As tablets containing 0.5/1/3/5 mg of a racemic mixture of warfarin sodium.

Main Action   Anticoagulation.

Mode of Action   Warfarin prevents the synthesis of the vitamin K-dependent clotting factors (II, VII, IX and X) in the liver. The formation of fully active clotting factors is dependent on the carboxylation of their precursor proteins; during this reaction vitamin K is oxidised to vitamin K 2,3-epoxide; warfarin prevents the reduction of this episode back to vitamin K. This results in vitamin K depletion and a decrease in the rate of formation of complete clotting factors. The S enantiomer is 2–5 times more potent than the R enantiomer.

Route of Administration/Dose   The adult oral dose is usually 3–9 mg/day, according to response as measured by the prothrombin time. The maximum anticoagulant effect occurs 18–72 hours after the administration of a loading dose.

Effects   Warfarin has no clinically significant effects other than its anticoagulant effect.

Toxicity/Side Effects   Haemorrhage is the most frequent side effect. Hypersensitivity reactions and gastrointestinal upsets may occur. The drug appears to be teratogenic if taken during pregnancy.

Kinetics

Absorption   The drug is rapidly and completely absorbed from the stomach and upper gastrointestinal tract and has an oral bioavailability of 100%.

Distribution   Warfarin is 99% protein-bound in the serum, predominantly to albumin. The V_D is 0.1–0.16 l/kg.

Metabolism   Warfarin is virtually completely metabolised in the liver by oxidation (of the L-form) and reduction (of the D-form); these metabolites are then conjugated with glucuronide.

Excretion   The metabolites are excreted in the faeces and urine. The clearance is 3.26–3.8 ml/min/kg and the elimination half-life of warfarin ranges from 35 to 45 hours; this is decreased in patients with renal impairment.

Special Points The response to warfarin treatment is monitored in the laboratory by the one-stage prothrombin time, which is particularly sensitive to the activity of factors II, VII and X. The INR should be maintained at 2–4.5 times the control value. Many factors may affect warfarin control; in particular, the drug may exhibit significant interactions with many other drugs. The activity of warfarin may be potentiated by alcohol, amiodarone, cimetidine, sulphonamides, salicylates and other NSAIDs and many antibiotics, including co-trimoxazole, erythromycin, chloramphenicol, metronidazole and tetracyclines. The activity of warfarin may be decreased by many drugs, including barbiturates, the oral contraceptive pill and carbamazipine.

Control of anticoagulation in the peri-operative period requires special attention. This is usually achieved by transferring the patient to heparin prior to and immediately after surgery; the INR should ideally be less than 2 for routine surgery. Acute reversal of the effects of warfarin can be achieved by the administration of fresh frozen plasma. Alternatively, 1 mg of vitamin K will reverse its effects within 12 hours and 10 mg will prevent re-warfarinisation due to the saturation of liver stores.

Spinal and epidural anaesthesia are contraindicated in patients anticoagulated with warfarin.

Zidovudine

Uses   Zidovudine is used to reduce the incidence of neoplasia and opportunistic infections in patients with the acquired immunodeficiency syndrome (AIDS) or AIDS-related complex (ARC).

Chemical   A thymidine analogue.

Presentation   As capsules containing 100/250/300 mg, a syrup containing 10 mg/ml of zidorudine and as intravenous solution 10 mg/ml which needs dilution prior to infusion.

Main Action   Antiviral.

Mode of Action   The drug is initially phosphorylated to an active form which becomes incorporated into intracellular viral DNA by acting as a substrate for, and inhibitor of, viral reverse transcriptase. It thereby prevents the uptake of thymidine into viral DNA. Once incorporated, it terminates the viral DNA chain.

Route of Administration/Doses   The adult oral dose is 200–300 mg (3.5 mg/kg) 4-hourly; the dosage interval should be increased to 8 hours if the haemoglobin level decreases or neutropenia occurs and the drug should be discontinued if the haemoglobin falls to below 7.5 g/dl or the neutrophil count falls to less than 0.75×10^9/litre.

Effects
Metabolic/Other   The use of zidovudine is associated with significant weight gain, increased well-being and improved survival rates in patients with AIDS or ARC. The drug produces a decrease in the incidence of opportunistic infections and an increased tendency to clear these when they do occur. Zidovudine appears to slow the rate of neurological deterioration in this group of patients.

Toxicity/Side Effects   Severe haematological disturbances (anaemia, leucopenia and neutropenia) occur in 45% of patients receiving zidovudine. Headache; nausea, insomnia and myalgia occur more commonly than in patients receiving placebo.

Kinetics

Absorption   The drug is well absorbed with an oral bioavailability of 60–70%.

Distribution   Zidovudine is 34–38% protein-bound in the plasma; the V_D is 1.4 l/kg.

Metabolism   Occurs in the liver by glucuronidation.

Excretion   10–20% appears unchanged in the urine, the remainder is excreted by renal tubular secretion as the glucuronide metabolite. The clearance is 21.67 ml/min/kg and the elimination half-life is 1–1.5 hours.

Special Points There is a theoretical risk of an interaction between nitrous oxide and zidovudine, since both may cause decreased availability of thymidine-5-triphosphate for DNA synthesis.

Accumulation of the drug is likely (although unproven) in patients with renal or hepatic impairment.

The combination of acyclovir and zidovudine appears to increase significantly long-term survival in patients with AIDS or ARC.

Index of drug derivation

Index of drug derivation

Index of medical uses